Contents

An Introduction to

Child Care
and **Education**

Carolyn Meggitt • Jessica Walker

Second Edition

Orders: please contact Bookpoint Ltd, 130 Milton Park, Abingdon, Oxon OX14 4SB. Telephone: (44) 01235 827720. Fax: (44) 01235 400454. Lines are open from 9.00 – 6.00, Monday to Saturday, with a 24-hour message answering service. You can also order through our website www.hodderheadline.co.uk.

British Library Cataloguing in Publication Data
A catalogue record for this title is available from the British Library

ISBN 0 340 81398 9

This edition published 2004
Impression number   10 9 8 7 6 5 4 3 2 1
Year   2007 2006 2005 2004

Typeset by Fakenham Photosetting Limited, Fakenham, Norfolk
Printed in Italy for Hodder & Stoughton Educational, a division of Hodder Headline, 338 Euston Road, London NW1 3BH

Acknowledgements

We gratefully acknowledge the help of Mrs Allum, Headteacher, and the staff and pupils of Millbrook Infant School, Kettering in allowing us to take photographs of their school; Sarah Kettle, Nursery Manager, Vicky Kaur and Lee Griffiths, nursery nurses and all the staff and children at Millbrook Day Nursery, Kettering for allowing us to take photographs in their nursery. We would also like to thank Alexandra Tattersall and the staff at Building Blocks Christian Day Nursery for their interest and support; Brenda Swaddle, Headteacher, and all the staff and parents at Eastwood Nursery School for allowing us to take photographs.

We would like to say a particular thank you to Tina Bruce, for her insightful contribution to the first edition of this book; also to Gerald Sunderland for his patience and skill in taking the specially commissioned photographs.

The following photo agencies supplied photographs: p. 5 Karen Robinson/ Photofusion; p. 155, p. 268 and p. 272 John Walmsley/Education Photos; p. 157 Nik Wheeler/CORBIS; p. 161 and p. 262 (a) and (c) Sally and Richard Greenhill; p. 238 Craig Lovell//CORBIS; p. 262 (b) Jacky Chapman/Photofusion.

Foreword

It is very heartening to see how the text in this second edition of the popular text *An Introduction to Child Care and Education* has been developed, so that it remains relevant and up-to-date. At the same time, it has kept the time-honoured principles and values which ensure that practitioners working with young children and their families constantly strive to offer quality of experience. This matters whether they are working with children in home-care or group settings.

This book introduces students to the subject matter, knowledge and understanding they need at the beginning of their studies. It begins, and leads them forward in, their journey learning the important aspects of children's development, growth and learning that they will find in the more advanced text *Child Care & Education, 3rd edition*.

The section on physical care and development stresses sequences of development. Observation is seen as a crucial skill to be developed in practitioners. Readers will learn about the physical safety and health needs of babies, toddlers and young children in ways which are practical, but the text also gives explanations and reasons for working in particular ways.

Play is emphasised as crucial in the development and learning of young children, and I am delighted with the way the importance of childhood play is highlighted throughout the book.

The intellectual, emotional and social aspects of the development of young children are approached so that those reading the book are encouraged to work in ways which are respectful and which build on the interests of babies, toddlers and young children, whilst giving children and families what they need.

The sections which focus on working with babies are invaluable, especially at a time when out-of-home care for very young children is increasing.

Professor Tina Bruce
University of Surrey Roehampton

Foreword

I am delighted to write the foreword for this new book supporting the revised CACHE level 2 Certificate in Child Care and Education which is listed as an approved qualification on the National Qualifications framework. At this time when there is a considerable expansion of child care and education provision there is a clear need for an informed and competent workforce at all levels. This new text will support candidates very effectively, either as new entrants to the occupational area or for existing workers as they study to improve their knowledge and skills.

Children and families deserve the very best care and education available and we know that the quality of provision is a crucial aspect of how effectively children's needs are met. Part of quality provision is training and the achievement of nationally recognised qualifications which motivate candidates to think about their practice and learn fundamental skills such as how to support children's learning or how to provide effectively for their physical needs. National qualifications need high quality supporting materials and textbooks to support tutors and candidates and Introduction to Child Care and Education helps to meet that requirement.

Introduction to Child Care and Education is a thorough, wide-ranging, well-researched and up-to-date text written by respected authors, that will not only support the learning for the CACHE level 2 Certificate in Child Care and Education, but will be useful for a variety of level 2 qualifications. It provides a good indication of the breadth and depth of knowledge and understanding required to underpin competent level 2 practice. The content is also designed to take the candidate further as it introduces them to higher level skills and concepts which can be used as reference points as candidates enter employment. As candidates develop their practice at level 2, having a text which actively encourages further learning and development will enrich their knowledge and competence and ultimately improve their service to children and families.

Maureen Smith
Former Director of Curriculum and Assessment
CACHE and co-founder of Duo Consulting.

(This foreword is written in a personal capacity and does not imply CACHE endorsement.)

Course Overview

Information about your course

Starting points

The CACHE Level 2 Certificate in Child Care and Education is an excellent foundation, or starter, course for anyone wanting to work with young children. The children's age range covered is 0 to 7 years 11 months.

The course usually runs as a one-year, full-time course in schools or colleges of further education. Institutions which offer the course are called **study centres** and the way training is provided can vary. Some may organise training programmes on a part-time basis to meet local needs.

You must be at least 16 years old to begin the course. In practice, the course often attracts some older students who find it an ideal programme for them to ease back into an education environment and to provide a recognised qualification.

CACHE does not state any prescribed entry qualifications but individual study centres are likely to have their own guidelines. Although the course is vocational rather than academic, the amount of written work involved usually leads centres to ask for some evidence of your ability to communicate well both orally and in writing. When discussing your suitability for this course (and its suitability for you!) they will also be looking for personal qualities which are essential for a career in this field (more about these later!). They may expect you to have completed a period of 'work experience' involving children or to have helped with children's holiday activities or clubs. This would show that you have some idea of what to expect and that you already know that you enjoy being with children. You may also have had experience through babysitting. **Remember *working* with children as a professional involves much more than looking after them**.

Structure

There are different elements in the course and each one is important and supports the others. The 'theory' part – what you are taught in the classroom – is often referred to as **underpinning knowledge**. The 'practical' part – what you actually do in your training placement – is detailed in a list of **competencies**. These are tasks which you must show you are able to carry out competently (capably and effectively). You must show your competence in practical skills in both **core age ranges**. When you are in your placement you will learn *how* to do things (e.g. set out play materials, supervise outdoor play, prepare snacks etc.) but the underpinning knowledge explains why they are done that way.

The content – *what* you have to know, understand and be able to do – is divided into units. You must complete **four Core Units** (which everyone must study) and, in addition, **one Option Unit**. CACHE has 2 options in the course programme but it is not usual for you to be able to choose yourself. For practical reasons most study centres offer one or the other, not both.

As a vocational course it is **multi-disciplinary** (i.e. it covers a wide range of subject areas) and includes health-related modules, education-related modules and some dealing with social studies. As part of these modules you should get the opportunity to carry out practical activities in the classroom as well as in your training placements. You are likely to be taught two, or even three, modules at the same time so personal organisation – of your time and your paperwork – is important.

Patterns of study vary and while some students will have alternate weeks in placement and school/college, others will have set days (usually two or three) each week so there is a weekly mix of school/college and placement. **The minimum number of training placement days for the course is 65**: 30 with children aged 1 to 3 years 11 months, 20 with children aged 4 to 7 years 11 months and 15 to cover whichever option module is taken. In some cases additional days may be required (see Assessment, below).

Assessment

* **Attendance record** – perhaps this is the form most easily overlooked. CACHE recommends that you achieve 80% attendance for each and every taught module. A lower level of attendance suggests that you are unlikely to have gained sufficient understanding and knowledge across the whole course. Attendance at your training placement is also recorded to ensure that you fulfil the requirements detailed above.

* **Unit Assignments** – You must complete an externally set assignment for each of the four core units (1–4). You will need to produce one major piece of work for the assignment – the exact word length will vary according to the individual assignment. Each assignment will be graded Pass, Merit or Distinction, and you will be told what you need to do to achieve each grade. If you complete the assignment for a core unit, you can get an individual unit certificate for that unit. You must also complete a similar assignment for your option unit.

* **Practice Evidence Record (PER)** – This is a booklet made up of three sections, which you must complete by the end of the course. First is a placement summary record, which must be signed by your tutor as an accurate record of your work placements. Second there are PER summaries which will help you keep track of which elements you have still to complete. Thirdly there are PER sheets, which set out the list of competencies you must achieve. These must be individually signed by your placement supervisor or tutor when they know you can do them.

* **Personal Development Profile (PDP)** – You must achieve satisfactory graded reports from your placement supervisors (at least two reports at grade C or above) in order to gain your Certificate.

* **Multiple Choice Question Test** – This test will assess your knowledge of Units 1 to 4 and will be sat under exam conditions. There are three set dates each year in November, March and June – your study centre will arrange your entry, which will normally be once you have studied all four units. The test lasts for one hour, and contains 40 questions. You can be awarded a grade of Distinction, Merit, Pass or Fail, according to the number of marks you achieve.

Key Skills

You might also be working towards Key Skills certification in the following areas: communication, application of number, information technology, working with others, improving own performance and/or problem solving. Suggestions for where you might find evidence for your Key Skills Portfolio are highlighted within the CACHE syllabus, and also within the set assignment for each unit.

Failure in any part of the assessment means that you cannot be awarded the Certificate without undertaking further training and/or resubmitting written work (this may involve submitting additional work). Your study centre will explain what is required in your own

individual circumstances, what grading can be achieved and whether or not the MCQ paper must be taken on another occasion.

Progression

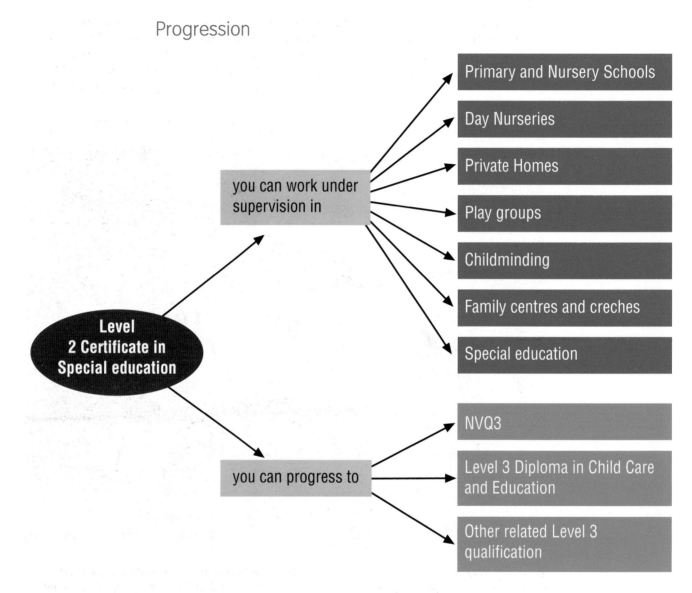

Organisation

Being well-organised will make the many separate demands of the course easier to cope with. Your training placement time is very precious and you need to ensure that the coursework you carry out is spread across the whole age range – your tutor will probably set each task to be implemented within a particular setting. It is easy to put off doing an activity because your supervisor has arranged something else for you to do or because you delay asking when would be convenient. The result can be lack of evidence for your PER! Planning how you can achieve what is required and discussing it in advance with your supervisor will help you to 'pace' yourself. This requires you to know what is needed. A record sheet can help you keep track of tasks as they are set and, importantly, ensures that you remember any pieces which have been given a referral grade and need resubmitting. Avoid allowing a 'backlog' of work to build during the early part of the course as assignments and MCQ paper loom menacingly from the mid-point onwards.

In conclusion

It is important to view your experiences positively, including those at placements where you have felt unsettled. Every work setting will be different depending on staff, premises, function, attitude, outlook and, of course, the children! There is plenty to learn from those who have experience and are willing to share their expertise with you and offer advice. You will have the opportunity to decide if you have a preferred age range which may be useful when you seek employment.

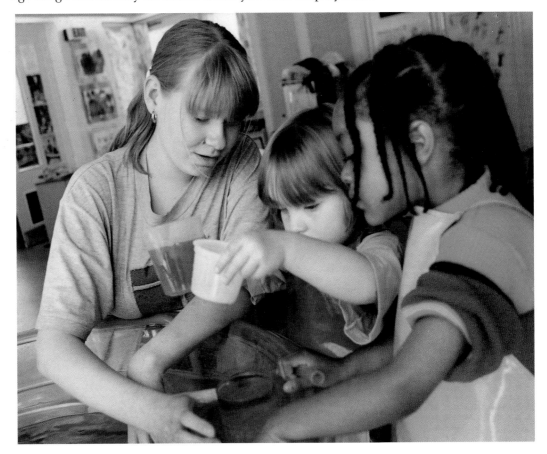

Similarly you may feel more comfortable and confident in some staff teams than others. It may be because of organisational factors or attitudes – try to analyse what makes the difference.

If you are following the career path which is right for you, then it is probable (and preferable) that you enjoy your training placement time more than your study centre time! If this is not the case, think carefully about your choices for now and the future. This is one field in which you cannot achieve through written work alone. Students who show little initiative, have poor communication and display little interest in placement are unlikely to receive satisfactory PDPs and so will not succeed, whereas those who are very good in their placements usually can be given the necessary support to complete written tasks successfully to achieve the award.

Using this book

How this book will help you gain your qualification – your pathway to success

This book contains all the underpinning knowledge required to gain the Certificate in Child Care and Education. Features include:

Activities

Throughout the book there are suggested activities, shown in boxes, many of which can be carried out during your practical placements.

Signposts

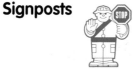

At the end of each unit we provide specific tasks, which we have called **Signposts**. These **Signposts** will:

1 Make sure that you have read and understood the material in the Unit

2 Prepare you for the **Unit Assignments** (which will be set by your tutor) for all **Core Units** and the two **Option Units**. (NB You only have to do *one* Option Unit.)

Multiple choice questions (MCQS)

Forty multiple-choice questions – and their answers – can be found in the Appendix on pages 361–372.

Photocopiable forms

Photocopiable forms needed throughout the **Signpost** tasks may be found in the Appendix at the end of the book.

The Physical Care and Development of the Child

1

The sequence of physical development

- the stages and sequence of the physical development of the child from 1 to 7 years 11 months
- how physical development relates to other aspects of development
- how different aspects of physical development relate to each other

Physical development

There are wide variations in the ages at which children acquire physical skills, such as sitting, standing and walking. The rate at which children develop these skills will have an effect on all the other areas of development: for example, on the development of language, understanding, self-confidence and social skills. Once a child has learnt to crawl, to shuffle on her bottom – or to be mobile in other ways – she will be more independent and be able to explore things that were previously out of reach. Adults will make changes to the child's environment now that she is mobile, by putting reachable objects out of her way and making clear rules and boundaries.

Three 4-year-olds – children grow at different rates

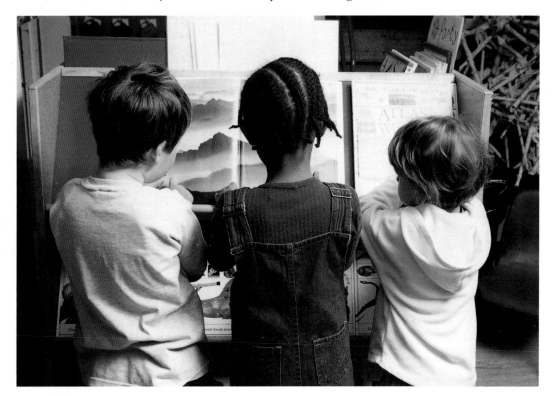

🧸 Physical growth

Physical growth is different from physical **development**. Physical growth means that children grow in height and weight, whereas physical development means that children gain **skills** through being able to control their own bodies. How children grow depends on the **genes** and **chromosomes** which they inherit from their parents. Up until adolescence, children's growth has two distinct phases:

1   **From birth to two years:** During the first two years of life, children grow very rapidly (about 25–30 cm in length) and triple their birth weight in the first year.

2   **From two years to adolescence:** This is a slower but steady period of growth; each year the child gains between 5 and 8 cm in height and about 3 kg in weight.

Growth charts (or centile charts) are used to plot the growth measurements of babies and children.

Girls' height-for-age and weight-for-age percentiles

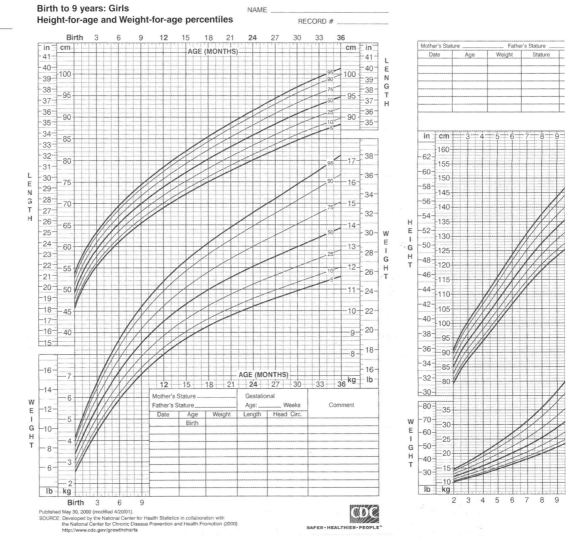

Boys' height-for-age and
weight-for-age percentiles

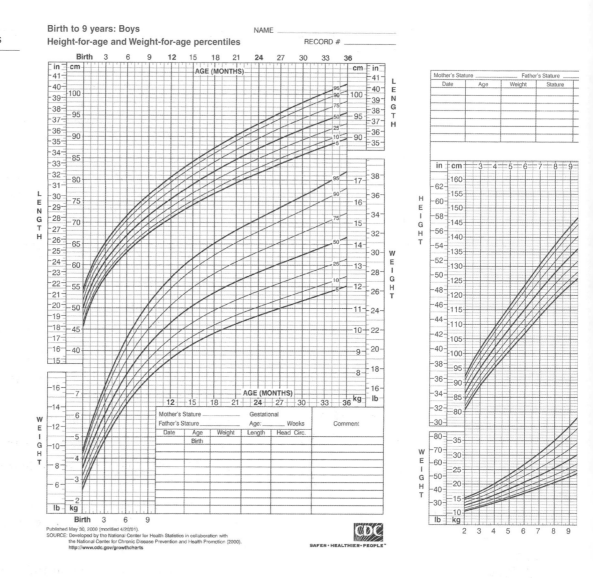

Birth to 9 years: Boys
Height-for-age and Weight-for-age percentiles

NAME _____

RECORD # _____

Published May 30, 2000 (modified 4/20/01).
SOURCE: Developed by the National Center for Health Statistics in collaboration with
the National Center for Chronic Disease Prevention and Health Promotion (2000).
http://www.cdc.gov/growthcharts

SAFER · HEALTHIER · PEOPLE™

The pattern of development

Children's development follows a pattern:

✳ **From simple to complex**: a child will stand before he can walk, and walk before he can skip or hop.

✳ **From head to toe:** physical control and co-ordination begins with a child's head and works down the body through the arms, hands and back and finally to the legs and feet.

✳ **From inner to outer:** a child can co-ordinate his arms using **gross motor skills** to reach for an object before he has learned the **fine motor skills** necessary to pick it up.

✳ **From general to specific:** a young baby shows pleasure by a massive general response (eyes widen, legs and arms move vigorously etc.); an older child shows pleasure by smiling or using appropriate words or gestures.

Physical development is the way in which the body increases in skill and becomes more complex in its performance. There are two main areas:

✱ **gross motor skills:** these use the large muscles in the body and include walking, squatting, running, climbing etc.;

✱ **fine motor skills:** these include:
> **gross manipulative skills** which involve single limb movements, usually the arm, for example throwing, catching and sweeping arm movements, and
> **fine manipulative skills** which involve precise use of the hands and fingers for pointing, drawing, using a knife and fork, writing, doing up shoelaces etc.

The following pages outline the main features of childhood development, the ages shown being those at which the **average child** performs the specific tasks. **Remember, however, that children develop at different rates and some may be faster or slower to learn certain skills than others may.**

Sequence of physical development

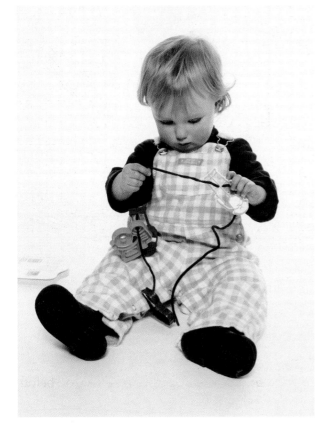

Twelve months

Gross motor skills: Babies:

- rise to a sitting position from lying down
- rise to standing without help from furniture or people
- crawl on hands and knees, bottom-shuffle or 'bear-walk' rapidly about the floor
- stand alone for a few moments
- 'cruise' along using furniture as a support
- probably walk alone, with feet wide apart and arms raised to maintain balance – or walk with one hand held

Note: *By 13 months, half of all children walk, but tend to fall over frequently and sit down rather suddenly.*

Fine motor skills: Babies:

- hold a crayon in palmar grasp and turn several pages of a book at once
- show a preference for one hand over the other, but use either
- drop and throw toys deliberately – and look to see where they have fallen
- pick up small objects with a fine pincer grasp, between thumb and tip of index finger
- point with index finger at objects of interest

Your role in promoting development

- Provide a wheeled push-and-pull toy to promote confidence in walking
- Read picture books with simple rhymes
- Provide stacking toys and bricks
- Talk to the baby about everyday activities, but always allow time for a response
- Provide an interesting, varied environment which contains pictures, music, books and food which all stimulate the senses

Fifteen months

Gross motor skills: Babies:

- crawl upstairs safely and may come down stairs backwards

- are generally able to walk alone

- kneel without support

- seat themselves in a small chair

Fine motor skills: Babies:

- can put small objects into a bottle

- grasp a crayon with either hand in a palmar grasp and imitate to and fro scribble

- may build a tower of two cubes after demonstration

- turn several pages of a picture book at once

- hold and drink from a cup using both hands

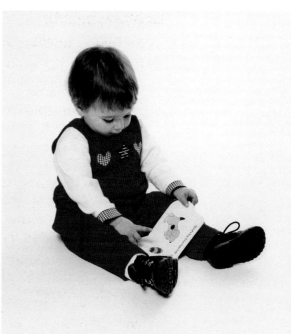

Your role in promoting development

- Arrange a corner of the kitchen or garden for messy play, involving the use of water, play dough or paint

- Encourage creative skills by providing thick crayons and paint brushes and large sheets of paper (e.g. wall lining paper)

- Join in games of 'let's pretend' to encourage imaginative skills; for example, pretending to be animals or to drive a bus

- Think about attending a mother and toddler group or a one o'clock club

Eighteen months

Gross motor skills: Children:

- walk steadily and stop safely, without sitting down suddenly

- climb forward into an adult chair and then turn round and sit

- move from squatting position to standing without support

- climb up stairs and down stairs with hand held or using rail for balance; puts two feet on each step before moving on to the next step

- crawl backwards (on their stomachs) down stairs alone

- kneel upright without support

- run steadily but are unable to avoid obstacles in their path

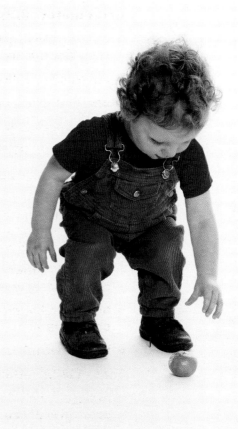

Gross manipulative skills: Children:

- point to known objects

- build a tower of three or more bricks

Fine manipulative skills: Children:

- use a delicate pincer grasp to pick up very small objects

- use a spoon when feeding themselves

- hold a pencil in whole hand or between thumb and the first two fingers (this is called the primitive tripod grasp)

- thread large beads on a lace or string

- control wrist movement to manipulate objects, e.g. turn door knobs and handles

Your role in promoting development

- Continue to provide walker trucks, pull-along animals etc.

- Encourage play with messy materials, e.g. sand, water, play dough

- Provide low stable furniture to climb on

- Provide pop-up toys, stacking toys and peg or shape bashing toys which are useful for hand eye coordination skill development

- Provide balls to roll, kick or throw

- Use action rhymes, singing games and other children to promote conversation and confidence

Two years

Gross motor skills: Children:

- can run safely, avoiding obstacles, and are very mobile
- can climb up onto furniture
- can throw a ball overhand but cannot yet catch it
- push and pull large wheeled toys
- walk up and down stairs, usually putting two feet on each step

By 2½ years, children:

- stand on tiptoe when shown
- climb nursery apparatus
- jump with both feet together from a low step
- kick a large ball, but gently and lopsidedly

Fine motor skills

- draw circles, lines and dots using preferred hand
- pick up tiny objects using a fine pincer grasp
- build a tower of six or more blocks with a longer concentration span
- enjoy picture books and turn pages singly
- copy a vertical line and sometimes a 'V' shape

By 2½ years, children:

- hold pencil in preferred hand, with an improved tripod grasp
- build a tower of 7 or more cubes using preferred hand

Your role in promoting development

- Provide toys to ride and climb on and space to run and play
- Take children on outings to the park or countryside to encourage them to learn about the natural world
- Encourage use of safe climbing frames and sandpits, always supervised
- Encourage ball play (throwing and catching) to promote co-ordination skills
- Provide bricks, hammer and peg toys and jigsaw puzzles to improve co-ordination and motor skills

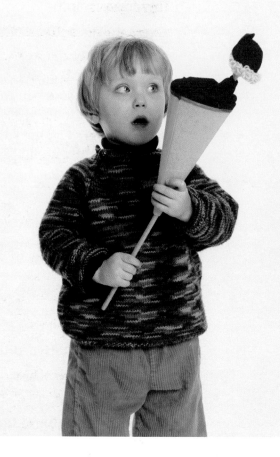

Three years

Gross motor skills: Children:

- can jump from a low step
- can stand and walk on tiptoe and stand on one foot
- ride a tricycle using pedals
- climb stairs with one foot on each step – downwards with two feet to each step
- can throw a ball overhand and can catch a large ball with arms outstretched
- use their whole body to kick a ball with force

Fine motor skills: Children:

- control a pencil using thumb and first two fingers – the dynamic tripod grip
- draw a person with head, and sometimes with legs and (later) arms coming out from the head; squiggles inside the head represent a face
- can cut paper with scissors
- can thread large beads onto a lace
- can eat using a fork or spoon and enjoy taking part in family mealtimes

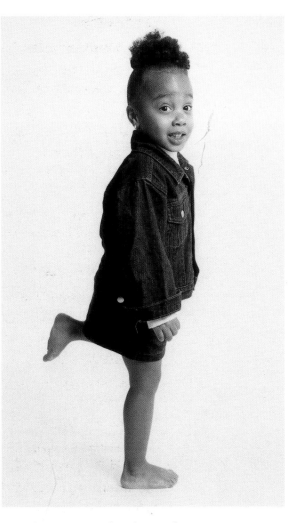

Your role in promoting development

- Provide a wide variety of playthings – balls for throwing and catching, sand, jigsaw puzzles etc
- Encourage play with other children
- Provide a variety of art and craft activities: thick crayons, stubby paint brushes, paper, paint, dough for modelling or play cooking
- Encourage swimming, trips to the park, maybe even enjoy longer walks
- Promote independence by teaching them how to look after and put away their own clothes and toys

Four years

Gross motor skills: Children:

- develop a good sense of balance and may be able to walk along a line
- stand, walk and run on tiptoe
- catch, kick, throw and bounce a ball
- bend at the waist to pick up objects from the floor
- ride a tricycle with skill and can make sharp turns easily

Fine motor skills: Children:

- can build a tower of ten or more cubes
- copy a model of three steps using six cubes
- are able to thread small beads on a lace
- hold and use a pencil in adult fashion

Your role in promoting development

- Provide plenty of opportunity for exercise; use rope swings and climbing frames
- Encourage play with small construction toys, jigsaw puzzles and board games
- Provide art and craft materials for painting, printing and gluing and sticking activities
- Encourage sand and water play and play with dough or modelling clay
- Play lotto and other matching games e.g. pairs. Teach children how to dress and undress themselves to prepare for school games lessons
- Encourage independence when going to the toilet

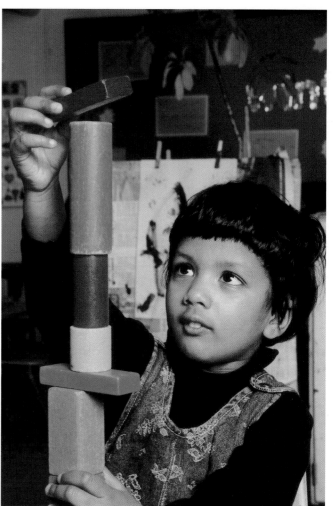

Five years

Gross motor skills: Children:

- have increased agility; they can run and dodge, run lightly on their toes, climb and skip
- show good co-ordination, playing ball games and dancing rhythmically to music
- can bend and touch their toes without bending at the knees
- use a variety of play equipment – slides, swings, climbing frames

Fine motor skills: Children:

- may be able to thread a large-eyed needle and sew with large stitches
- draw a person with head, body, legs, nose, mouth and eyes
- have good control over pencils and paintbrushes
- count the fingers on one hand using the index finger on the other
- do puzzles with interlocking pieces

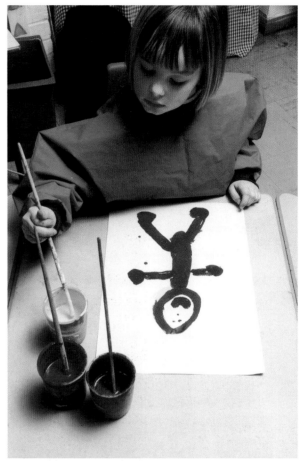

Your role in promoting development

- Provide plenty of outdoor activities
- Teach children to ride a two-wheeled bicycle
- Encourage non-stereotypical activities e.g. boys using skipping ropes and girls playing football
- Encourage the use of models, jigsaws, sewing kits and craft activities as well as drawing and painting

Six years

Gross motor skills: Children:

- are gaining in both strength and agility; they can jump off apparatus at school with confidence

- run and jump and kick a football up to six metres away

- catch and throw balls with accuracy

- ride a two-wheeled bike, usually using stabilisers at first

- skip in time to music, alternating feet

Fine motor skills: Children:

- build a tower of cubes which is virtually straight

- hold a pencil in a similar hold to an adult – the **dynamic tripod grip**

- are able to write a number of letters of similar size

- write their last name as well as their first name

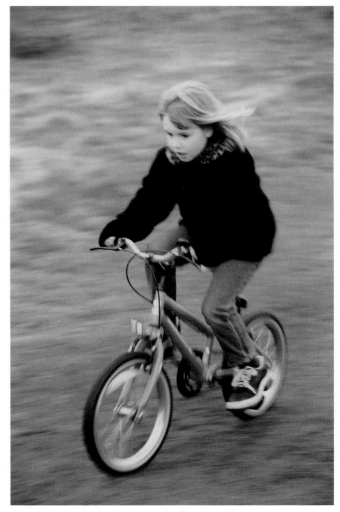

Your role in promoting development

- Provide opportunity for vigorous exercise

- Allow children to try a new activity or sport, e.g. football, dancing, judo or gymnastics

- Encourage writing skills by providing lots of examples of things written for different purposes, e.g. shopping lists, letters, recipes etc.

Seven years

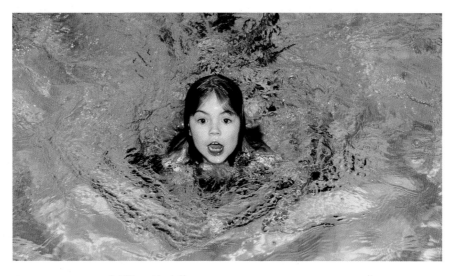

Gross motor skills: Children:

- may be expert at riding a two-wheeled bike or using roller skates
- have increased stamina, shown in activities such as swimming, skating, gymnastics and martial arts
- are able to control their speed when running and swerve to avoid collision
- are skilful in ball catching and throwing, using one hand only

Fine motor skills: Children:

- can build tall straight towers with cubes
- are more competent in their writing skills – individual letters are more clearly differentiated now and capital and small letters are in proportion
- draw people with heads, bodies, hands, hair, fingers and clothes
- use a large needle to sew with thread

Your role in promoting development

- Encourage vigorous outdoor play – on swings, climbing frames and skipping and hopping games such as hopscotch
- Take children swimming, skating, riding or to a dancing or martial arts class
- Arrange an obstacle course for children to navigate bikes around
- Provide a range of drawing and craft materials, such as charcoal, paint, clay and materials for collage

Measuring development

The stages (or milestones) of development described in these charts are **normative measurements** of development; this means that they only show what most children can do at a particular stage. They can only indicate general trends in development in children across the world. There are, inevitably, some drawbacks in using normative measurements. It may cause unnecessary anxiety when children do not achieve 'milestones' which are considered normal for their age. But the child's performance could be affected by a number of factors, for example, by tiredness, anxiety or illness.

Developmental reviews

Children's **holistic** (or all-round) development is reviewed by doctors and health visitors either in the child's home or in health clinics; the areas looked at are:

☐ gross motor skills: sitting, standing, walking, running;

☐ fine motor skills: handling toys, stacking bricks, doing up buttons and tying shoelaces (gross and fine manipulative skills);

☐ speech and language: including hearing;

☐ vision, including squint;

☐ social behaviour: how the child interacts with others – e.g. family and friends.

Developmental reviews give parents an opportunity to say what they have noticed about their child. They can also discuss anything that concerns them about their child's health and behaviour. Most parents in the UK are given a **Child Health Record book**, which they can use to chart milestones in development and immunisations. Parents are usually invited to a developmental review when their child is:

☐ 6 to 8 weeks old;

☐ 6 to 9 months old;

☐ 18 to 24 months old;

☐ 3 to 3½ years old;

☐ 4½ to 5½ years old (before or just after their child starts school).

Sample page from a Personal Child Health Record

REVIEW AT 8 MONTHS						
Child Health Promotion Areas discussed 						
General health		SPOTRN	Feeding/nutrition discussed	☐ Yes		☐ No
Fine motor development		SPOTRN	Language development discussed	☐ Yes		☐ No
Gross motor development		SPOTRN	Hearing questionnaire: Please fill in page 10			
Hips	Left	SPOTRN	Distraction test (where appropriate)			
	Right	SPOTRN				
Testes *(If not previously documented)*		SPOTRN				
Sleep/behaviour		SPOTRN	Immunisation discussed	☐ Yes		☐ No
Visual behaviour & Corneal reflex		SPOTRN	Dental care discussed	☐ Yes		☐ No
Any other comments			Referral required	☐ Yes		☐ No
			Review required	☐ Yes		☐ No
Signed			*Date* .... / .... /			
S = satisfactory P = problem O = observe T = treatment R = referral N = not examined						

In some parts of the country, the age that children are reviewed may vary slightly from those given above, especially after the age of three.

Some health visitors may ask parents or carers questions about their baby or ask the child to do little tasks such as building with blocks or identifying pictures. Others may simply watch the child playing or perhaps drawing, and get an idea from this observation, and your comments, of how the child is doing. If the child's first language isn't English, parents may need to ask if development reviews can be carried out with the help of someone who can speak their child's language.

After the child has started school, the School Health Service takes over these reviews.

2

Providing a safe and secure environment

- ways to promote a safe and secure environment
- potential hazards and safety measures – indoors and outdoors
- health and safety requirements
- the importance of the adult as a role model
- encouraging learning through the physical layout of the environment
- the importance of daily routines
- the involvement of parents
- planning and preparing outings

The care and education environment

Children need both care and education. It is impossible to separate the two. In the United Kingdom, children receive care and education in a variety of settings. These include:

- **Their own homes:** Parents are the first carers and educators of children and often their relatives and friends share in early child care. Children are also cared for in their own homes by **nannies**. Some nannies care for children from more than one family.

- **Childminders:** Childminders use their own homes to care for other people's children; they also often care for older children after school.

- **Nursery classes, Nursery Units and Kindergartens:** The Local Education Authority is responsible for provision of care and education in nursery classes and nursery units. A **nursery class** is attached to a primary school; the class teacher will be a trained nursery teacher who will work alongside a fully qualified nursery nurse. **Nursery units** are usually in a separate building with a separate co-ordinator. They are larger than a nursery class but will have the same adult:child ratio as the nursery, which is 1:15. There are also many **private nursery schools** and kindergartens; these may be staffed by qualified people, but not always. There tends to be pressure within private nursery schools to introduce children early to formal academic learning.

- **Centres of Early Years Excellence:** These provide integrated provision in education, care and health according to each family's needs. Many of these centres emerged from being nursery schools and typically offer year-round all-day care. They are staffed by nursery teachers and nursery nurses.

- **Family Centres:** These are jointly funded by the Education, Social Services and Health departments. All staff in Family Centres are qualified; the team may include teachers trained for the relevant age group, nursery nurses, social workers and health visitors. Family Centres take a very wide catchment of children, and the provision they offer is as much for the parents as it is for the children.

- **Day Nurseries and Children's Centres:** These offer full-time provision and often work with families who may be facing many challenges. They also work closely with the Social Services and Health departments and often make strong links with the nursery schools within their area. The staff are usually trained nursery nurses.

- **Community Nurseries:** These are often funded by voluntary organisations such as Barnardo's. They function in a similar way to family centres, but usually offer part-time rather than full-time care.

- **Pre-schools (playgroups):** Pre-schools are non-profit-making groups which are usually part-time; children under five attend two or three half-day sessions a week, often in a church hall. Parents pay a small charge per session. Sometimes pre-school groups are the only form of provision available for young children in isolated rural areas.

- **Infant and Primary Schools:** Children can attend either
  > one primary school from the age of 5–11 years;
  > an infant school at 5–7 years and a junior school from 7–11 years, or
  > a first or lower school at 5–8 years and then a middle school at 9–13 years.

Although the legal requirement is for children aged 5 years and over to attend school, in England more than 80% of four-year-old children are now in reception classes in primary schools. In the private sector, there are pre-preparatory and preparatory schools which exist alongside the state nursery schools and primary schools, but which charge fees.

- ✽ **Extended Day Care in Schools:** After-school clubs provide help to working parents. Children stay on after a session in the nursery or school, in a home-like atmosphere and with different staff. They will have tea and recreational activities.

- ✽ **Workplace nurseries and crèches:** Some workplaces offer nursery provision for employees' children; there are also crèches in shopping centres, where children under the age of eight can be looked after while their parents shop.

- ✽ **Holiday play schemes:** These offer care for children of school age during the school holidays and are usually staffed by playleaders, volunteers and community workers. They are often used by working parents.

Working as a team

It is important that within any work setting all staff share the same values and attitudes towards the environment and the children in their care. There will be some responsibilities which are the role of particular individuals while others lie with everyone. Maintaining the environment so that it is safe, hygienic, reassuring and attractive is part of everyone's role and may include jobs shared out on a rota basis e.g. cleaning toilets, preparing snacks, washing and sterilising equipment etc. However, it is every individual's responsibility to deal with any health and/or safety hazard which arises. This may be something straightforward such as mopping up a spillage or more serious such as glass from a broken window. Immediate steps should be taken to make the surrounding area safe by clearing away fragments, keeping children away and then reporting the situation to the appropriate person. Where children are able to see that the care of their environment is important and shared between all adults they are provided with positive role models to influence their own attitudes.

Children learn about themselves, others, and the world through play. As adults, it's our responsibility to make sure play is as safe as possible. You have an important role in ensuring that the environment where children play, learn and are cared for is as safe as possible. To achieve this you should follow this **10-point plan**:

10 Understand child protection policies – see pp. 101–103

9 Understand your role and responsibility in reporting accidents

8 Learn First Aid techniques

7 Understand the importance of immunisation and other preventative health measures

6 Follow the setting's health and safety policies

5 Teach children how to play safely

4 Check equipment regularly

3 Identify potential hazards

2 Be a good role model

1 Understand safety issues relevant to child care

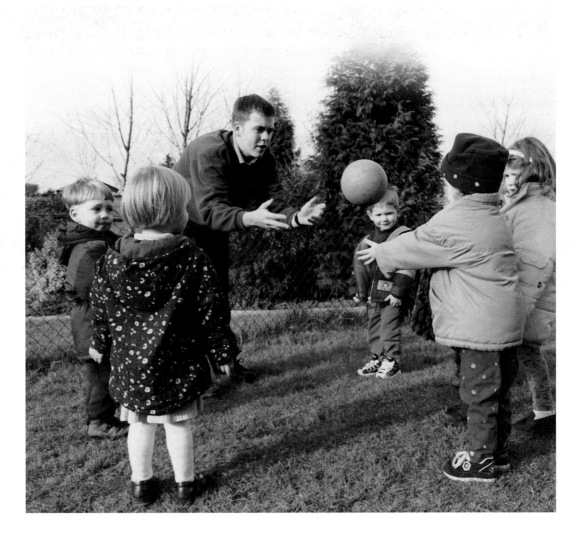

Understanding safety issues relevant to child care

Accidents are the most common cause of death in children between the ages of 1 and 14 years old. The pattern of accidents varies with the child's age, in keeping with:

* the child's stage of development, and

* their exposure to new hazards.

The table below shows the most common injuries to children and the age group which is most vulnerable to them.

Choking and suffocation	High-risk age	Burns and scalds	High-risk age
Use of pillows Unsupervised feeding and play with small parts of toys Plastic bags Peanuts Cords and ribbons on garments	Babies under 1 year	Matches, lighters, cigarettes Open fires and gas fires Baths Kettles and irons Cookers Bonfires and fireworks	From 9 months on (when children are newly mobile)
Falls	**High-risk age**	**Poisoning**	**High-risk age**
Stairs Unlocked windows Bouncing cradles left on worktops or tables Push chairs and high chairs Climbing frames	Children under 5 years	Household chemicals, e.g. bleach & disinfectant Medicines Berries and fungi Waste bins Vitamins	1 to 3 years
Electric shocks	**High-risk age**	**Road accidents**	**High-risk age**
Uncovered electric sockets Faulty wiring	Children under 5 years	Running into the road Not wearing child restraints in cars Playing in the road	All ages up to age 14 years
Drowning	**High-risk age**	**Cuts**	**High-risk age**
Unsupervised in the bath Ponds, water butts Swimming pools, rivers & ditches	Children under 4 years	Glass doors Knives, scissors and razor blades Sharp edges on doors and furniture	1 to 8 years old

Be a good role model

To be a good role model for children, you need:

❋ to set a **good example** to children and to others. Children unconsciously imitate the adults they are with. If you show a real concern for safety issues, then children will pick up on this and behave as you do.

❋ to be **vigilant** at all times. When supervising children in a group setting, you need to be aware of their moods and to anticipate any problems.

❋ to follow **safety procedures**: for example, you should learn the **Green Cross Code** and make sure that you always adhere to the rules when you are out with children

❋ to keep the environment as **safe** and **hygienic** as possible: mop up spills straightaway, clear up after activities with children etc.

Identify potential hazards

You need to be able to identify potential hazards whether you are in the home setting or in a group setting. Make the home, garden and nursery setting as accident-proof as possible:

The following guidelines apply to the home setting, but are equally applicable to nursery and other group settings:

A Safety guidelines for playing indoors

✓ Try to keep very young children out of the kitchen, even when an adult is there.

✓ Put them in a playpen or high chair if there is no alternative; or you could try putting a stairgate in the doorway.

✓ Put safety film over glass doors and beware of children playing rough and tumble games near glass doors or low windows.

✓ Encourage children not to play on the stairs or in the main walkways in group settings

In a flat or maisonette:

✓ Always supervise children on balconies – they may be tempted to climb up or over the railings.

Playing with toys:

✓ Keep toys and other clutter off the floor so that no one trips up – use a toy box e.g. a large, strong cardboard box.

✓ Choose toys suitable for the child's age and stage of development. Keep toys for older children away from younger brothers or sisters to prevent them from choking on small parts.

Guidelines for choosing suitable toys for children

Choosing and using toys wisely is an essential part of helping children to get the most out of toys and play. The National Toy Council gives guidelines on ensuring that all play is safe play.

1 **Make sure that the toys you buy conform to safety standards** and will not present a risk to children. Most toys on the UK market today are carefully made and safe to play with.

2 **Always go to a reputable shop**, ideally one that is a member of the British Association of Toy Retailers (BATR). You are more likely to get useful help and advice if you go to a specialist toy shop, the toy department of a large store or the toy section of a major chain.

3 **Check out the packaging.** There are three things you should look for:
- *Small parts:* Young children can easily choke on small objects. Children under 3 years old are particularly at risk because they put everything into their mouths to explore the shape and texture. A safety message such as 'not suitable for children under 36 months because of small parts', therefore must be taken literally.
- *Age advice:* Messages such as 'recommended for children aged 3–4' or 'play age 5–7' are discretionary guidelines. It is sensible to obey the age guidelines as they can help you decide if the toy will be fun for the child to play with, if it will prove stimulating, and above all, if it is safe for the child.
- *The Lion Mark:* This is a symbol of quality, backed by a Code of Practice, and used only by members of the British Toy & Hobby Association (BTHA). Toys bearing the Lion Mark have been made to the highest standards currently in force in Britain and the European Community.
- *The CE mark:* **This is NOT an indication of safety.** When looking for a mark of safety and quality, you should always turn to the **Lion Mark**.

4 **Check the toy:** Ask to see the toy out of the box and check that it's sturdy and well made. It is especially important to look over toys for babies and toddlers to make sure there are no small pieces that come loose or seams that come apart.

5 **Choose the right toy for the right child:** Often a toy is well designed and safe but causes problems when it gets into the wrong hands. A building brick that is safe, interesting and educational for an older child can be lethal if a toddler chokes on it. Likewise, a toddler who can only just sit up won't cope with a sit-and-ride truck and will just keep falling off. The table on p. 28 gives guidelines on which toys may prove dangerous for certain age groups and suggests safe alternatives.

Safety symbols on children's toys

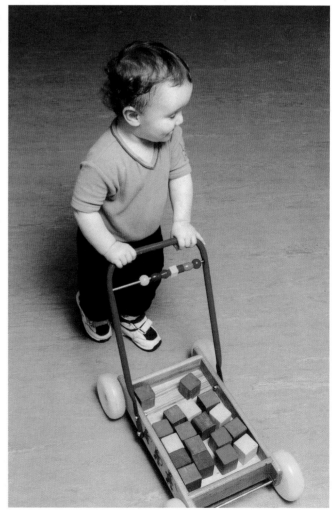

A child with a push-along truck

Approximate age	Toys to avoid	Choose instead
0–1 year	sit-in babywalkers sit-and-ride trucks motorised toys hairy and furry toys	push along toys toys with smooth fabric covers, or solid plastic toys
1–3 years	little toys or little pieces including thin, breakable crayons or pencils toys you can bite such as foam balls	large toys and drawing materials (that can't be swallowed or put into ears or up noses) tough toys that you can chew
3–6 years	deflated balloons	balloons that are already blown up (as long as you are watching), or balls
6–8 years	chemistry sets or other kits with chemicals	science kits with no chemicals, such as magnets or prisms

B Safety guidelines for playing outdoors

If there is a garden or outdoor play area

✓ Make sure the children can't get out on their own: block up gaps in the fence and keep the gates locked.

✓ Set up garden toys properly and check they are stable and with no loose nuts and bolts.

✓ Have something soft under climbing frames – regularly watered grass is fine, but dried earth can be as hard as concrete.

✓ Watch children at all times in the paddling pool and empty it straight away after use –

Small children can drown in just a few inches of water

✓ Cover, fence off or fill in the garden pond to keep small children away.

Playgrounds are good places for children to run around and play, but some are safer than others. You should always:

✓ Teach children to use the equipment properly – make sure they understand your instructions; e.g. teach children never to run in front or behind children using swings

✓ **Keep a close eye on very young children at all times**.

✓ Avoid old, damaged or vandalised equipment which could hurt a child.

✓ Try to keep to playgrounds with safety surfaces like bark chippings – they are not completely safe but may mean a less serious injury.

✓ Check for rubbish such as broken glass or even syringes, particularly if older children or adults meet there. If these problems persist, report them to the playground owners.

✓ Watch out for nearby hazards such as roads and streams.

✓ **Remember that playing should be fun and is an important part of growing up. Your role is to make sure that it stays fun and doesn't lead to a serious accident.**

Check equipment regularly

✓ **Check the toys** in family homes and group settings. Go through the toy box regularly and clear out any broken and damaged toys. Don't hand them on to jumble sales or charity shops, where they could cause injury to another child.

✓ **Check for objects which stick out** on equipment and could cut a child or cause clothing to become entangled, e.g. screws or bolts on trucks or playground equipment

✓ **Sandpits** should be covered overnight or brought indoors to prevent contamination from animals, such as cats; they should also be checked for hazardous litter – such as sharp sticks or broken glass – and insects

✓ Check metal equipment, such as **tricycles**, **pushchairs** and **prams** for rust and/or broken hinges or sticking-out screws etc.

✓ Check wooden equipment, such as **wooden blocks** or **wheeled carts** for splinters and rough edges; remove any which are damaged and report it to your supervisor

✓ Plastic toys and equipment can be checked for splits and cracks when you clean them; plastic toys such as Duplo bricks should be washed weekly

✓ Clean all toys and playthings which are used regularly by children and check them for safety at the same time.

Teach children how to play safely

✓ Make sure that children understand how dangerous it is to play in the road. Playing in the road, even just outside the front door, is *not* safe – even if you live in a quiet street, cars will still be coming and going.

✓ Teach children never to play near or stray onto railway lines or embankments and never to dangle or throw things from railway bridges. Playing on or near railway lines is extremely dangerous – children can be electrocuted or hit by a train.

✓ Police officers are often willing to come into schools and talk to young children about road and railway safety.

✓ Learn about **sun safety**: Strong sun can easily burn the skin. For people with fair skin, the more sun that you get, the more likely you are to get skin cancer later on. Sunburn is especially bad; it hurts a lot at the time, and sunburnt children may be especially prone to skin cancer later in life. Follow these guidelines:
- Keep children out of the sun between 11 am and 2 pm. This is the time to let them read, do some drawing, watch a video or play with toys and games.
- Cover the children up. It's better to wear some clothes than nothing at all. The most protection comes from clothes that are loose; are long sleeved; and are made of tightly woven materials like T-shirts
- Provide floppy sun hats. Try to shade the head, face, neck and ears
- Coat children with sun cream. Choose a high sun protection factor (SPF), anything less than 8 is no help at all. It won't last all day so put more on from time to time especially if the children are in and out of the water.

NB Babies under 6 months old should be kept out of direct sunlight altogether.

Sun safety code

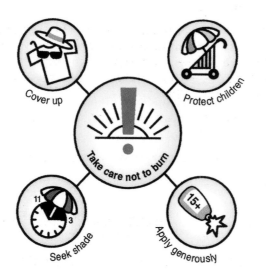

If a child does get sunburnt – move the child out of the sun and follow the guidelines on page 49 (First Aid for burns and scalds).

Children need an environment which is safe, hygienic, healthy, caring and stimulating. There is far more to creating a positive environment for children than just meeting the basic needs of children. The early childhood setting must meet all the needs of the child; these needs can be considered under the following headings:

- **Safety and security**
- **Hygiene and health**
- **Providing for children's developmental and particular needs**
- **Feeling valued**
- **A sense of belonging**
- **A comfortable child-friendly environment**

A Safety and security

A safe environment is one in which the child or adult has a low risk of becoming ill or injured. Safety is a basic human need.

❑ Children should be supervised at all times.

❑ The nursery environment and all materials and equipment should be in a safe condition.

❑ There must be adequate first aid facilities and staff should be trained in basic first aid.

❑ Routine safety checks should be made daily on premises, both indoors and outdoors.

❑ Fire drills should be held twice a term in schools and nurseries and every 6 weeks in day nurseries.

❑ Children should only be allowed home with a parent or authorised adult.

B Hygiene and health

Children need a clean, warm and hygienic environment in order to stay healthy. Although most large early years settings employ a cleaner, there will be many occasions when you have to take responsibility for ensuring that the environment is kept clean and safe; for example if a child has been sick or has had a toileting accident. You can help in the following ways:

- Be a good role model by, for example, always looking neat and tidy, washing your hands, wearing an apron during messy activities etc.

- Encourage children to cover their mouths when coughing.

- Make sure that food is stored at the correct temperature and snacks are prepared hygienically.

- Find out about the more common childhood illnesses (such as infectious diseases and asthma) and how to deal with a child who is ill.

- Prevent accidents by keeping the environment clean, tidy and uncluttered.

Providing a stimulating environment

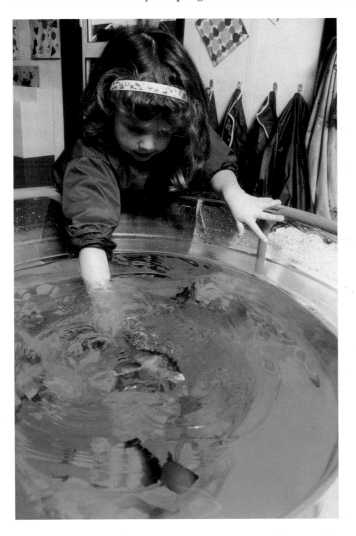

C Providing for children's developmental and particular needs

To provide for all children's needs (i.e. their physical needs, intellectual and language needs, emotional and social needs), the early years environment should:

☐ take account of each child's **individual needs** and provide for them appropriately;

☐ be **stimulating**; it should offer a wide range of activities which encourage experimentation and problem-solving;

☐ provide opportunities for all types of **play**.

D Feeling valued

Children and their families need to feel that they matter and that they are valued for themselves. You can help by:

☐ establishing a good relationship with parents; always welcoming and listening to them.

☐ squatting down or bending down to the children's level when you are talking with them.

☐ praising, appreciating and encouraging children.

☐ being responsive to children's needs.

☐ using positive images in the setting.

☐ provide **support** for children who may be experiencing strong feelings, e.g. when settling in to a new nursery or when they are angry or jealous;

☐ encourage children who use them to bring in their comfort objects, e.g. a favourite teddy or a piece of blanket;

☐ encourage the development of self-reliance and independence;

☐ ensure that children who have special needs are provided with appropriate equipment and support.

✎ ACTIVITY

Look at the layout of your own work placement. What physical changes would be necessary to include (a) a child in a wheelchair; (b) a partially sighted child; and (c) a child who uses elbow crutches.

Children with particular needs should have the same opportunities for playing and learning as other children. Early childhood settings may need to adapt their room layout to improve access, for example for children who use wheelchairs or for children with visual impairment. They may need to work with parents to find out how the child can be encouraged to participate fully with other children within the nursery or school.

E A sense of belonging

Children and their families need an environment which is reassuring and welcoming; children also need to feel that they **belong**. You can help to promote a sense of belonging by:

- greeting children individually by name and with a smile when they arrive;

- marking their coat pegs with their names and their photographs;

- naming their displayed work;

- ensuring that their cultural backgrounds are represented in the home corner, in books, displays and interest tables;

- providing **routines** for children; children like their environment to be predictable. They feel more secure and comfortable when their day has some sort of shape to it. Most early years settings have a daily routine, with fixed times for meals, snack times and outdoor play.

An organisational chart

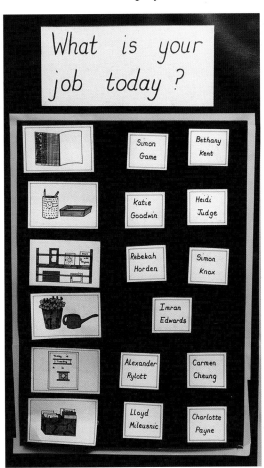

F Creating a comfortable child-friendly environment

Children who are cared for at home, in a child-minder's home or in an isolated rural pre-school group will probably not have access to special child-sized equipment or the range of activities that can be provided in a purpose-built nursery setting. Many pre-school groups have to clear away every item of equipment after each session because the hall or room is used by other groups.

In purpose-built nurseries and infant schools, there are child-sized chairs, basins, lavatories and low tables. Such provision makes the environment safer and allows children greater independence. Creating a comfortable child-friendly environment means planning both the **physical layout** and the organisation of **activities**: It involves:

✱ considering **health and safety** before anything else; for example, fire exits and doors should be kept clear at all times;

✱ giving children the maximum space and freedom to explore; rooms should be large enough to accommodate the numbers of children and be uncluttered;

✱ ensuring that the room temperature is pleasant – neither too hot nor too cold (between 18° and 21°C);

✱ making maximum use of natural light; rooms should be bright, airy and well-lit;

✱ enabling access to outdoors; this should not be restricted to certain times and seasons;

✱ ensuring displays are clearly visible and interest tables are at child height where possible, and include items which can be safely handled and explored;

✱ available space being divided appropriately to suit the range of activities offered.

The physical layout of the environment

There are certain aspects of arranging the space which are decided already by some fixed features. The electric sockets will dictate, to a certain extent, where you can site the computer, and where you can use a television/video recorder. Remember it is dangerous to have wires and leads trailing across the floor. There may need to be similar consideration for audio/tape players. Washable flooring is likely to be near the sinks and taps and messy activities need to be arranged in this area. Quieter activities and the book 'corner' will be best suited to a carpeted area although a natural light source is important. Equipment should be stored close to the area where it will be used – construction resources and 'small world' may be in tubs or crates near a large carpeted floor space where children can spread out. Pencils, paper, puzzles and table top games need to be near tables and chairs.

Furniture

The furniture in any work setting should:

* be appropriately child-sized – in all dimensions;

* comply with safety standards with regard to materials;

* be well-designed to suit its intended purpose or function;

* be stable but not too heavy – this allows items to be moved to create flexibility in layout;

* be hard-wearing;

* be easily washed/cleaned;

* have safe 'corners' (rounded or moulded) and edges;

* be attractive – perhaps through use of colour.

Provision of equipment

* *Sand – wet and dry:* equipment in boxes on shelves nearby, labelled and with a picture of contents – these may be 'themed' e.g. things with holes in/clear plastic/red items.

* *Water:* activities which require water or hand-washing should be near the sink and with aprons nearby. Equipment can be stored as for sand.

* *Clay and playdough:* cool, airtight storage; selection of utensils for mark-making, moulding, cutting.

* *A quiet area:* for looking at books and reading stories; doing floor puzzles; ideally carpeted with floor cushions.

* *Puzzles, small blocks and table-top games:* stored accessibly close to tables and carpeted area.

* *Technology:* computer, weighing balance, calculators, tape recorders etc.

* *Cookery:* with measuring equipment, bowls, spoons and baking trays

* *Art work:* with tabards/aprons, brushes, paints and other materials within easy reach.

* *Domestic play:* with dolls, cots, telephones, kitchen equipment etc.

* *Make-believe play:* box of dressing-up clothes – these should be versatile and have simple fastenings.

❋ *Small world toys:* animals, cars, people, farms, dinosaurs, train and track etc.

❋ *Construction:* blocks for building, small construction blocks e.g. Duplo; Mobilo; Stickle Bricks, etc.; a woodwork area.

❋ *Writing/graphics:* with a variety of paper and different kinds of pencils and pens.

❋ *Workshop:* with found materials e.g. cardboard from boxes, egg-boxes etc. glue, scissors, masking tape etc.

❋ *Interest table:* with interesting objects for children to handle.

❋ *Growing and living things:* fish aquarium, wormery, growing mustard and cress etc.; ensure conditions suit e.g. away from direct sunlight.

A variety of outdoor play equipment is needed:

● *Outdoor space:* with safe equipment for climbing and swinging, a safety floor surface, wheeled toys, balls and bean bags

● *Garden:* plants and a growing area, a wild area to encourage butterflies, a mud patch for digging

Supervision is important and separate areas can be divided at child height so that they can focus attention and not be distracted yet still be overseen by an adult. Storage units, low level screens and display surfaces can all be used to divide space effectively without 'shutting off ' some activities. The 'role play' area can get quite noisy and needs to be set up away from similar activities – 'small world' play, train track, construction etc. In school settings, particularly, where there will be more 'directed' and 'structured' activities this can lead to rising noise levels and causes disruption. (See pp.108–171 for detailed information about Play.)

Different types of display

☐ **Wall display:** the most usual type of display which you will find in work settings is a straightforward wall display. Boards of varying shapes and sizes are often placed on otherwise plain walls so displays can be created and changed frequently to provide interest.

☐ **Window display:** the use of windows for displays is also common. Paint (with a little washing-up liquid added so it can be easily washed off) is used to create colourful window displays – often of well-known characters from cartoons, stories or television or of animals or seasonal pictures. Sometimes pieces of art or craft work may also be attached to windows, particularly if the materials lend themselves to having light behind them – e.g. 'stained glass' windows or tissue paper pictures. Remember that the sunlight will fade the colours after a short time.

☐ **'Mobile' or 'hanging' display:** mobile or hanging displays can be used effectively, especially in very large rooms. Hanging or suspending shapes or pictures from a hoop or the ceiling needs careful thought. For them to be at an appropriate height for the children may cause difficulties for staff! Also you may have to consider security/alarm systems which can be set off by moving objects. Such displays can be useful in identifying particular areas of a work setting e.g. story characters over the book area, solid or flat shapes over the maths/number area etc.

☐ **Table top (often 'interactive') display:** table top displays (sometimes referred to as interactive displays) give you the opportunity to use objects or artefacts which will engage the children's interest. Ideas for appropriate items are given in Unit 2. Interest objects should be attractively and appealingly displayed to encourage children to interact with them. Posing a question – e.g. 'How many blue shapes can

A mobile or hanging display

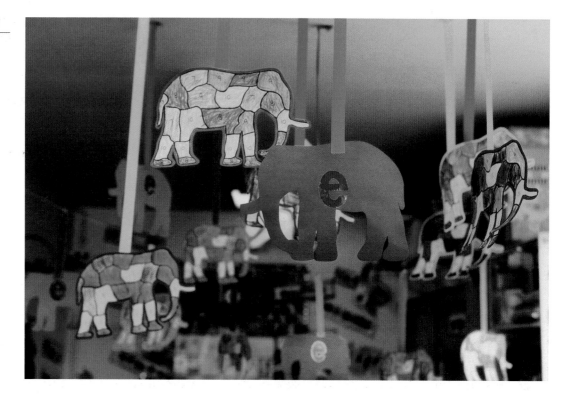

you find?' will invite children to use the display as an extra activity (if working with very young children then you must explain what they might do and, perhaps, take them to the display and handle the objects with them). These displays are often accompanied by an upright board or display space which can be used for interesting pictures, photographs or posters and your own titles to add interest. Older children may appreciate related fact and story books to use for research.

Displays

Work settings would be dull and uninteresting places without displays. They can give a lot of information to children, parents and visitors about the setting's values and **curriculum**. Displays are created for a range of purposes and, sometimes for different audiences. Most settings have a notice or display board for parents and carers, usually sited near the entrance. This is used to update general information and news about usual routine and forthcoming events. Often there will be named photographs of staff members and, perhaps, the week's menus.

Most displays reflect the activities and learning that take place. Some will be used as learning resources – alphabet and number friezes, days of the week, word banks (lists of commonly used words to consolidate reading and support writing, particularly in school settings), children's birthdays etc. – and remain on display indefinitely. Others will be of work done by the children themselves showing their ideas, of their own or about a topic or different materials – e.g. string painting, finger painting, collage etc. These displays show that we value all the children's efforts.

Displaying children's work

Creating attractive displays needs careful consideration and can be time consuming. Factors to take into account: size of space available, themes/materials/colour schemes of adjacent displays, location of space (some are very tricky, having thermostat controls or pipes in awkward places or involve going round corners!), availability of materials, age and stage of development of children – this affects content and what labels/titles/ lettering you use.

Some general points to bear in mind when you are creating displays:

DO

✓ name individual children's work (correctly), preferably top left-hand corner (unless you are labelling underneath);

✓ let children see you handle their work with respect;

✓ use appropriate language and symbols;

✓ check that work is trimmed and properly aligned (straight!);

✓ make sure titles and labels are clearly legible;

✓ arrange any objects at a good viewing height for children;

✓ mount the exhibits – use clean backgrounds and think carefully about colours;

✓ talk to the children about your display and, where appropriate, let them help in selecting work;

✓ allow space and margins around each piece of work;

✓ use appropriate lettering for age and stage of development of children.

DO NOT

✗ use drawing pins (unless instructed to do so by your placement) – they are dangerous and unsightly;

✗ display things where they can be easily damaged or splashed (or picked at!);

✗ make spelling mistakes;

✗ overcrowd your display space;

✗ waste resources;

✗ leave paper cutters and/or your materials lying around.

REMEMBER Good lettering enhances a display – poor lettering spoils it!

A wall display

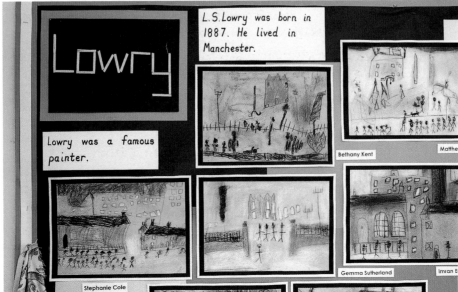

✎ ACTIVITY

Create two displays. It is a good idea to do them in different settings for different age ranges and to produce different types – e.g. one of individual children's work and one 'whole class' display or one hanging and one table-top display. You will need permission from your supervisor(s) and signature(s) to them. When writing your display 'reports' you should include a photograph of the finished display or an accurate, labelled sketch. Your tutor will guide you for your written work but your report could include:

- A description of the theme or subject of your display – explain your choice (or why you carried it out – e.g. Supervisor's request to fit with current work etc.).

- Descriptions (or if possible samples) of the materials you used in creating the display. This includes the backing paper, borders etc. Give reasons for your choice e.g. range of textures, appropriate colours.

- Information about the factors you needed to consider in creating your display? Some examples may be siting/position/size or availability of resources, consideration of children's age/background etc.

- Information about the decisions you made about lettering, titles, children's names etc. Think about size/upper or lower case/style. Give reasons for your choices.

- The value of the display to the children, the environment, visitors etc.? How has the display been used or referred to in the work setting?

- Your own learning – were you happy with the end result? How did the children and other staff/visitors respond? What might you have done differently and why?

An interactive table display

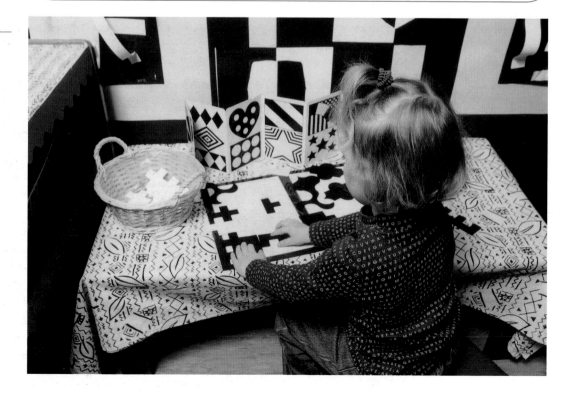

✏ ACTIVITY

Plan an activity which teaches children about one aspect of safety, for example:

- safety in the outdoor area or playground
- road safety

The activity should be appropriate for the age of the children you will carry it out with. Ideas include a story, an action rhyme, a board game or a simple computer game. You could write to **The Child Accident Prevention Trust** for some ideas. See Addresses list at the end of the book. (Don't forget to enclose a stamped addressed envelope.)

🧸 Follow the setting's health and safety policies

Every workplace must follow Government guidelines for health and safety. The relevant Acts for child care settings are **The Children Act 1989**, **The Health and Safety at Work Act 1974**, and **The Food Safety Regulations Act 1995**.

The safety of children on group outings

Children sometimes get the chance to go on organised trips with schools or nurseries. These outings include trips to farms, parks, museums and theatres. Many schools now employ an Educational Visit Coordinator to oversee the safety of school trips. The need for safety of children is the primary concern. Each setting must consider the following points:

☐ **Planning:** you may need to visit the place beforehand and to discuss any particular requirements, for example – what to do if it rains, or specific lunch arrangements.

☐ **Permission:** The manager or head teacher must give permission for the outing, and a letter should be sent to all parents and guardians of the children.

☐ **Help:** usually help is requested from parents so that adequate supervision is ensured.

☐ **Informing parents:** about what is involved on the outing – what the child needs to bring – e.g. packed meal, waterproof coat etc.; emphasise NO glass bottles and NO sweets; spending money if necessary – state the advised maximum amount.

☐ **Supervision:** arrange adequate adult supervision. There should always be trained staff on any outing, however local and low-key. The adult:child ratio should never exceed 1:4. If the children are under 2 years old or have special needs, then you would expect to have fewer children per adult. Swimming trips should only be attempted if the ratio is 1 adult to 1 child for children under 5 years. The younger the children, the more adults are required, particularly if the trip involves crossing roads, when an adult must be available to hold the children's hands.

☐ **Transport:** if a coach is being hired, check whether it has seat belts for children. New laws require all new minibuses and coaches to have seat belts fitted and minibus drivers have to have passed a special driving test.

Safety at home times

Any early childhood setting or school should be secure so that children cannot wander off without anyone realising. There should also be a policy which guards against strangers being able to wander in without reason. Many child care settings now have door entry phones, and staff wear name badges. It is a matter of courtesy and security for all visitors for them to give advance notice of their visit.

CASE STUDY

Rachel is a three-year-old child who attends a nursery group three mornings a week. Her parents recently separated and now live apart. Rachel is usually collected at the end of the nursery session by her mother, but occasionally, usually on a Friday, her father and his new female partner collect her because she stays with them at weekends. Rachel's mother has spoken to the nursery manager about this arrangement and has agreed that she will always inform the staff on the days when Rachel's father will be collecting her. One Friday, Rachel's father turns up unexpectedly – and ten minutes early – to collect her from nursery and explains that it was a last-minute arrangement between himself and Rachel's mother that he should collect Rachel because they were going away on holiday. Rachel seems very excited about going away. Her father insists that Rachel's mother is happy about it and is clearly angry to be questioned and impatient to get away as they have a train to catch.

Discuss the scenario above in class and answer the following questions;

1　Should the staff at the nursery consent to Rachel's father taking Rachel from the nursery?

2　What are the main issues involved in this case study?

3　What would you do if you were in charge?

Try to think around the problem, e.g. if you decide to contact Rachel's mother, what if you can't get in touch? etc.

Find out how your training placement deals with issues of safety at home times.

Understand the importance of immunisation and other preventative health measures

Another important part of protecting children and keeping them safe is to protect them from the **spread of infection**. You can help to minimise the spread of infection by:

- learning about childhood immunisation;
- understanding how **cross-infection** occurs and taking appropriate measures;
- developing routines which ensure **good hygiene**;
- **caring for animals** in the work setting in a safe and hygienic manner.

Childhood immunisation

In the UK parents can decide whether or not to have their children immunised against the common childhood infectious diseases. In group settings, children come into contact with a number of bacteria and viruses for the first time. Immunisation is a good way of ensuring that the more common childhood infections, such as measles, mumps and rubella (German measles) are prevented. The current schedule for immunisation in the UK is:

Birth	bcg	to those in high-risk groups – i.e. likely to be in close contact with a case of tuberculosis
8 weeks	Diphtheria Tetanus Pertussis	Given as a single injection
	Hib	Haemophilus influenza type b
	Polio	Given orally
12 weeks	Diphtheria Tetanus Pertussis	Given as a single injection
	Hib	Given in another site
	Polio	Given orally
16 weeks	Diphtheria Tetanus Pertussis	Given as a single injection
	Hib	Given in another site on the body
	Polio	Given orally
12–18 months	Measles Mumps Rubella	MMR – given as a single injection
4–5 years	Diphtheria Tetanus	Given as a single injection
	Polio	Given orally

The immunisation schedule

Health and hygiene in the child care setting

All child care and education settings must have a written policy for dealing with health and hygiene issues:

✱ Always wear disposable latex gloves when dealing with blood, urine, faeces or vomit.

✱ Always wash your hands after dealing with spillages – even if gloves have been worn.

✱ Use a dilute bleach (hypochlorite) solution to mop up any spillages.

✱ Make sure paper tissues are available for children to use.

✱ Always cover cuts and open sores with adhesive plasters.

✱ Food is stored and prepared hygienically

✱ Parents are asked to keep their children at home if they are feeling unwell or if they have an infection.

✱ Children who are sent home with vomiting or diarrhoea must remain at home until at least 24 hours have elapsed since the last attack.

✱ Parents must provide written authorisation for child care workers to administer medications to children.

Caring for animals in child care settings

Small pets can provide a homely atmosphere in nurseries and schools. They can extend children's knowledge and skills as well as giving enjoyment to everyone. However, a number of infectious diseases can be acquired from contact with animals, so good pet care and attention to hygiene is very important.

Parents choosing a pet for their children should accept that they (the parents themselves) are totally responsible for its well-being and survival, however keen the children themselves are.

A young child cannot be expected to judge when the animal has played long enough, whether its diet is suitable or how often its cage needs cleaning.

The most popular animals to keep in child care settings are:

✱ Guinea pigs

✱ Gerbils

✱ Rabbits

✱ Hamsters

Playing with a hamster in a nursery setting

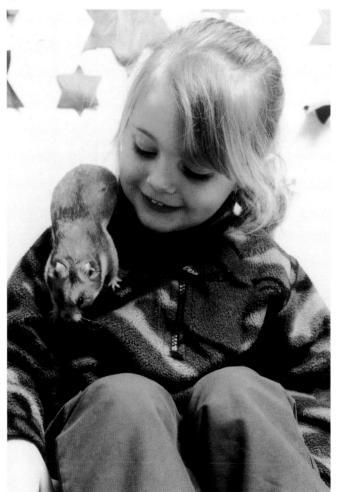

The **RSPCA** (the Royal Society for the Prevention of Cruelty to Animals) advises child care settings to explore alternatives to keeping pets in the workplace. They recommend, for example, taking children on walks to observe animals and birds in their natural habitat, or inviting people to bring their pets in to the nursery for a special session.

Pet safety and hygiene

If pets are kept in the setting, the following safety and hygiene rules should be followed:

✓ Always make sure that animals are well cared for – regular cleaning of cages and feeding bowls, adequate rest and sleep periods, and good care during holidays and weekends

✓ Children and adults should always wash their hands after handling pets

✓ Make sure that children do not put their fingers in cages or come into contact with the food, bowls and litter trays of pets

✓ Keep cutlery and crockery for animals separate from those for the children in the setting

✓ Never leave babies and young children alone in a room with any uncaged animal

✓ Always supervise children when handling a small pet.

3

Basic First Aid

- recording accidents and emergencies
- basic first aid procedures
- basic accident procedures
- getting emergency help
- the contents of the first aid box and the procedures for replacing used materials
- giving accurate information to parents without causing undue alarm

Everyone who works with children should attend a first aid course. There are now specialist courses, such as the St John's Babies and Children Lifesaver Awards. (See addresses section at the end of this book.) Once you have learnt how to respond to an emergency you never lose that knowledge, and knowing how means that you could save a life one day.

The following charts explain the major first aid techniques, but should not be used as a substitute for attending a first aid course with a trained instructor.

ABC of resuscitation: babies up to one year old

If a baby appears unconscious and gives no response

A Airway – open the airway

✱ Place the baby on a firm surface.

✱ Remove any obstruction from the mouth.

✱ Put one hand on the forehead and one finger under the chin, and gently tilt the head backwards VERY SLIGHTLY. (If you tilt the head too far back, it will close the airway again.)

If there is no pulse, or the pulse is slower than 60 beats per minute, and the baby is not breathing, start **chest compressions**.

1 Find a position one finger's width below the line joining the baby's nipples, in the centre of the breastbone.

2 Place the tips of two fingers on this point and press to a depth of about 2 cm (¾ inch) at a rate of 100 times per minute.

B Breathing – check for breathing

- Put your ear close to the baby's mouth.
- Look to see if the chest is rising and falling.
- Listen and feel for the baby's breath on your cheek.
- Do this for five seconds.

If the baby is **not** breathing

1 Start MOUTH TO MOUTH-AND-NOSE RESUSCITATION:
   - Seal your lips around the baby's mouth and nose.
   - Blow GENTLY into the lungs until the chest rises.
   - Remove your mouth and allow the chest to fall.

2 Repeat five times at the rate of one breath every three seconds.

3 Check the pulse.

4 After five compressions, blow gently into the lungs once.

5 Continue the cycle for one minute.

6 Carry the baby to a phone and dial 999 for an ambulance.

7 Continue resuscitation, checking the pulse every minute until help arrives.

If the baby is **not** breathing but **does** have a pulse

1 Start **MOUTH TO MOUTH-AND-NOSE RESUSCITATION**, at the rate of one breath every three seconds.

2 Continue for one minute, then carry the baby to a phone and dial 999 for an ambulance.

C Circulation – check the pulse

Lightly press your fingers towards the bone on the inside of the upper arm and hold them there for five seconds.

If the baby **does** have a pulse and **is** breathing

1 Lay the baby on its side, supported by a cushion, pillow, rolled-up blanket or something similar.

2 Dial 999 for an ambulance.

3 Check breathing and pulse every minute, and be prepared to carry out resuscitation.

ABC of resuscitation: children aged 1 to 10

A Airway – open the airway

☐ Lay the child flat on their back.

☐ Remove clothing from around the neck.

☐ Remove any obstruction from the mouth.

☐ Lift the chin and tilt the head back slightly to open the airway.

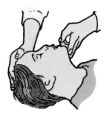

If the child is **not** breathing and does **not** have a pulse

1 Begin a cycle of five chest compressions (see chest compression) and one breath (see mouth-to-mouth resuscitation). Continue for one minute.

2 Dial 999 for an ambulance.

3 Continue at the rate of one breath to five compressions until help arrives.

If the child is **not** breathing but **does** have a pulse

1 Give 20 breaths (see mouth-to-mouth resuscitation) in one minute.

2 Dial 999 for an ambulance.

3 Continue mouth-to-mouth resuscitation, rechecking the pulse and breathing after each set of 20 breaths, until help arrives or until the child starts breathing again. When breathing returns, place the child in the recovery position.

B Breathing – check for breathing

- Keep the airway open and place your cheek close to the child's mouth.
- Look to see if their chest is rising and falling.
- Listen and feel for their breath against your cheek.
- Do this for five seconds.
- If the child is not breathing, give five breaths (see mouth-to-mouth resuscitation), then check the pulse.

Mouth-to-mouth resuscitation:

1 Open the airway by lifting the chin and tilting back the head. Check the mouth is clear of obstructions.

2 Close the child's nose by pinching the nostrils.

3 Take a deep breath and seal your mouth over the child's.

4 Blow firmly into the mouth for about two seconds, watching the chest rise.

5 Remove your mouth and allow the child's chest to fall.

6 Repeat until help arrives.

C Circulation – check the pulse

Find the carotid pulse by placing your fingers in the groove between the Adam's apple and the large muscle running down the side of the neck

Do this for five seconds.

Chest compression:

1 Make sure the child is lying on their back on a firm surface (preferably the ground).

2 Find the spot where the bottom of the ribcage joins on to the end of the breastbone, and measure one finger's width up from this point.

3 Using one hand only, press down sharply at a rate of 100 times a minute, to a depth of about 3 cm (1¼ inches). Counting aloud will help you keep at the right speed.

4 Continue until help arrives.

Choking

Check inside the baby's mouth. If the obstruction is visible, try to hook it out with your finger, but don't risk pushing it further down. If this doesn't work, proceed as follows:

- Lay the baby face down along your forearm with your hand supporting her head and neck, and her head lower than her bottom. OR:
- An older baby or toddler may be placed face down across your knee with head and arms hanging down.
- Give five brisk slaps between the shoulder blades.
- Turn the baby over, check the mouth and remove any obstruction.
- Check for breathing.
- If the baby is not breathing, give five breaths (see **MOUTH TO MOUTH-AND-NOSE RESUSCITATION**).
- If the airway is still obstructed, give five **CHEST COMPRESSIONS**.
- If the baby is still not breathing, repeat the cycle of back slaps, mouth to mouth-and nose breathing and chest compressions.
- After two cycles, if the baby is not breathing, dial 999 for an ambulance.

NB: Never hold babies or young children upside down by the ankles and slap their back – you could break their neck.

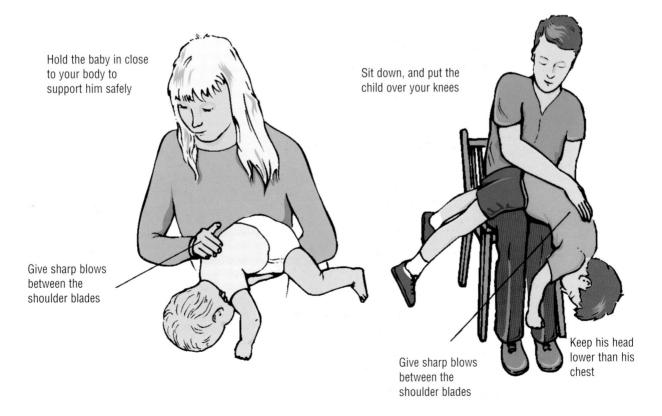

Hold the baby in close to your body to support him safely

Give sharp blows between the shoulder blades

Sit down, and put the child over your knees

Give sharp blows between the shoulder blades

Keep his head lower than his chest

Head injuries

Babies and young children are particularly prone to injury from falls. Any injury to the head must be investigated carefully. A head injury can damage the scalp, skull or brain.

Symptoms and signs

If the head injury is mild, the only symptom may be a slight headache and this will probably result in a crying baby. More seriously, the baby may:

- lose consciousness even if only for a few minutes;
- vomit;
- seem exceptionally drowsy;
- complain of an ache or pain in the head;
- lose blood from her nose, mouth or ears;
- lose any watery fluid from her nose or ears;
- have an injury to the scalp which might suggest a fracture to the skull bones.

Treatment

If the baby or young child has any of the above symptoms: **dial 999 for an ambulance or go straight to your nearest A&E department.**

Meanwhile:

- if the child is unconscious, follow the **ABC routine** described on page 44–46;
- stop any bleeding by applying direct pressure, but take care that you are not pressing a broken bone into the delicate tissue underneath; if in doubt, apply pressure around the edge of the wound, using dressings;
- if there is discharge from the ear, position the child so that the affected ear is lower and cover with a clean pad; do not plug the ear.

Burns and scalds

Burns are injuries to body tissues caused by heat, chemicals or radiations. Scalds are caused by wet heat, such as steam or hot liquids.

Superficial burns involve only the outer layers of the skin, cause redness, swelling, tenderness and usually heal well. Intermediate burns form blisters, can become infected, and need medical aid. Deep burns involve all layers of the skin, which may be pale and charred, may be pain free if the nerves are damaged, and will ALWAYS require medical attention.

Treatment for severe burns and scalds

- Lay the child down and protect burnt area from ground contact
- Check ABC of resuscitation and be ready to resuscitate if necessary
- Gently remove any constricting clothing from the injured area before it begins to swell

- Cover the injured area loosely with a sterile un-medicated dressing or use a clean non-fluffy tea-towel or pillowcase

DO NOT remove anything that is sticking to the burn

DO NOT apply lotions, creams or fat to the injury

DO NOT break blisters

DO NOT use plasters

- If the child is unconscious, lay the child on her side, supported by a cushion, pillow, rolled-up blanket or something similar
- Send for medical attention

Treatment for minor burns and scalds

- Place the injured part under slowly running water, or soak in cold water for 10 minutes
- Gently remove any constricting articles from the injured area before it begins to swell
- Dress with clean, sterile, non-fluffy material

DO NOT use adhesive dressings

DO NOT apply lotions, ointments or fat to burn or scald

DO NOT break blisters or otherwise interfere

- If in doubt, seek medical aid

Treatment for sunburn

- Remove the child to the shade and cool the skin by gently sponging the skin with tepid (lukewarm) water
- Give sips of cold water at frequent intervals
- If the burns are mild, gently apply an after-sun cream
- For extensive blistering, seek medical help

Drowning

If a baby or small child is discovered under water, either in the bath or a pool, follow these guidelines:

✓ Call for emergency medical attention. Dial 999

✓ Keep child's neck immobilized as you remove him/her from the water.

✓ Restore breathing and circulation first.

✓ If child is unconscious or you suspect neck injuries, do not bend or turn neck while restoring breathing.

✓ Give rescue breathing if the child is not breathing but has a pulse. Breathe forcefully enough to blow air through water in the airway. Do not try to empty water from child's lungs.

✓ Do not give up. Give cardio-pulmonary resuscitation (CPR) if the child does not have a pulse. Continue until child is revived, until medical help arrives, or until exhaustion stops you.

Signs and symptoms

Look for one or more of the following:

- unconsciousness; no pulse
- no visible or audible breath
- bluish-coloured skin
- pale lips, tongue, and/or nail bed

Immediate treatment

1 Lie child on flat surface, or begin first aid in the water.

2 Check ABC (Airway, Breathing, Circulation)

3 If child is not breathing, open airway and start rescue breathing.

4 Check pulse and continue CPR if necessary to restore circulation.

5 When breathing and pulse have been restored, treat for shock.

6 Have child lie down on his/her side to allow water to drain from the mouth.

7 Restore child's body heat by removing wet clothing and covering child with warm blankets.

8 Do not give up if breathing and pulse are not restored. Continue CPR until help arrives.

Cuts and bleeding

Young children often sustain minor cuts and grazes. Most of these occur as a result of falls and only result in a very small amount of bleeding.

NB Always wear disposable gloves if in an early years setting to prevent cross infection.

For minor cuts and grazes:

- Sit or lie the child down and reassure him or her
- Clean the injured area with cold water, using cotton wool or gauze
- Apply a dressing if necessary
- Do not attempt to pick out pieces of gravel or grit from a graze; just clean gently and cover with a light dressing

Record the injury and treatment in the **Accident Report Book** and make sure the parents/carers of the child are informed.

For severe bleeding:

1 Summon medical help – dial 999 or call a doctor.

2 Try to stop the bleeding:

- Apply direct pressure to the wound. Wear gloves and use a dressing or a non-fluffy material, such as a clean tea-towel
- Elevate the affected part if possible

3 Apply a dressing. If the blood soaks through, DO NOT remove the dressing, apply another on top and so on.

- Keep the child warm and reassure him or her
- DO NOT give anything to eat or drink
- Contact the child's parents or carers.
- If the child loses consciousness, follow the ABC procedure for resuscitation.

NB Always record the incident and the treatment given in the Accident Report Book

How to get emergency help

1 **Assess the situation:** stay calm and don't panic

2 **Minimise any danger** to yourself and to others; e.g. make sure someone takes charge of other children at the scene

3 **Send for help.** Notify a doctor, hospital, parents etc. as appropriate. If in any doubt: call an ambulance: dial 999

Be ready to assist the emergency services by answering some simple questions:

❑ your name and the telephone number you are calling from;

❑ the location of the accident. Try to give as much information as possible, e.g. familiar landmarks such as churches or pubs nearby;

❑ explain briefly what has happened: this helps the paramedics to act speedily when they arrive;

❑ tell them what you have done so far to treat the casualty.

Understand your role and responsibility in reporting and recording accidents

Reporting to parents

All accidents, injuries or illnesses which occur to children in a group setting must be reported to the child's parents or primary carers. If the injury is minor – e.g. a bruise or a small graze to the knee – the nursery or school staff will inform parents when the child is collected at the end of the session; or they may send a notification slip home if the child is collected by someone else. The parents are notified about

- the nature of the injury or illness;
- any treatment or action taken;
- the name of the person who carried out the treatment.

In the case of a major accident, illness or injury then the child's parents or primary carers must be notified as soon as possible. Parents need to know that the staff are dealing with the incident in a caring and professional manner and to be involved in any decisions regarding treatment.

Accident Report Book

Every workplace is, by law, required to have an Accident Report Book and to maintain a record of accidents. Information recorded includes:

* Name of person injured.

* Date and time of injury.

* Where the accident happened, e.g. in the garden.

* What exactly happened, e.g. Kara fell on the path and grazed her left knee.

* What injuries occurred, e.g. a graze.

* What treatment was given, e.g. graze was bathed and an adhesive dressing applied.

* Name and signature of person dealing with the accident.

* Signature of witness to the report.

* Signature of parent or guardian.

One copy of the duplicated report form is given to the child's parent or carer; the other copy is kept in the Accident Report book at the child care setting.

If you are working in the family home as a nanny, you should follow the same reporting procedure, even though you do not have an official Accident Report Book.

The first aid box

Every place of work must, by law, have an accessible First Aid box with the following recommended basic contents:

* 20 individually-wrapped sterile adhesive dressings – in assorted sizes

* 2 sterile eye pads

* 6 individually-wrapped triangular bandages

* 6 safety pins

* 6 medium-sized individually-wrapped sterile wound dressings

* 2 large individually-wrapped sterile wound dressings

* 3 extra-large individually-wrapped sterile wound dressings

* 2 pairs of disposable gloves

* 1 pair of blunt-ended scissors.

Large nurseries and schools may have more than one first aid box and the contents will vary according to individual needs; for example, a nursery setting will have a larger number of small adhesive dressings or plasters.

* The first aid box must be a strong container which keeps out both dirt and damp.

* It should be kept in an accessible place, but one that is out of reach of children.

* All employees should be informed where the first aid box is kept and it should only be moved from this safe place when in use.

* Supplies must be replaced as soon as possible after use.

* Some first aid boxes also contain a small first aid manual or booklet.

4

The physical care and development of children

- basic needs of children
- preventing cross infection
- basic care of children
- choosing and caring for appropriate clothing and footwear
- the role of rest and sleep
- personal hygiene routines for each stage of development
- caring for all children including those with special needs

The basic needs of children

To achieve and maintain healthy growth and development, (that is physical, intellectual and emotional), certain basic needs must be fulfilled. These basic needs are:

- food
- shelter, warmth, clothing
- cleanliness
- fresh air and sunlight
- sleep, rest and activity
- love and consistent and continuous affection
- protection from infection and injury
- stimulation
- social contacts
- security

It is difficult to separate these basic needs in practical care, as they all contribute to the holistic development of a healthy child.

Caring for children's skin and hair

As children grow and become involved in more vigorous exercise, especially outside, a daily bath or shower becomes necessary. Most young children love bath-time and adding bubble bath to the water adds to the fun of getting clean. **NB Children should never be left alone in the bath or shower, because of the risk of drowning and scalding.**

Caring for children's skin and hair

- Wash face and hands in the morning (NB Muslims always wash under running water).

- Always wash hands after using the toilet and before meals; dry hands thoroughly – young children will need supervision.

- After using the toilet, girls should be taught to wipe their bottom from front to back to prevent germs from the anus entering the vagina and urethra.

- Wash hands after playing outside or after handling animals.

- Nails should be scrubbed with a soft nailbrush and trimmed regularly by cutting straight across; never cut into the sides of the nails as this can cause sores and infections.

- Find out about any special skin conditions, such as eczema or dry skin and be guided by the parents' advice concerning the use of soap and creams.

- Hair usually only needs washing twice a week; children with long or curly hair benefit from the use of a conditioning shampoo which helps to reduce tangles. Hair should always be rinsed thoroughly in clean water and not brushed until it is dry – brushing wet hair damages the hair shafts. A wide-toothed comb is useful for combing wet hair.

- Afro-Caribbean hair tends to dryness and may need special oil or moisturisers; if the hair is braided (with or without beads), it may be washed with the braids left intact, unless otherwise advised.

- Rastafarian children with hair styled in dreadlocks may not use either combs or shampoo, preferring to brush the dreadlocks gently and secure them with braid.

- Children should have their own flannel, comb and brush which should be cleaned regularly.

- Skin should always be dried thoroughly, taking special care of such areas as between the toes and under the armpits; black skin tends to dryness and may need massaging with special oils or moisturisers.

Care of children's teeth

After the child's first birthday, children can be taught to brush their own teeth; but they will need careful supervision. You can help by following these guidelines:

- Teach children to brush their teeth after meals.

- Show them how to brush up and away from the gum when cleaning the lower teeth and down and away from the gum when cleaning the upper teeth.

- Younger children will need help in brushing the back teeth.

- Provide a diet with foods rich in calcium, vitamins and with good textures for chewing.

- Clean teeth thoroughly after sugary drinks or sweets to avoid tooth decay.

- Take children regularly to the dentist so that they get used to the idea of having their mouth looked at.

Teeth care routine in a nursery

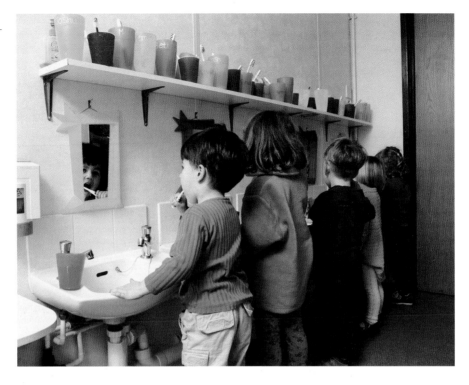

Supporting hygiene routines

All children benefit from regular routines in daily care. You need to encourage children to become independent by helping them to learn how to take care of themselves. Ways of helping children to become independent include:

- ❑ teaching children how to wash and to dry their hands before eating or drinking;

- ❑ making sure that children always wash and dry their hands after going to the toilet and after playing outdoors;

- ❑ providing children with their own combs and brushes and encouraging them to use them every day;

- ❑ providing a soft toothbrush and teaching children how and when to brush their teeth;

- ❑ ensuring that you are good role models for children; for example, when you cough or sneeze, you always cover your mouth;

- ❑ devise activities which develop an awareness in children of the importance of hygiene routines; for example, you could invite a dental hygienist or dental nurse to the setting to talk to children about daily teeth care;

- ❑ make sure that children are provided with a healthy diet and that there are opportunities for activity, rest and sleep throughout the nursery or school day.

Equipment for physical care

There is a wide variety of equipment which may be used when physically caring for children. Children will find it easier to be independent in their hygiene routines if they are provided with suitable equipment, e.g. a stool that enables them to reach the washbasin or a child-sized toothbrush.

✏️ ACTIVITY

In groups of three or four, make a list of items that you think would be helpful when caring for two children, aged 2 and 4 years, at home and in a nursery school. You could look at advertisements for children's toiletries and equipment in parenting magazines or use a store catalogue. Use the following headings:

- items for washing and bathing;
- items for caring for teeth;
- items for caring for children's hair;
- items to encourage independence during toilet training.

Under each heading list the item, your reason for choosing it and its cost.

The importance of rest and sleep

Rest and sleep are important for our health and well being. **Sleep** has the following functions:

- it rests and restores our bodies;
- it enables the brain and the body's **metabolic** processes to recover;
- during sleep, **growth hormone** is released; this renews tissues and produces new bone and red blood cells;
- dreaming is believed to help the brain sort out information stored in the memory during waking hours.

Children vary enormously in their need for sleep and rest. Some children seem able to rush around all day with very little rest; others will need to recharge their batteries by having frequent periods of rest. You need to be able to recognise the signs that a child is tired; these may include:

- ☐ Looking tired – dark rings under the eyes and yawning
- ☐ Asking for their comfort object
- ☐ Constant rubbing of the eyes
- ☐ Twiddling their hair and fidgeting with objects
- ☐ Showing no interest in activities and in their surroundings
- ☐ Being particularly emotional – crying or being stubborn
- ☐ Withdrawing into themselves – sucking thumb and appearing listless

Establishing a routine

Children will only sleep if they are actually tired, so it is important that enough activity and exercise is provided. Some children do not have a nap during the day but should be encouraged to rest in a quiet area.

When preparing children for a daytime nap, rest or bedtime sleep, you need to:

- ☐ Treat each child uniquely; every child will have their own needs for sleep and rest.
- ☐ Find out all you can about the individual child's sleep habits; for example, some children like to be patted to sleep, whilst others need to have their favourite comfort object.

❑ Be guided by the wishes of the child's parents or carers; some parents, for example, prefer their child to have a morning nap but not an afternoon nap, as this routine fits in better with the family's routine.

❑ Reassure children that they will not be left alone and that you or someone else will be there when they wake up.

❑ Keep noise to a minimum and darken the room; make sure that children have been to the lavatory – children need to understand the signals which mean that it is time for everyone to have a rest or sleep.

❑ Provide quiet, relaxing activities for children who are unable, or who do not want to sleep; for example, jigsaw puzzles, a story tape or reading a book.

When preparing children for the night-time sleep, you need to follow the guidelines above and also to:

● Warn the child that bedtime is approaching (e.g. after the bath and story) and then follow a set routine.

A bedtime routine

✓ Take a family meal about 1½ hours before bedtime. This should be a relaxing, social occasion.

✓ After the meal, the child could play with other members of the family.

✓ Make bath-time a relaxing time to unwind and play with the child; this often helps the child to feel drowsy.

✓ Give a final bedtime drink followed by teeth cleaning. (Never withhold a drink at bedtime when potty-training – see below.)

✓ Read or tell a story; looking at books together develops a feeling of closeness between the child and their carer.

✓ Settle the child in bed, with curtains drawn and nightlight on if desired, and then say goodnight and leave.

ACTIVITY

Sleep and rest

This task actually requires **two observations**. One should be carried out in your reception class and the other at a later stage in your nursery placement.

For each observation:

1 Complete a front sheet and ensure you have your supervisor's signature.

2 Write an introduction (see below).

3 Present your information in a chart format (the method is called a time sample).

4 Write an evaluation or conclusion (see below).

When you have done all of the above you must then make a comparison between the two children referring to theories about children's sleep requirements. Include a bibliography.

Introduction

In this section you need to explain how the placement timetable allows periods of activity and rest. It is unlikely that children at school actually sleep/take naps, but there are playtimes when they can be energetic and take exercise and also quieter periods when they can sit and be still. If the child you are observing has only recently started attending for whole days you should make this clear in this section. When you focus on the nursery age child the attendance may be only for half-day sessions. You need to make this clear too.

Time	Activity	What child is doing	Other information
9.00	Register time	Sitting quietly on carpet with rest of class	Smiling and looking at teacher
9.40	Drawing pictures and writing in news book	Sitting at table drawing picture and talking to another child	Fidgeting and looking up from work
10.20	Playtime – in playground	Running around at one corner of playground – game with three other children	Smiling and stopping sometimes to shout to friend
etc.			

Evaluation or conclusion

Use the information from your chart to see if there is a pattern of rest/activity. Can you tell when the child is restless and wants to be active or is tired and needs a period of rest? Does this child's day offer enough of each at the right times? What do you know about the importance of rest and/or sleep for health and to aid concentration?

Comparison

Try to note similarities and differences between the two and try to explain them. Refer to what you know about children's needs at different ages and stages of their development – do these children fit the patterns you would expect?

Bibliography

List the books you have read and/or used in writing your conclusions.

The development of bowel and bladder control

Newborn babies pass the waste products of digestion automatically; in other words, although they may go red in the face when passing a stool or motion, they have no conscious control over the action. Parents used to boast with pride that all their children were potty trained at nine months, but the reality is that they were just lucky in their timing! Up to the age of about 18 months, emptying of the bladder and bowel is still a totally automatic reaction – the child's central nervous system (CNS) is still not sufficiently mature to make the connection between the action and its results. There is no point in attempting to start toilet training until the child shows that he or she is ready, and this rarely occurs before the age of 18 months. The usual signs that children are ready to make the move from nappies to using the potty or toilet are when they:

show increased interest when passing urine or a motion; they may pretend play on the potty with their toys;

✱ may tell their carer when they have passed urine or a bowel motion or look very uncomfortable; sometimes a child will anticipate a bowel motion by calling for you and clutching themselves;

✱ may start to be more regular with bowel motions or the wet nappies may become rarer.

Toilet training

Toilet training should be approached in a relaxed, unhurried manner. If the potty is introduced too early, or if a child is forced to sit on it for long periods of time, they may rebel and the whole issue of toilet training becomes a battleground.

Toilet training can be over in a few days or may take some months. Becoming dry at night takes longer, but most children manage this before the age of 5.

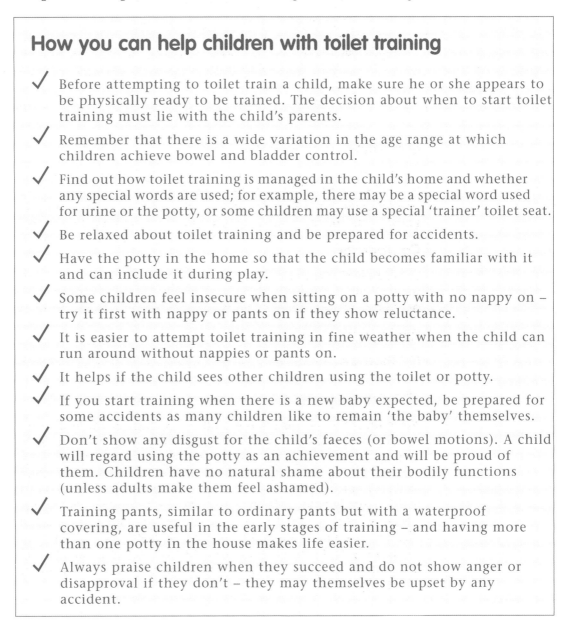

How you can help children with toilet training

✓ Before attempting to toilet train a child, make sure he or she appears to be physically ready to be trained. The decision about when to start toilet training must lie with the child's parents.

✓ Remember that there is a wide variation in the age range at which children achieve bowel and bladder control.

✓ Find out how toilet training is managed in the child's home and whether any special words are used; for example, there may be a special word used for urine or the potty, or some children may use a special 'trainer' toilet seat.

✓ Be relaxed about toilet training and be prepared for accidents.

✓ Have the potty in the home so that the child becomes familiar with it and can include it during play.

✓ Some children feel insecure when sitting on a potty with no nappy on – try it first with nappy or pants on if they show reluctance.

✓ It is easier to attempt toilet training in fine weather when the child can run around without nappies or pants on.

✓ It helps if the child sees other children using the toilet or potty.

✓ If you start training when there is a new baby expected, be prepared for some accidents as many children like to remain 'the baby' themselves.

✓ Don't show any disgust for the child's faeces (or bowel motions). A child will regard using the potty as an achievement and will be proud of them. Children have no natural shame about their bodily functions (unless adults make them feel ashamed).

✓ Training pants, similar to ordinary pants but with a waterproof covering, are useful in the early stages of training – and having more than one potty in the house makes life easier.

✓ Always praise children when they succeed and do not show anger or disapproval if they don't – they may themselves be upset by any accident.

✓ Offer the potty regularly so that the child becomes used to the idea of a routine, and get used to the signs that a child needs to use it.

✓ Encourage good hygiene right from the start; wipe the child's bottom (wipe girls from front to back to prevent infection); wash (or help the child to wash) their hands after every visit to the potty.

✓ Some children are frightened when the toilet is flushed; be tactful and sympathetic and wait to flush until the child has left the room.

✓ Cover the potty and flush the contents down the toilet. Always wear disposable gloves.

✓ The child may prefer to try the 'big' toilet seat straight away; a trainer seat fixed onto the normal seat makes this easier. Boys need to learn to stand in front of the toilet and aim at the bowl before passing any urine; you could try putting a piece of toilet paper in the bowl for him to aim at.

Dealing with accidents

Even once a child has become used to using the potty or toilet, there will inevitably be occasions when they have an 'accident', that is, they wet or soil themselves. This happens more often during the early stages of toilet training, as the child may still lack the awareness or the control to allow enough time to get to the potty. Older children may become so absorbed in their play that they simply forget to go to the toilet.

You can help children when they have an accident by:

✓ Not appearing bothered; let the child know that it is not a big problem, just something that happens from time to time.

✓ Reassure the child by using a friendly tone of voice and offering a cuddle if they seem distressed.

✓ Be discreet; deal with the matter swiftly – wash and change them out of view of others and with the minimum of fuss.

✓ If older children want to manage the incident themselves, encourage them to do so, but always check tactfully afterwards that they have managed.

✓ Always follow safety procedures in the setting; e.g. wear disposable gloves and deal appropriately with soiled clothing and waste.

Other developmental areas and gaining control

As we have seen before, all the areas of development are closely linked with each other and the stages of development reached in one area will have an effect on the way in which independence in toilet needs is reached.

✱ **Physical development:** a child with a spinal injury or other physical disability may not receive the messages to the brain that tells them that their bladder is full; independence is therefore restricted.

✱ **Cognitive and language development:** Children who have communication difficulties may need the support of a signed language such as Makaton or Signalong in order to signal their toilet needs.

✱ **Emotional and social development:** If a child is feeling insecure or under stress, this may affect the rate at which they gain control over their bladder and bowel function. Sometimes, children who have previously been both dry and clean may begin to have more 'accidents'. This is known as regression and is usually a temporary response to an emotional upset, e.g. the birth of a sibling in the family.

Signs of illness or abnormality

When you help children to use the potty or the toilet you should always be alert to any problems they may have. All observations should be reported to the child's parents, or, if not appropriate, to your immediate supervisor. Some of the signs to look for are:

* **Diarrhoea:** some nursery-age children are prone to bouts of diarrhoea, which is not usually a sign of infection but a result of the immaturity of the nervous system affecting the speed of digestion.

* **Constipation:** a child may have difficulty and feel pain when passing a motion.

* **Pain when passing urine:** this may be caused by a bladder infection (cystitis) and will require treatment.

* **Rashes around the nappy and genital area:** Nappy rash or thrush may cause red spots around the nappy area (see Option A Babies).

* **Bruising or other marks:** These could indicate abuse (see pages 101–103 for further information).

Footwear and clothing for children

Footwear

Parents and carers should always go to a shoe shop where trained children's shoe fitters can help them choose from a wide selection of shoes. Second-hand shoes should never be worn as all shoes take on the shape of the wearer's foot.

Choosing footwear for children

- When shoes are fitted, there should be at least 1 cm between the longest toe and the inside of the shoe.

- Both feet should be measured for length, width and depth.

- The soles of the shoes should be flexible and hard-wearing; non-slip soles are safer.

- Leather is the ideal material for shoes that are to be worn every day as it lets the feet 'breathe' and lets moisture out.

- Padders – soft corduroy shoes – keep a baby's feet warm when crawling or toddling, but should not be worn if the soles become slippery with wear.

- Shoes should never be bought a size too large as they could cause friction and blistering.

Wellington boots should not be worn routinely because they do not allow the feet to breathe; they are very useful for outdoor play, with socks worn underneath.

- Socks should have a high cotton content so that moisture from the feet can escape.

- Always check that socks fit properly and do not stretch too tightly over the toes or sag and ruck up around the heels.

- Make sure that toenails are cut regularly. Always cut nails straight across, not down at the edges.

Clothing

Parents and carers should expect children to become dirty as they explore their surroundings and should not show disapproval when clothes become soiled. Clothes for children need to be:

✓ Hard-wearing

✓ Comfortable

✓ Easy to put on and take off, especially when going to the toilet

✓ Washable

- **Underwear** should be made of cotton, which is comfortable and sweat-absorbent.

- **Sleepsuits** – all-in-one pyjamas with hard-wearing socks – are useful for children who kick the bedcovers off at night (NB These must be the correct size to prevent damage to growing feet).

- **Daytime clothes** should be adapted to the stage of mobility and independence of the child; for example, a dress will hinder a young girl trying to crawl; dungarees may prove difficult for a toddler to manage when being toilet trained. Suitable daytime wear includes: cotton jersey track suits, T-shirts and cotton jumpers.

- **Outdoor clothes** must be warm and loose enough to fit over clothing and still allow freedom of movement; a shower-proof anorak with a hood is ideal as it can be easily washed and dried.

- **Choose clothes that are appropriate for the weather:** for example, children need to be protected from the sun with wide brimmed hats with neck shields; they need warm gloves, scarves and woolly or fleece hats in cold, windy weather and waterproof coats and footwear when out in the rain.

Caring for children's clothes

Many nannies have total responsibility for the care of children's clothes and bed linen. When caring for clothes, you should:

❑ look at the laundry care labels on each garment and make sure that you are familiar with the different symbols;

❑ check and empty all pockets before laundering;

❑ be guided by the parents regarding choice of washing powder; some detergents can cause an adverse skin reaction in some children;

❑ dry clothes thoroughly before putting away;

❑ label children's clothes with name tapes before they go into group settings.

✎ ACTIVITY

Children's clothing

Plan a wardrobe of clothes for a child aged three years throughout a year. For each item, give:

- the reason you have chosen it;

- how it should be cared for – washed and ironed;

- how it may promote the child's independence.

If possible, find out how much it would cost to provide the basic wardrobe you have chosen.

Caring for children with special needs

Whenever you are caring for children, you should always treat each child as an individual. This means that you should be aware of their **individual needs** at all times. Sometimes a child may have **special needs**. Children may need specialist equipment or extra help with play activities. For further information, see page 183.

5

Providing food and drink for children

- requirements of a balanced diet
- effects of dietary deficiencies and common food allergies
- diets associated with different cultures and religions
- hygiene requirements for preparing, eating and storing food
- the effects of illness on appetite and behaviour
- social and educational role of food and mealtimes
- understanding families' requirements for the child

The principles of good nutrition

Food is the body's fuel. During childhood we develop food habits that will affect us for life. Establishing healthy eating patterns will help to promote normal growth and development and protect against disease. As carers of children you need to know what constitutes a healthy diet and how it can be provided. Although food comes in many forms, it all has the same basic chemical functions:

- to supply body cells with a source of energy;
- to provide material for the **growth** of body cells; and
- to enable **repair and replacement** of damaged body tissues.

The substances in food that fulfil these functions are called **nutrients**.

Basic food requirements

A healthy diet consists of a wide variety of foods to help the body to grow and to provide energy. It must include enough of these nutrients: proteins, fats, carbohydrates, vitamins, minerals, and fibre – as well as water, to fuel and maintain the body's vital functions.

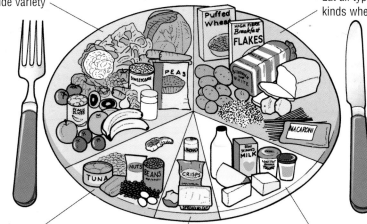

Fruit and vegetables
Choose a wide variety

Bread, other cereals and potatoes
Eat all types and choose high fibre kinds whenever you can

Meat, fish and alternatives
Choose lower fat alternatives whenever you can

Fatty and sugary foods
Try not to eat these too often, and when you do, have small amounts

Milk and dairy foods
Choose lower fat alternatives whenever you can

nutrient/food & use

Proteins: essential for growth and repair of body cells. Also form enzymes, hormones and important parts of the blood.

Fats: fats supply concentrated energy. Also contain essential vitamins & conserve body heat.

Carbohydrates: sugars & starches are broken down to provde energy. Also aid the digestion of other foods.

Vitamins: used in many cell activities. Aid the release of energy from glucose & assist growth & repair mechanisms.

Minerals: sixteen different minerals help growth and repair mechanisms, the release of energy from nutrients, and help form new tissues.

Fibre: also known as roughage, fibre adds bulk to food and helps prevent constipation.

Table 1.1   Basic food requirements

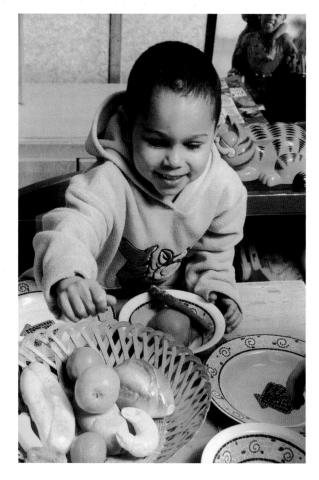

🧸 Planning a healthy diet for children

Children need a varied energy-rich diet for good health and growth. For balance and variety, choose from the five main food groups. (See Table 1.2.)

Food groups	Main nutrients	Types to choose	Portions per day	Suggestions for meals and snacks
1. Bread, other cereals and potatoes All types of bread, rice, breakfast cereals, pasta, noodles, and potatoes (beans and lentils can be eaten as part of this group)	Carbohydrate (starch), fibre, some calcium and iron, B-group vitamins	Wholemeal, brown. Wholegrain or high-fibre versions of bread; avoid fried foods too often (e.g. chips). Use butter and other spreads sparingly	FIVE All meals of the day should include foods from this group	One portion = ● 1 bowl of breakfast cereal ● 2 tabs pasta or rice ● 1 small potato Snack meals include bread or pizza base
2. Fruit and vegetables Fresh, frozen and canned fruit and vegetables, dried fruit, fruit juice (beans and lentils can be eaten as part of this group)	Vitamin C, carotenes, iron, calcium, folate, fibre and some carbohydrate	Eat a wide variety of fruit and vegetables; avoid adding rich sauces to vegetables, and sugar to fruit	FOUR/FIVE Include 1 fruit or vegetable daily high in Vitamin C, e.g. tomato, sweet pepper, orange or kiwi fruit	One portion = ● 1 glass of pure fruit juice ● 1 piece of fruit ● 1 sliced tomato ● 2 tabs of cooked vegetables ● 1 tab of dried fruit – e.g. raisins
3. Milk and dairy foods Milk, cheese, yoghurt and fromage frais (this group does not contain butter, eggs and cream)	Calcium, protein, B-group vitamins (particularly B12), vitamins A and D	Milk is a very good source of calcium, but calcium can also be obtained from cheese, flavoured or plain yogurts and fromage frais	THREE Children require the equivalent of one pint of milk each day to ensure an adequate intake of calcium	One portion = ● 1 glass of milk ● 1 pot of yogurt or from age frais ● 1 tabs of grated cheese, e.g. on a pizza Under 2s – do not give reduced-fat milks, e.g. semi-skimmed – they do not supply enough energy
4. Meat, fish and alternatives Lean meat, poultry, fish, eggs, tofu, quorn, pulses – peas, beans, lentils, nuts and seeds	Iron, protein, B-group vitamins(particularly B12), zinc and magnesium	Lower-fat versions – meat with fat cut off, chicken without skin etc. Beans and lentils are good alternatives, being low in fat and high in fibre	TWO Vegetarians will need to have grains, pulses and seeds; vegans avoid all food associated with animals	One portion = ● 2 fish fingers (for a 3 year old) ● 4 fish fingers (for a 7 year old) ● baked beans ● chicken nuggets or a small piece of chicken
5. Fatty and sugary foods Margarine, low-fat spread, butter, ghee, cream, chocolate, crisps, biscuits, sweets & sugar, fizzy soft drinks, puddings	Vitamins and essential fatty acids, but also a lot of fat, sugar and salt	Only offer small amounts of sugary and fatty foods. Fats and oils are found in all the other food groups	NONE Only eat fatty and sugary foods sparingly, e.g. crisps, sweets and chocolate	Children may be offered foods with extra fat or sugar – biscuits, cakes or chocolate – as long as they are not replacing food from the four main food groups

Table 1.2　Food groups

By the age of five, children should be enjoying a healthy diet. The diet should contain plenty of starchy foods, five portions of fruit and vegetables daily, with low-fat milk and dairy products, small amounts of meat, fish or alternatives and the occasional treat (i.e. foods that are high in fat and sugar).

✎ ACTIVITY

Observation

Choose three children in your placement for this observation. Ask your supervisor's permission to carry out this observation. (NB You must complete all sections of a front sheet – ensure you have your supervisor's signature.)

Your observation needs an *introduction* which explains the usual meal patterns and times, together with any rules about what types of food may be brought for snacks (some schools do not allow crisps, chocolate bars or sweets). Without identifying the children by name give a brief description of the physical build, complexion and general health. Include any information you may have about any of their food allergies.

On both placement days of one week make a list of the food items each child brings/has for snack or break time and for lunch – it does not matter whether it is a packed lunch or a cooked school meal. Ask the children to tell you what they have had for breakfast on those days and what they had for tea/evening meal on the previous nights.

Use a *checklist* to present your information showing the foods and identifying the recognised food groups i.e.

Produce a separate chart for each child. In addition find out which foods each child likes and dislikes.

food item	carbohydrate	protein	fats	vitamins	minerals	high in salt	high in sugar
Coco Pops	✓			✓	✓		
Milk		✓	✓	✓	✓		
Etc.							

Conclusion

Using the information in your charts, state whether each child appears to have a healthy, balanced diet taking into account 'servings' and essential dietary needs (e.g. vitamin C, fibre etc.). Explain any important items which are missing and suggest what could be added or substituted to improve the overall diet. Explain what effects the child's diet might have on his/her overall health and development. Use textbooks to support what you say and list them in a bibliography.

Nutritional values of foods

Scientists have identified a range of nutrients that must be present in the diet. The amounts that should be taken every day are called RDAs (Recommended Daily Amounts). These terms may be seen on all packaged foods in the UK.

Children need to obtain energy from the food they eat. Food energy is measured in calories (kcal) or kilojoules (kj).

1 kcal = 4.2 kj
1000kj = 1MJ (megajoule) = 239 kcal

Different foods contain different amounts of energy per unit of weight; foods which contain a lot of fat and sugar, e.g. jam doughnuts, have high energy values. A balanced diet (see Table 1.3) will contain all the nutrients they need for growth and energy.

Meal or snack	Monday	Tuesday	Wednesday	Thursday	Friday
Breakfast	Orange juice Weetabix + milk 1 slice of buttered toast	Milk Cereal e.g. corn or wheat flakes Toast and jam	Apple juice 1 slice of toast with butter or jam	Milk Cereal with slices of banana or Scrambled egg on toast	Yoghurt Porridge Slices of apple
Morning snack	Diluted apple juice 1 packet raisins	Blackcurrant & apple drink Cheese straws	1 glass fruit squash 1 biscuit	Peeled apple slices Wholemeal toast fingers with cheese spread	Diluted apple juice Chapatti or pitta bread fingers
Lunch	Chicken nuggets or macaroni cheese Broccoli Fruit yoghurt Water	Thick bean soup or chicken salad sandwich Green beans Fresh fruit salad Water	Vegetable soup or fish fingers/cakes Sticks of raw carrot Kiwi fruit Water	Sweet potato casserole Sweetcorn Spinach leaves Chocolate mousse Water	Bean casserole (or chicken drumstick) with noodles Peas or broad beans Fruit yoghurt Water
Afternoon snack	Diluted fruit juice Cubes of cheese with savoury biscuit	Milk shake Fruit cake or chocolate biscuit	Diluted fruit juice Thin-cut sandwiches cut into small pieces	Hot or cold chocolate drink 1 small packet dried fruit mix e.g. apricots, sultanas etc.	Lassi (yogurt drink) 1 banana 1 small biscuit
Tea or supper	Baked beans on toast or ham & cheese pasta Lemon pancakes Milk or yoghurt	Fish stew or fish fingers Mashed potato Fruit mousse or fromage frais Milk or yoghurt	Baked potatoes with a choice of fillings Steamed broccoli Ice cream	Home-made beefburger or pizza Green salad Pancakes Milk	Lentil & rice soup Pitta or wholegrain bread Rice salad Milk

Table 1.3　Providing a balanced diet

✎ ACTIVITY

The balanced daily diet

1 Look at the following daily diet:

- Breakfast: A glass of milk + scrambled egg and toast

- Mid-morning: A packet of crisps + a glass of blackcurrant squash

- Lunch: A cheese and egg flan + chips + baked beans + apple fritters and ice cream + apple juice

- Snack: Chocolate mini roll + orange squash

- Tea: Fish fingers + mashed potatoes + peas + strawberry milk shake

Arrange the portions or servings into five columns (see example on page 66) – i.e. the four food groups and one extra column for extra fat and sugar. Count the number of portions from each food group and assess the nutritional content of the diet.

2 How could you improve the menu to ensure a healthy balanced diet?

How much food should children be given?

Children's appetites vary enormously, so common sense is a good guide on how big a portion should be. Always be guided by the individual child:

- do not force them to eat when they no longer wish to, but

- do not refuse to give more if they really are hungry.

Some children always feel hungry at one particular mealtime. Others require food little and often. You should always offer food that is nourishing as well as satisfying their hunger.

Meals and snacks

Some children really **do** need to eat between meals. Their stomachs are relatively small and so they fill up and empty faster than adult stomachs. Sugary foods should not be given as a snack, because sugar is an appetite depressant and may spoil the child's appetite for the main meal to follow. Healthy snack foods include:

☐ pieces of fruit – banana, orange, pear, kiwi fruit, apple or satsuma;

☐ fruit bread or wholemeal bread with slice of cheese;

☐ milk or home-made milk shakes;

☐ sticks of carrot, celeriac, parsnip, red pepper, cauliflower;

☐ dried fruit and diluted fruit juices, and

☐ wholegrain biscuits, oatcakes or sesame seed crackers.

Enjoying a healthy snack

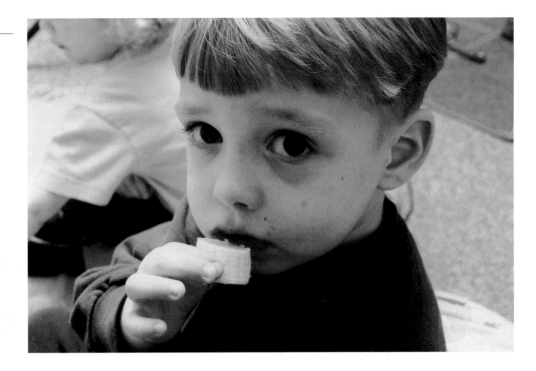

Iron, calcium and vitamin D in children's diets

Iron is essential for children's health. Lack of iron leads to **anaemia**, which can hold back both physical and mental development. Children who are poor eaters or on restricted diets are most at risk.

Iron comes in two forms, either:

☐ found in foods from animal sources (especially meat), which is easily absorbed by the body; or

☐ found in plant foods, which is not quite so easy for the body to absorb.

If possible, children should be given a portion of meat or fish every day, and kidney or liver once a week. Even a small portion of meat or fish is useful because it also helps the body to absorb iron from other food sources.

If children do not eat meat or fish, they must be offered plenty of iron-rich alternatives, such as egg yolks, dried fruit, beans and lentils, and green leafy vegetables. It is also a good idea to give foods or drinks that are high in **vitamin C** at mealtimes, as this helps the absorption of iron from non-meat sources.

Calcium and vitamin D

Children need **calcium** for maintaining and repairing bones and teeth. Calcium is:

• found in milk, cheese, yoghurt and other dairy products;

• only absorbed by the body if it is taken with vitamin D.

The skin can make all the vitamin D that a body needs, when it is exposed to gentle sunlight. Sources of vitamin D include:

✱ milk

✱ fortified breakfast cereals

* oily fish

* meat

* fortified margarine

* soya mince, soya drink

* tahini paste*, tofu

(*Tahini is made from sesame seeds, and these may cause an allergic reaction in a small number of children.)

Vitamin drops provide vitamins A, C and D. Children under the age of five should be given vitamin drops as a safeguard **only** when their diets may be insufficient.

Providing drinks for children

You need to offer children drinks several times during the day. The best drinks for young children are water and milk:

* Water is a very under-rated drink for the whole family as it quenches thirst without spoiling the appetite; if bottled water is used it should be still, not carbonated (fizzy) which is acidic. More water should be given in hot weather in order to prevent dehydration.

* Milk is an excellent nourishing drink. Reduced-fat milks should not normally be given to children under the age of five because of their lower energy and fat-soluble content; however semi-skimmed milk may be offered from 2 years of age, provided that the child's overall diet is adequate.

Other drinks

All drinks that contain sugar can be harmful to teeth and can also take the edge off children's appetites. Examples are:

* flavoured milks

* flavoured fizzy drinks

* fruit squashes

* fruit juices (containing natural sugar)

Unsweetened diluted fruit juice is the best drink – other than water or milk – for children, but should ideally only be offered at mealtimes. The low-sugar or diet fruit drinks contain artificial sweeteners and are best avoided.

Tea and coffee should not be given to children under five, as they prevent the absorption of iron from foods. They also fill children easily without providing nourishment.

Nutritional disorders in children

Nutritional disorders may be caused by an excess or a deficiency of one or more nutrients. Most disorders respond to treatment, by special diets; these work by adding or subtracting the relevant nutrient in the child's diet.

- **Obesity (fatness):** obesity results from taking in more energy from the diet than is used up by the body. It can lead to physical problems, such as being more prone to infection, as well as emotional and social problems caused by the negative attitudes of others. A diet low in fat and sugar is prescribed and the child will need a lot of support and encouragement.

- **Coeliac disease:** coeliac disease is a condition in which the lining of the small intestine is damaged by **gluten**, a protein found in wheat and rye. In babies, it is usually diagnosed after they have been weaned onto solid foods containing gluten, but some children do not show any symptoms until they are older. Treatment for coeliac disease is by gluten-free diet and is lifelong.

- **Failure to thrive:** failure to thrive is a term used when a child does not conform to the usual pattern of weight gain and growth. It could occur as a result of intolerance to a newly introduced food or after a severe bout of **gastro-enteritis** or whooping cough.

- **Diabetes (mellitus):** diabetes develops when the **pancreas** fails to make enough **insulin**, which is needed to regulate sugar levels within the body. Children with diabetes often need insulin injections and regular meals containing carbohydrate. Children are advised to carry glucose sweets whenever they are away from home in case of **hypoglycaemia**.

- **Cystic fibrosis:** the majority of children with cystic fibrosis have difficulty in absorbing fats; they need to eat 20% more protein and calories than children without the disorder, and so require a diet high in fats and carbohydrates.

A summary of deficiency disorders

Disorder	Shortage	Effect
Anaemia	Iron or vitamin B12	Fatigue, weight loss, headaches, breathlessness
Beriberi	Thiamine (vitamin B1)	Wasting of the heart muscles, heart failure
Kwashiorkor	Protein or calories	Severe malnutrition, swollen tummies, sparse brittle hair
Marasmus	Severe lack of protein and calories	Emaciation, stunted growth and dehydration
Night blindness	Vitamin A	Inability to see in dim light
Pellagra	Niacin (a vitamin)	Soreness and cracking of the skin; mental disturbances
Rickets	Calcium or vitamin D	Bones do not form properly, resulting in bow legs
Scurvy	Vitamin C	Wounds are slow to heal; gums loose and bleeding

Table 1.4 A summary of deficiency disorders

Establishing healthy eating habits

Some children can be choosy about the food they eat, and this can be a source of anxiety for parents and for those who work with children. However, as long as children eat some food from each of the five food groups – even if they are the same old favourites – there is no cause for worry.

Guidelines for making mealtimes healthy and fun

✓ Set an example: children imitate both what you eat and how you eat it. Be relaxed, patient and friendly.

✓ Be prepared for messy mealtimes! Present the food in a form that is fairly easy for children to manage by themselves (e.g. not difficult to chew).

✓ Be imaginative with presentation, e.g. cut slices of pizza into interesting shapes. Use ideas from children's food manufacturers.

✓ Encourage children to feed themselves, either with a spoon or by offering suitable finger foods.

✓ Some families prefer to eat with their fingers, while others use chopsticks or cutlery. Whatever tool is preferred, be patient as children need time to get used to them.

✓ Try not to pass on your own personal dislikes; children are very quick to notice an expression of disgust!

✓ Limit in-between meal snacks to, for example, a milk drink and a small cracker with a slice of cheese

✓ Offer a wide variety of different foods. Give young children a chance to try a new food more than once; any refusal on first tasting may be due to a dislike of the new rather than of the food itself.

✓ If a child prefers drink to food, cut down on the amount of drinks you give just before mealtimes.

Lunchtime in a day nursery

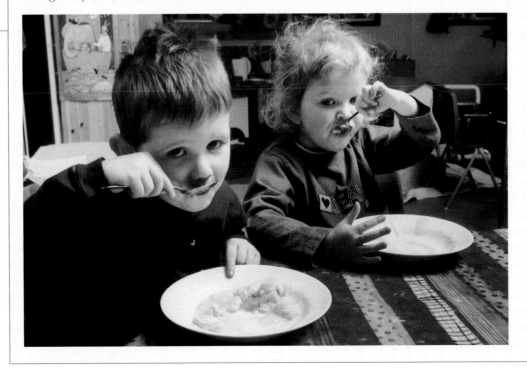

✗ Avoid adding salt to any food at the table

✗ *Never give a young child whole nuts to eat* – particularly peanuts. Children can very easily choke on a small piece of the nut or even inhale it, which can cause a severe type of pneumonia. Rarely, a child may have a serious allergic reaction to nuts.

✗ If a child rejects the food, don't ever force-feed him. Simply remove the food without comment. Give smaller portions next time and praise the child for eating even a little.

✗ Don't use food as a punishment, reward, bribe or threat. For example, don't give sweets or chocolates as a reward for finishing savoury foods. To a child this might be saying, 'here's something nice after eating those nasty greens'. Reward them instead with a trip to the park or a story session.

Vegetarian and vegan diets

Vegetarians do not eat meat or fish, but most will eat eggs and dairy produce. Vegans avoid all animal products, including eggs, milk, milk products and honey. Some people are partial vegetarians, excluding red meat from their diet, but including fish and perhaps poultry.

A vegetarian diet may not provide enough **calories** for normal growth, so more dairy produce should be offered to provide the extra energy needed.

Food hygiene

Young children are particularly vulnerable to the **bacteria** which can cause food poisoning or **gastro-enteritis**. Bacteria multiply rapidly in warm, moist foods and can enter food without causing the food to look, smell or even taste bad. So it is very important to store, prepare and cook food safely, and to keep the kitchen clean.

The prevention of food poisoning

Storing food safely

❑ Keep food cold. The fridge should be kept as cold as it will go without actually freezing the food (1–5°C or 34–41°F)

❑ Cover or wrap food with foodwrap or microwave clingfilm

❑ Never refreeze food which has begun to thaw

❑ Do not use foods that are past their sell-by or best-before date

❑ Always read instructions on the label when storing food

❑ Once a tin is opened, store the contents in a covered dish in the fridge

☐ Store raw foods at the bottom of the fridge so that juices cannot drip onto cooked food

☐ Thaw frozen meat completely before cooking

Preparing and cooking food safely

- Always wash hands in warm water and soap and dry on a clean towel: before handling food and after handling raw foods, especially meat

- Wear clean protective clothing which is solely for use in the kitchen

- Keep food covered at all times

- Wash all fruits and vegetables before eating. Peel and top carrots and peel fruits such as apples.

- Never cough or sneeze over food

- Always cover any septic cuts or boils with a waterproof dressing

- Never smoke in any room that is used for food

- Keep work surfaces and chopping boards clean and disinfected; use separate boards for raw meat, fish, vegetables etc.

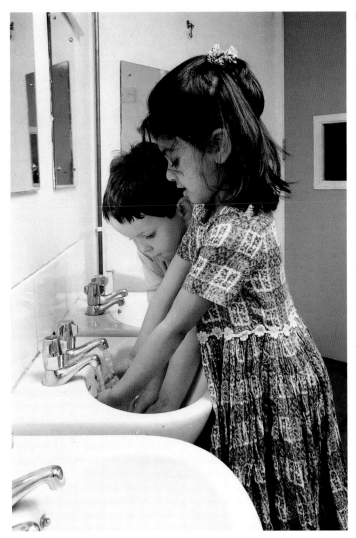

Washing hands before a meal

- Make sure that meat dishes are thoroughly cooked

- Avoid raw eggs. They sometimes contain *Salmonella* bacteria, which may cause food poisoning. (Also avoid giving children uncooked cake mixture, home-made ice creams, mayonnaise, or desserts that contain uncooked raw egg.) When cooking eggs, the egg yolk and white should be firm.

- When re-heating food, make sure that it is piping hot all the way through, and allow to cool slightly before giving it to children. When using a microwave, always stir and check the temperature of the food before feeding children, to avoid burning from hot spots.

- Avoid having leftovers – they are a common cause of food poisoning

Keeping the kitchen safe

- [ ] Teach children to wash their hands after touching pets and going to the toilet, and before eating.
- [ ] Clean tin-openers, graters and mixers thoroughly after use
- [ ] Keep flies and other insects away – use a fine mesh over open windows
- [ ] Stay away from the kitchen if you are suffering from diarrhoea or sickness
- [ ] Keep the kitchen clean – the floor, work surfaces, sink, utensils, cloths and waste bins should be cleaned regularly.
- [ ] Tea towels should be boiled every day and dishcloths boiled or disinfected
- [ ] Keep pets away from the kitchen
- [ ] Keep all waste bins covered, and empty them regularly
- [ ] Keep sharp knives stored safely where children cannot reach them

Poverty and diet

There is a clear link between poverty and health. Families on a low income may be unable to provide their children with a healthy, nourishing diet for various reasons:

- [ ] Healthy food is relatively expensive. Lean meat costs more than fattier cuts, and wholemeal bread can cost 25% more than white bread.
- [ ] Fuel costs are variable; it is cheaper to cook chips than jacket potatoes.
- [ ] Supermarkets are often sited on the outskirts of towns; this has meant that shops in inner city areas are smaller and more expensive. Parents may not have transport to get to the supermarkets.
- [ ] Cooking facilities may be inadequate for preparing healthy foods, e.g. if the family has to share a kitchen in bed and breakfast accommodation.

Ideas for providing a healthy diet on a tight budget include:

- Use less meat and more pulses and lentils in stews and casseroles.
- Use as little oil or fat in cooking as possible.
- Cut down on meat and fill up on potatoes, rice and starchy vegetables
- Avoid highly processed foods which contain high levels of sugar and salt, and also often fail to provide protein or vitamin C.

Providing food in a multicultural society

The UK is the home of a multicultural and multi-ethnic society. Food is an important part of the heritage of any culture. Providing food from a wide range of cultures is an important way of celebrating this heritage. Children learn to enjoy different tastes and to respect the customs and beliefs of people different from themselves.

The largest ethnic minority group in the UK belongs to the Asian community – about 1.25 million people. Asian dietary customs are mainly based on three religious groups: Muslims (or Moslems), Hindus and Sikhs.

Hindus

Orthodox Hindus are strict vegetarians as they believe in **Ahimsa** – non-violence towards all living beings – and a few of them are vegans. Some will eat dairy products and eggs, while others will refuse eggs on the ground that they are a potential source of life. Even non-vegetarians do not eat beef as the cow is considered a sacred animal. It is also unusual for pork to be eaten, as the pig is considered unclean. Wheat is the main staple food eaten by Hindus in the UK; it is used to make chapattis, puris and parathas. Ghee (clarified butter) and vegetable oil are used in cooking. Three festivals in the Hindu calendar are observed as days of **fasting**, which lasts from dawn to dusk and during which Hindus eat only 'pure' foods such as fruit and yoghurt:

1   Mahshivrati – the birthday of Lord Shiva (March)

2   Ram Naumi – the birthday of Lord Rama (April)

3   Jan Mash Tami – the birthday of Lord Krishna (late August)

Muslims

Muslims practise the Islamic religion, and their holy book, the Koran, provides them with their food laws. Unlawful foods (called haram) include pork, all meat which has not been rendered lawful (halal), alcohol and fish without scales. Halal meat has been killed in a certain approved way and must be bought from a Halal butcher. Wheat, in the form of chapattis, and rice are the staple foods. During the lunar month of **Ramadan**, Muslims fast between sunrise and sunset. Children under 12 and elderly people are exempt from fasting.

Sikhs

Most Sikhs will not eat pork or beef. Some Sikhs are vegetarian, but many eat chicken, lamb and fish. Wheat and rice are staple foods. Devout Sikhs will fast once or twice a week, and most will fast on the first day of the **Punjabi** month or when there is a full moon.

Afro-Caribbean diets

The Afro-Caribbean community is the second largest ethnic minority group in the UK. Dietary customs vary widely. Many people include a variety of European foods in their diet alongside the traditional foods of cornmeal, coconut, green banana, plantain, okra and yam. Although Afro-Caribbean people are generally Christian, a minority are Rastafarians.

Rastafarians

Dietary customs are based on laws, laid down by Moses in the Bible, which state that certain types of meat should be avoided. The majority of followers will only eat 'Ital' foods, which are considered to be in a whole or natural state. Most rastafarians are vegetarians and will not eat processed or preserved foods.

Jewish diets

Jewish people observe dietary laws which state that animals and birds must be killed by the Jewish method to render them kosher (acceptable). Milk and meat must never be cooked or eaten together, and pork in any form is forbidden. Shellfish are not allowed as they are thought to harbour disease. The most holy day of the Jewish calendar is **Yom Kippur** (the Day of Atonement) when Jewish people fast for 25 hours.

Food and festivals

There are often particular foods which are associated with religious festivals, e.g. mince pies at Christmas and pancakes on Shrove Tuesday. Providing foods from different cultures within an early childhood setting is a very good way of celebrating these festivals. Parents of children from ethnic minority groups are usually very pleased to be asked for advice on how to celebrate festivals with food, and may even be prepared to contribute some samples. (See also pages 155–157.)

Some festivals from different cultures	
Rastafarian New Year	7th January
Chinese New Year	late January/early February
Holi (Hindu spring festival)	February or March
Shrove Tuesday/Mardi Gras	40 days before Easter
Rosh Hoshanah (Jewish New Year)	usually September
Diwali (Hindu New Year)	October or November
Shichi-go-san (Japanese festival for young children)	15th November
Id Al Fitr (major Muslim festival)	end of Ramadan

Chinese New Year – Parade of the Dragon

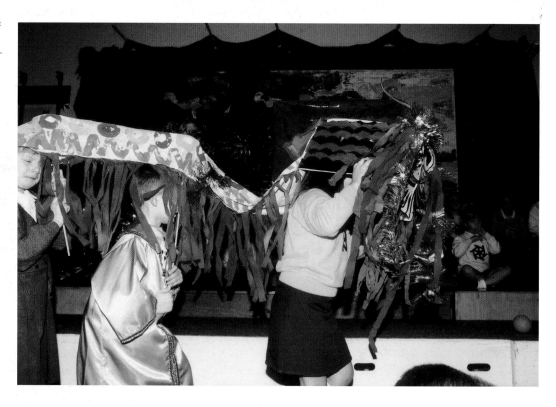

The social and educational role of food and mealtimes

Passing a drink

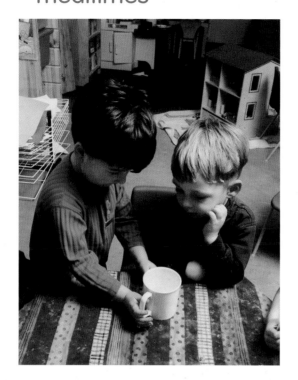

Promotes:

* hand–eye co-ordination – using cutlery and other tools

* sensory development – taste, touch, sight & smell

* language development – increased vocabulary

* development of concepts of shape and size, using food as examples

* learning through linked activities e.g. cookery, weighing food, stories about food, where food comes from etc.

* independence – skills of serving food and taking responsibility

* listening skills

* courtesy towards others and turn-taking

* sharing experience – a social focus in the child's day

* self-esteem – child's family and cultural background are valued

* self-confidence – through learning social skills, taking turns and saying 'please' and 'thank you'

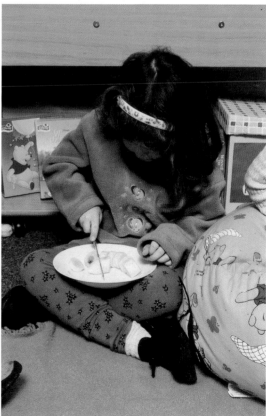

Using a knife to slice bananas

Contact with families

When parents register their child at nursery or school they are asked to detail any special dietary requirements that their child may have. Some children may need special diets because of an underlying medical condition; others may require a vegetarian or vegan diet. It is important that all child care settings are aware of any particular allergies or problems with eating that a child may have. If a parent or carer expresses any concern to you about the food provided within your nursery or school, refer them to the person in charge or the child's key worker for guidance.

Caring for a child who is not well

6

- signs and symptoms of common childhood illnesses
- procedures for reporting and recording illness
- caring for a child who is not well
- games and activities for children who are not well
- maintaining hygiene and preventing cross infection

General signs and symptoms of illness

Young children often can't explain their symptoms when they feel ill. They may not have the language to be able to describe what is wrong, although parents – and other people who know them well – can almost always tell when their child is 'off-colour'. It is important for you to be able to recognise some of the more general signs of childhood illness so that you can get appropriate help for the child. Sometimes, these non-specific signs and symptoms are a warning that a child is **incubating** an illness. These signs may include some or several of the following:

- loss of appetite
- lethargy or listlessness
- lack of interest in play
- irritability and fretfulness
- sleepy more of the time
- dark rings around eyes

- unusual crying or screaming bouts
- flushed cheeks
- pale face – a black child may have a paler area around the lips and the conjunctiva may be pale pink instead of red

More specific signs that a child is ill include:

❋ fever (see below)

❋ diarrhoea and **vomiting**

❋ dehydration – any illness involving fever or loss of fluid through vomiting or diarrhoea may result in dehydration; the mouth and tongue become dry and parched and cracks appear on the lips. (The first sign in a baby is a **sunken anterior fontanelle**)

❋ abdominal pain – a baby with **colic** or abdominal pains will draw her knees up to her chest in an instinctive effort to relieve the pain

❋ specific signs and symptoms of disease such as a **rash**. NB the darker a child's skin colour, the more pimples or a red rash will show merely as raised areas. Only when the skin is affected by scratching will the spots become noticeably red.

When a child has a high temperature (or fever) it usually means that they have an infection.

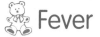 # Fever

A fever is defined as a body temperature above 37°C. The only sure way to tell if a child has a high fever is to take his or her temperature with a thermometer. All family first aid kits should contain a thermometer, either:

- a plastic strip which is placed on the child's forehead, or
- a digital thermometer which can safely be placed in a child's mouth, or
- a clinical thermometer which can be used in the child's armpit

Condition (and cause)	Signs and symptoms	Role of the carer
Colic	This occurs in the first 12 weeks. It causes sharp spasmodic pain in the stomach, and is often at its worst in the late evening. Symptoms include inconsolable high-pitched crying, drawing her legs up to her chest, and growing red in the face.	Try to stay calm! Gently massage her abdomen in a clockwise direction, using the tips of your middle fingers. Sucrose solution (3 x 5ml teaspoons of sugar in a cup of boiling water and left to cool) is said to have a mild pain-killing effect on small babies. Dribble 2 ml of this solution into the corner of the baby's mouth twice a day. If the problem persists, contact the doctor.
Diarrhoea	Frequent loose or watery stools. Can be very serious in young babies, especially when combined with vomiting, as it can lead to severe dehydration.	Give frequent small drinks of cooled, boiled water containing glucose and salt or a made-up sachet of rehydration fluid. If the baby is unable to take the fluid orally, she must be taken to hospital urgently and fed intravenously, by a 'drip'. If anal area becomes sore, treat with a barrier cream.
Gastro-enteritis virus or bacteria	The baby may vomit and usually has diarrhoea as well; often has a raised temperature and loss of appetite. May show signs of abdominal pain i.e drawing up of legs to chest and crying.	Reassure the baby. Observe strict hygiene rules. Watch out for signs of dehydration. Offer frequent small amounts of fluid, and possibly rehydration salts.
Neonatal cold injury – or hypothermia	The baby is cold to the touch. Face may be pale or flushed. Lethargic, runny nose, swollen hands and feet. Pre-term infants and babies under 4 months are at particular risk.	Prevention (see Option A) Warm slowly by covering with several light layers of blankets and by cuddling. No direct heat. Offer feeds high in sugar and seek medical help urgently.
Reflux	Also known as gastro-intestinal reflux (GIR) or gastro-oesophageal reflux GOR). The opening to the stomach is not yet efficient enough to allow a large liquid feed through. Symptoms include grizzly crying and excessive possetting after feeds.	Try feeding the baby in a more upright position and bring up wind by gently rubbing her back. After feeding leave the baby in a semi-sitting position. Some doctors prescribe a paediatric reflux suppressant or antacid mixture to be given before the feed.
Tonsillitis virus or bacteria	Very sore throat, which looks bright red. There is usually fever and the baby will show signs of distress from pain on swallowing and general aches and pains. May vomit.	Encourage plenty of fluids – older babies may have iced lollies to suck. Give pain relief, e.g. paracetamol. Seek medical aid if no improvement and if fever persists.

Table 1.5 Illnesses in babies

Disease and cause	Spread	Incubation	Signs and symptoms	Rash or specific sign	Treatment	Possible complications
Common cold (coryza) Virus	Airborne/droplet, hand-to-hand contact	1–3 days	Sneeze, sore throat, running nose, headache, slight fever, irritable, partial deafness		Treat symptoms, Vaseline to nostrils	Bronchitis, sinusitis, laryngitis
Chickenpox (varicella) Virus	Airborne/droplet, direct contact	10–14 days	Slight fever, itchy rash, mild onset, child feels ill, often with severe headache	Red spots with white centre on trunk and limbs at first; blisters and pustules	Rest, fluids, calamine to rash, cut child's nails to prevent secondary infection	Impetigo, scarring, secondary infection from scratching
Dysentery Bacillus or amoeba	Indirect: flies, infected food; poor hygiene	1–7 days	Vomiting, diarrhoea, blood and mucus in stool, abdominal pain, fever, headache		Replace fluids, rest, medical aid, strict hygiene measures	Dehydration from loss of body salts, shock; can be fatal
Food poisoning Bacteria or virus	Indirect: infected food or drink	½ hour to 36 hours	Vomiting, diarrhoea, abdominal pain		Fluids only for 24 hours; medical aid if no better	Dehydration – can be fatal
Gastro-enteritis Virus	Direct contact. Bacteria or infected food/drink	Bacterial: 7–14 days. Indirect: ½ hr–36 hrs	Vomiting, diarrhoea. Viral: signs of dehydration		Replace fluids – water or Dioralyte; medical aid urgently	Dehydration, weight loss – death
Measles (morbilli) Virus	Airborne/droplet	7–15 days	High fever, fretful, heavy cold – running nose and discharge from eyes; later cough	Day 1: Koplik's spots, white inside mouth. Day 4: blotchy rash starts on face and spreads down to body	Rest, fluids, tepid sponging. Shade room if photophobic (dislikes bright light)	Otitis media, eye infection, pneumonia, encephalitis (rare)
Meningitis (inflammation of meninges which cover the brain) Bacteria or virus	Airborne/droplet	Variable – usually 2–10 days	Fever, headache, drowsiness, confusion, photophobia (or dislike of bright light), arching of neck	Can have small red spots or bruises	Take to hospital, antibiotics and observation	Deafness, brain damage, death
Mumps (epidemic parotitis) Virus	Airborne/droplet	14–21 days	Pain, swelling of jaw in front of ears, fever, eating and drinking painful	Swollen face	Fluids: give via straw, hot compresses, oral hygiene	Meningitis (1 in 400), orchitis (infection of testes) in young men
Pertussis (Whooping cough) Bacteria	Airborne/droplet; direct contact	7–21 days	Starts with a snuffly cold, slight cough, mild fever	Spasmodic cough with whoop sound, vomiting	Rest and assurance; feed after coughing attack; support during attack; inhalations	Convulsions, pneumonia, brain damage, hernia, debility
Rubella (German measles) Virus	Airborne/droplet; direct contact	14–21 days	Slight cold, sore throat, mild fever, swollen glands behind ears, pain in small joints	Slight pink rash starts behind ears and on forehead. Not itchy	Rest if necessary. Treat symptoms	Only if contracted by woman in first 3 months of pregnancy – can cause serious defects in unborn baby
Scarlet fever (or Scarlatina) Bacteria	Droplet	2–4 days	Sudden fever, loss of appetite, sore throat, pallor around mouth, 'strawberry' tongue	Bright red pinpoint rash over face and body – may peel	Rest, fluids, observe for complications, antibiotics	Kidney infection, otitis media, rheumatic fever (rare)
Tonsillitis Bacteria or virus	Direct infection, droplet		Very sore throat, fever, headache, pain on swallowing, aches and pains in back and limbs		Rest, fluids, medical aid – antibiotics, iced drinks relieve pain	Quinsy (abscess on tonsils), otitis media, kidney infection, temporary deafness

Taking children's temperature

☐ A **Clinical thermometer:** a glass tube with a bulb at one end containing mercury. This tube is marked with gradations of temperature in degrees Centigrade and Fahrenheit. When the bulb end is placed under the child's armpit or in the groin fold, the mercury will expand and so move up the tube until the temperature of the child's body is reached.

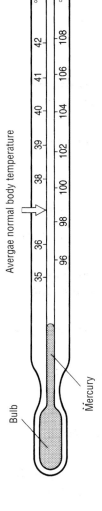
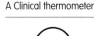

A Clinical thermometer

1 Check that the silvery column of mercury is shaken down to 35 degrees centigrade.

2 Place the bulb end of the thermometer in the child's armpit, holding her arm close to her side for two minutes.

3 Remove the thermometer, and holding it horizontally and in a good light, read off the temperature measured by the level of the mercury. **Record** the time and the temperature reading.

4 After use, wash the thermometer in tepid water, and shake the column of mercury down again to 35 degrees Centigrade. Dry carefully and replace in case.

NB A clinical thermometer should never be placed in a baby's mouth, because of the danger of biting and breaking the glass.

☐ B **Digital thermometer:** this is battery-operated and consists of a narrow probe with a tip sensitive to temperature. It is easy to read via a display panel and unbreakable.

1 Place the narrow tip of the thermometer under the child's arm as described above.

2 Read the temperature when it stops rising; some models beep when this point is reached.

☐ C **Plastic fever strip:** this is a rectangular strip of thin plastic which contains temperature sensitive crystals that change colour according to the temperature measured. It is not as accurate as the other thermometers but is a useful check.

1 Hold the plastic strip firmly against the child's forehead for about 30 seconds.

2 Record the temperature revealed by the colour change.

Other signs which indicate fever are:

● the child may appear 'feverish' – red, hot cheeks and bright, glittery eyes;

● the baby will be reluctant to feed and the older child will usually not want to eat;

● the child will usually appear fretful or restless, or may sleep a lot.

Whatever the cause of the high temperature, it is important to try to reduce it, as there is always the risk of a fever leading to **convulsions** or **fits**.

Bringing down a high temperature/reducing a fever

☐ Offer cooled boiled water and encourage the child to drink as much fluid as possible. Avoid fizzy or sweet drinks in case they make the child sick.

☐ Sponge the child down, using tepid water (see below) – or give a cool bath.

☐ Give the correct dose of paracetamol syrup. Follow the instructions on the bottle carefully. *

☐ Try to cool the air in the child's room – use an electric fan or open the window.

☐ Reassure the child who may be very frightened. Remain calm yourself and try to stop the child from crying, as this will tend to push the temperature higher still.

☐ If the temperature will not come down, then call the doctor.

NB: *Always consult a doctor if a high fever is accompanied by symptoms such as severe headache with stiff neck, abdominal pain or pain when passing urine.*

You must not give a child any medicine unless you have the written permission of their parent or guardian.

Tepid sponging to reduce a temperature

☐ Make sure the air in the room is comfortably warm – not hot, cold or draughty.

☐ Lay the child on a towel on your knee or on the bed and gently remove her clothes; reassure her by talking gently and explaining what you are doing.

☐ Sponge her body, limbs and face with tepid or lukewarm water – not cold; as the water evaporates from the skin, it absorbs heat from the blood and so cools the system.

☐ As the child cools down, pat her skin dry with a soft towel and dress her only in a nappy or pants; cover her with a light cotton sheet.

☐ Keep checking her condition to make sure that she does not become cold or shivery; if she does become cold, put more light covers over her.

☐ If the temperature rises again, repeat sponging every 10 minutes.

If you think the child's life is in danger, dial 999 if you are in the UK, ask for an ambulance urgently and explain the situation.

Contact the family doctor (GP) if the child has any of the following symptoms. If the doctor cannot reach you quickly, take the child to the Accident and Emergency department of the nearest hospital:

When to call a doctor

● Has a temperature of 38.6°C (101.4°F) which is not lowered by measures to reduce **fever**, or a temperature over 37.8°C (100°F) for more than one day.

● **Cannot be woken**, is unusually drowsy or may be losing consciousness.

● Has severe or persistent **vomiting** and/or **diarrhoea**, seems dehydrated or has projectile vomiting.

● Has been **injured**, e.g. by a burn which blisters and covers more than 10% of the body surface.

- Has symptoms of **meningitis**.
- Has **croup** symptoms.
- Is pale, listless, and **does not respond** to usual stimulation.
- **Cries or screams** inconsolably and may have severe pain.
- Has **convulsions**, or is limp and floppy.
- Develops purple-red rash anywhere on body.
- **Refuses** two successive feeds.
- Has jaundice.
- Passes bowel motions (stools) containing **blood**.
- Has difficulty in **breathing**.
- Has a suspected **ear infection**.
- Appears to have severe abdominal pain, with symptoms of **shock**.
- Has swallowed a **poisonous** substance, or an object, e.g. a safety pin or button.
- Has inhaled something, such as a peanut, into the air passages and may be **choking**.
- Has bulging **fontanelle** (soft spot on top of head) when not crying.
- Has bright pink cheeks and swollen hands and feet (could be due to **hypothermia**).

Supporting a child with asthma

About one in ten children in the UK has asthma. **Asthma** is an inflammatory condition of the airways of the lungs. When you have asthma the airways are extra sensitive to certain substances and events (known as **trigger factors**) which irritate them; these include:

* dust
* animal fur
* pollen
* exercise
* cigarette smoke
* colds, flu and other viral infections

Any contact with a trigger factor can cause the air passages to become narrower and a sticky mucus (phlegm) is then produced making it difficult for air to pass through. No one knows exactly what causes asthma, but an attack can be triggered by an allergy to a particular substance or by a non-allergic substance. It is clear that asthma often runs in families.

Prevention

* Where possible, avoid the likely **triggers** of asthma
* **Preventer inhalers:** Children who have been diagnosed with asthma are often issued with these; they are usually in a brown or orange case. and need to be taken every day, even when the child is feeling well. They act by reducing the inflammation and swelling in the airways.

Signs that a child is having an asthma attack

* Wheezing
* Dry persistent cough
* Difficulty in breathing
* Rapid breathing
* Sweating
* May be very frightened
* Becomes pale (a darker-skinned child may appear drained of colour, particularly around the mouth)

Using a preventer volumatic inhaler. Note: brown case

Using a reliever inhaler. Note: blue case

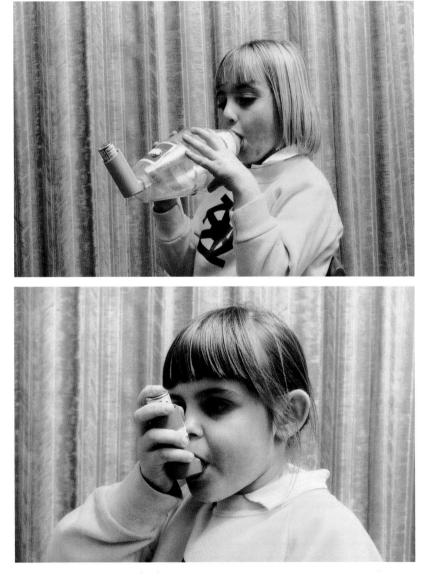

What to do if a child has an acute asthma attack

Not all asthma attacks can be prevented. During an acute attack, the child needs a reliever inhaler, which is usually in a blue case. Most children will have been shown how to use the inhaler. There are also nebulisers and spinhalers which act in the same way as the smaller inhalers but are more effective in some cases.

Helping a child with acute asthma

✓ If the attack is the child's first, then call a doctor and the parents

✓ Stay calm and reassure the child who may be very frightened

✓ Encourage the child to sit up to increase lung capacity

✓ If the child has a reliever inhaler or nebuliser, then supervise him while using the inhaler

✓ Never leave the child alone during an attack

✓ Try not to let other children crowd around

✓ If these measures do not stop the wheezing and the exhaustion caused by the attack, call a doctor. He or she will either give an injection of a drug to expand the child's airways or arrange admission to hospital.

ACTIVITY

In small groups, design and produce a colourful poster for use in a nursery or primary school to raise awareness of asthma; include the following information:

● a brief description of what asthma is;

● the main factors known to trigger an asthma attack;

● what to do when a child has an asthma attack.

Practical hints on nursing sick children at home

Wherever possible children should stay at home when ill, within the secure environment of their family and surroundings. **The child will want his or her primary carer available at all times.** The parents may need advice on how to care for their child and this is provided by the family GP and primary health care team – some health authorities have specialist paediatric nursing visiting services.

Bedrest

Children usually dislike being confined to bed and will only stay there if feeling very unwell. Making a bed on a settee in the main living room will save the carer the expense of extra heating and tiring trips up and down stairs; the child will also feel more included in family life and less isolated.

Preventing the spread of infection

If the illness is infectious, advice may be needed on how it spreads; visits from friends and relatives may have to be reduced. The most infectious time is during the incubation period but the dangers of infecting others remain until the main signs and symptoms e.g. a rash, have disappeared. A child attending nursery or school will usually be kept at home until the GP says he or she is clear of infection. You can help to prevent the spread of infection by following these guidelines:

- Wash your hands after touching any body fluids or their receptacles, e.g. vomit, urine etc.

- Empty and disinfect potties immediately after use.

- If the child has bouts of vomiting, pillows should be protected and a container should be kept close to the bed, emptied and rinsed with a disinfectant after use.

- Change wet or soiled bedlinen immediately and put dirty sheets directly in washing machine or in a covered container until they can be washed.

- Use paper tissues for minor spillages; these can be disposed of either by burning or by sealing in disposal bags.

Nutrition

Children who are ill often have poor appetites – a few days without food will not harm the child but fluid intake should be increased as a general rule.

❑ Provide a covered jug of fruit juice or water; any fluid is acceptable according to the child's tastes e.g. milk, meaty drinks or soups.

❑ NB if the child has **mumps**, do not give fruit drinks because the acid causes pain to the tender parotid glands.

❑ 'Bendy' straws or feeding beakers are useful.

❑ Drinks should be offered at frequent intervals to prevent dehydration – the child will not necessarily request drinks.

❑ Try to make food as attractive as possible; don't put too much on the plate at once and remember that weak patients often cope better with foods that do not require too much chewing e.g. egg custard, milk pudding, thick soups, chicken and ice cream.

Hygiene

All children benefit from having a routine and this need not be drastically altered during illness.

A hygiene routine for an ill child

- The sick room should be well ventilated and uncluttered. Open a window to prevent stuffiness but protect the child from draughts.

- Provide a potty to avoid trips to the lavatory.

- Protect the mattress by a plastic sheet.

- A daily bath is important, but during the acute phase this can be done in the form of an all-over wash in bed.

- Brush hair daily.

- Clean teeth after meals – apply Vaseline to sore, cracked lips.

- Crisp, clean sheets are very soothing – try to change sheets as often as you can.

- Keep the child's nails short and clean and prevent scratching of any spots.

- Dress the child in cool, cotton clothing.

Medicines

Every home should have a properly stocked medicine cabinet, preferably locked but always out of reach to children. The cabinet should contain:

- a pain reliever such as paracetamol syrup (e.g. Calpol). The different doses for children of different ages should be on the bottles;
- a hot-water bottle – when wrapped in a towel it can relieve the pain of an aching abdomen or bruised joint;
- a kaolin mixture for the relief of simple diarrhoea;
- zinc and castor oil cream – for nappy rashes;
- calamine lotion – for itchy spots and rashes;
- a clinical or digital thermometer/ fever strip;
- a teething ring (if appropriate);
- a measuring spoon or glass for liquid medicines;
- a small packet of cotton wool;
- a pack of assorted fabric plasters and one of hypo-allergenic plasters;
- crêpe bandages and conforming bandages;
- a small bottle of liquid antiseptic;
- any necessary prescription drugs.

Before stocking the medicine cabinet, discard all the half-empty, improperly labelled bottles and any medicines that are over 6 months old. Keep down costs by buying non-branded products.

Guidelines for giving medicine

Written permission from the parent, guardian or next-of-kin must always be obtained before you give any medicine to a child.

Oral medicine (to be taken by mouth) is usually dispensed in liquid form (elixir or suspension) and may be given to a baby by spoon or dropper. Most medicines for children are flavoured to make them easy to swallow. When giving a child medicine:

✓ Always check the label on the bottle and the instructions. If it has been prescribed by the doctor, check that it is for the child and follow the instructions exactly.

✓ Shake the bottle before measuring the dose. Always pour any medicine bottle with the label uppermost so that the instructions remain legible if the medicine runs down the side of the bottle.

✓ Put a bib on a baby and have some baby wipes or a flannel close at hand to wipe clean. Cradle the baby as if bottle-feeding, with her head tilted back.

✓ Use a 5ml medicine spoon to measure the dose; if using a dropper, measure the dose in a 5ml spoon and then suck it up with the dropper

✓ Spoon or squeeze the dose into the child's mouth

✓ If tablets or capsules are prescribed, these may be crushed between two spoons and given in fruit juice, jam or honey.

✓ Antibiotics may be prescribed for any infection or to prevent secondary infection (these sometimes cause diarrhoea) NB Some antibiotics may need to be kept in the fridge.

✓ When a course of antibiotics is prescribed it is vital that all the tablets/medicines are given, even if the child makes a speedy recovery.

ACTIVITY

Every child care group setting has a policy on the administration of medicines to children in their care. In your training placement, find out the following information:

1 Where are medicines stored and who is responsible for them?

2 Who gives the medicine? What happens when that person is away from work?

3 Do any children in the setting use inhalers and where are they kept?

4 What records are kept about the administration of medicines in your setting?

Procedures for reporting and recording illness

If a child becomes ill in the home environment, then the nanny or childminder must contact the parents directly. If you observe that a child is unwell in the nursery or school, you should report your concerns to a senior staff member, who will then decide whether to contact the child's parents or primary carers. It is useful to record in writing what you have observed, so that a doctor and the parents can build up an accurate picture of the nature of the illness. Record the following information about the child's symptoms, for example:

☐ **When** you first noticed something was wrong.

☐ **What** was wrong, e.g. Did the child complain of pain? Was he or she actually sick? Did the child have a high temperature? Did you notice a rash?

☐ **What** action you have taken, e.g. taking the temperature or giving sips of water.

☐ **How** the child's symptoms have progressed.

Any improvement or worsening in the child's condition should be noted down while you stay with the child and offer reassurance. Any change must be reported to a senior staff member.

Records in child care settings

Child care settings need to keep up-to-date records about each child to enable contacts to be made in the event of illness or emergency. Parents are asked to supply as much information about the child's health as they feel comfortable about. In general, the settings should have a record of each child's:

- ☐ full name and date of birth;
- ☐ current address and telephone number;
- ☐ names and addresses of the child's parents/carers;
- ☐ emergency contact telephone numbers;
- ☐ telephone numbers of the child's GP and health visitor.

If the child has a special health or dietary need, e.g. asthma or an allergy to wheat products, this should be recorded with the information above. Anyone using these records to telephone a parent or doctor must only pass on essential information. Confidentiality is a very important part of the relationship of trust which exists between parents and staff.

Play activities for sick children

After an illness children will need a period of convalescence to recover their strength and adjust to their daily routine. Most children regress when unwell; this means that they often need help with things that they could previously manage, such as using the toilet or washing themselves. They may appreciate games and activities usually considered suitable for a younger aged child. Some useful activities to relieve the boredom for a child who is in bed or resting:

- a large tray or bed-table with a favourite jigsaw;
- drawing and painting (protect bed-clothes first);
- a 'surprise' box containing previously discarded toys, pictures, paper-glue and a scrapbook, books, cut-out kits and scissors;
- reading stories aloud;
- card games and board games for older children;
- singing and listening to audio-tapes.

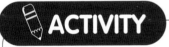 **ACTIVITY**

Invite a play specialist or nursery nurse working in hospital to come and talk about his or her job. Prepare a list of questions beforehand and collect as much information as you can about the needs of the child in hospital.

The needs of parents

There are a number of extra pressures on parents when their child is unwell. You can do much to help and support the parents of children in your care by recognising these additional worries:

Parents may feel

Guilty
because they
- have to work
- can't be with child
- feel helpless

Anxious
because they
- lack information
- fear the child will not improve
- fear they cannot cope

Tired
because they
- lack sleep
- are caring for other children

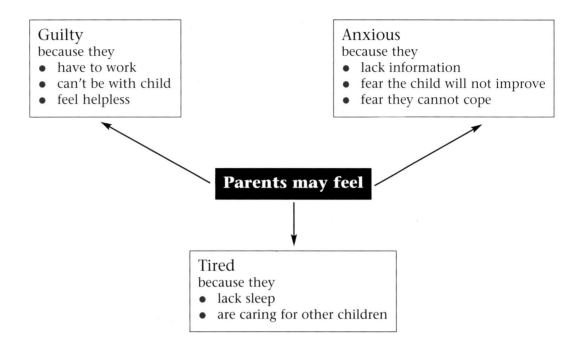

You can also help by:

* being calm and reassuring to parents;
* giving accurate information;
* offering practical help and support where possible;
* showing understanding and that you care.

If one of the common childhood infections has been diagnosed, e.g. rubella, chicken pox, measles etc. then the nursery manager or head teacher should inform parents (without mentioning names to preserve confidentiality).

The role of healthcare professionals

Health visitors

Health visitors are qualified nurses who work exclusively in the community. They see children up to the age of 5 years old in their homes and in community health clinics. As specialists in the area of child development, health visitors are ideally placed to advise and support parents with sick children.

Family doctors (General Practitioners – GPs)

Family doctors are trained to diagnose illnesses and to prescribe medicines. They can also refer parents and children to specialist doctors for further treatment.

School nurses

School nurses monitor children's health and development whilst they are of school age. They give advice to schools and to parents about all aspects of child health.

Practice nurses

Practice nurses are based in the GP's surgery. They give general health advice and also give immunisations and routine health checks.

District nurses/Community nurses

District nurses work as part of the **Primary Health Care** Team. They work with patients in their own homes. Some areas have specialist paediatric district nursing teams to help and support parents whose children have a long-term illness or who can be nursed at home with regular visits to hospital.

Paediatricians

Paediatricians are usually based in a hospital. They are qualified doctors who specialise in treating children.

Play specialists

Play specialists are employed in hospitals and are often qualified child care and education workers who have additional training and work with children who are sick in hospital.

- physical activities for stages of development
- the importance of supervision during physical exercise
- restrictions during outdoor play

Supporting a child in developing a new skill

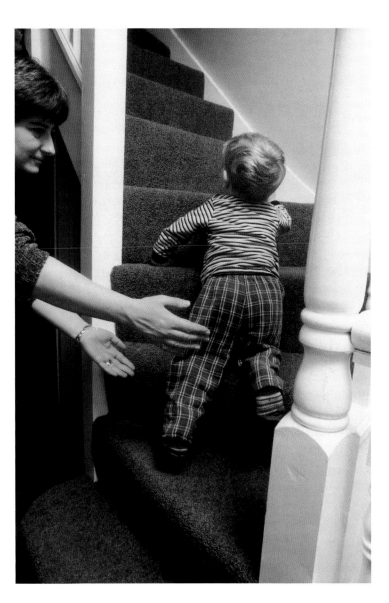

Why physical activity is important

Children need opportunities for physical activity or exercise. Exercise is important because it keeps people's bodies – and minds – healthy. Regular exercise reduces the risk of children developing heart disease in later life. **Physical activity** is essential for children because it:

✓ **Makes the heart strong:** The heart is a muscle, and it's the strongest muscle in the body. The heart needs **aerobic exercise** to keep bringing fresh **oxygen** to all the muscles in the body. The number of blood cells in the blood increases, so the blood can carry even more oxygen. Children need to do some kind of aerobic exercise two or three times a week, for 20 to 30 minutes at a time. Some excellent aerobic activities are swimming, basketball, running, jogging (or walking quickly), inline skating, soccer, and cycling. Dancing, skipping, and playing hopscotch are also good aerobic activities.

✓ **Develops the muscles:** Exercise makes the muscles stronger and sometimes larger. As the muscles become stronger, children can do more active things for longer periods of time. Strong muscles also help protect children from injuries when they exercise, because they give better support to the joints. Children can strengthen their arm muscles by using climbing equipment and by playing tug-of-war games. For strong leg muscles, they can run, ride a bike or try inline skating.

✓ **Makes children more flexible:** Most children are very flexible, which means that they can bend and stretch their bodies without too much trouble. But as people get older they tend to get less flexible; this is why it is important to exercise when you're a child – in order to stay flexible. Dancing, yoga, gymnastics and martial arts such as karate and tae-kwon-do are very good ways to become more flexible.

✓ **Keeps children at a healthy weight:** Every time you eat food, your body does the same thing: it uses some of the nutrients in the food as fuel. It burns these nutrients to give us energy or calories. But if the body isn't able to use all the **calories** that are coming from food, it stores them away as fat. Exercise helps keep a child at a weight that's right for their height, by burning up extra calories.

✓ **Makes children feel good:** Exercising is a very good way to feel happy, whether you're exercising on your own or with a group. This is because when you exercise, your body can release **endorphins**, which are chemicals that create a happy feeling in your brain. Also, when you are breathing deeply during exercise and bringing more air into your lungs, your brain is receiving extra oxygen.

✓ **Helps children to develop self-esteem and independence:** Exercise can make children feel better about themselves; when they have mastered a certain skill, such as climbing a rope ladder or swimming, they feel a sense of achievement and independence.

✓ **Helps to promote sleep:** children need to relax after physical activity; this does not necessarily mean that they will need to sleep more, but they will need to rest after exercise.

✓ **Promotes social skills and mutual understanding:** Children learn to share when using play equipment and to take turns. They also learn how to play and work together in team games and in cooperative play, e.g. pulling each other along in a cart.

Age/Stage of development	Activities	Benefits to child
Three Years + Walks with arms swinging Climbs upstairs with one foot on each step, and downwards with two feet on each step	● Provide balls and bean bags for throwing and catching ● Simple running games	● Develops muscles and hand/eye co-ordination ● Develops leg muscles
Four years + Good sense of balance Catches, throws and kicks a ball Runs up and down stairs, one foot per step	● Climbing frames, rope swings, slides, suitable trees ● Party games, e.g. musical statues ● Running to music – fast or slow, loudly or quietly according to the music	● Develops confidence and control; leg muscles and spatial awareness ● Promotes the idea of co-operation and learning rules of games ● Develops a sense of rhythm and confidence
Five years + Can run and dodge Runs lightly on the toes Climbs, skips and hops forwards on each foot separately Shows good co-ordination	● Climbing frames, rope swings etc. ● Skipping ropes and hoops ● Hopping and jumping ● Riding tricycles, bikes – with or without stabilizers ● Swimming	● Develops confidence and control; leg muscles and spatial awareness ● Stamina, sense of rhythm, co-ordination ● Balance, co-ordination, develops leg muscles ● Develops muscles, stamina, balance, hand-eye co-ordination, sense of speed ● Overall muscle development, stamina and co-ordination
Six to eight years Jumps off apparatus with confidence Runs and kicks a football Hops easily with good balance Catches and throws ball, using one hand	● Football, dancing, judo or gymnastics, bikes ● Swimming ● Hopping games, such as hopscotch ● Obstacle courses for bike riders	● Promotes social skills, independence, co-ordination ● Overall muscle development, stamina and co-ordination ● Balance, co-ordination, develops leg muscles ● Balance, co-ordination, control, stamina

Your role in promoting children's physical development

- Recognise the **skills** that children have developed
- Provide plenty of **opportunities** for children to practise their skills
- Make sure that children have the freedom to explore their environment **in safety**
- Be there for children; offer them **reassurance**, encouragement and praise
- Provide **access to a range of facilities** and equipment; this need not be expensive – a visit to the local park, a pre-school group (play group or one o'clock club) or an adventure playground will provide facilities not available in a small flat
- Promote **outdoor play** whenever possible; even in cold or windy weather, children will enjoy running around outside as long as they are warmly wrapped up. (If you are supervising, make sure that you are warmly wrapped up too)

Some helpful ideas:

- Avoid running races where children may feel discouraged if always last. Try imaginative running – e.g. where the children pretend to be jet planes zooming down the runway
- For children who have difficulty with throwing and catching, try using a small soft pillow, standing quite close at first and gradually stepping back as they gain control
- Always supervise climbing play carefully. For children who seem nervous when climbing, stand close by to encourage and help if they falter
- Children with a hearing impairment can often feel the vibrations from noisy toys and loud music, even though they cannot hear the sound
- Make an obstacle course using planks, barrels, ladders and boxes and rearrange them frequently. Children can climb up, over and under
- Make a 'hopping trail' using cut-out contact footprints that show hopping steps on one foot; then hopping on the other foot, tiptoeing and jumping

ACTIVITY

Observing children during physical activity

Select **one child** to observe during a period of physical activity, e.g. a gymnastics or dance class, outdoor play with climbing equipment, or ball games. Devise a **checklist** (see pp. 176–179 for guidelines on making observations) to record the child's use of:

- gross motor skills: e.g. running, squatting, climbing, etc., and
- fine motor skills: e.g. throwing and catching a ball, picking up equipment and carrying objects etc.

Write a conclusion to show how the particular session of physical activity benefited the individual child; note if there were ways that the session could be extended to improve the development of these skills.

Providing opportunities for physical activity

Young children's physical development is inseparable from all other aspects of development because they learn through being active and interactive. Children will develop physical skills if they have sufficient time to persevere and to learn from their mistakes. Confidence and self-esteem grow when children are successful, whether it is in climbing a tree, kicking a ball or moving to a favourite piece of music.

Where possible, children should be encouraged to move freely between indoor and outdoor environments. Children will improve their co-ordination, control and ability to move more effectively if they can run, climb, slide, tumble, throw, catch and kick when they want to, rather than at a set time of the day.

Providing opportunities for physical activity	
Plan activities that offer appropriate physical challenges	Provide sufficient space, indoors and outdoors, to set up relevant activities
Give sufficient time for each child to use a range of equipment	Provide resources that can be used in a variety of ways or to support specific skills
Introduce the language of movement to children, alongside their actions, e.g. up, over, slowly, quickly etc.	Provide time and opportunities for children with physical disabilities or motor impairments to develop their physical skills, working as necessary with physiotherapists and occupational therapists
Use additional adult help, indoors if necessary, to support individual children and to encourage increased independence in physical activities	

Using space and equipment effectively

It is often difficult to find space for outdoor exercise. Some settings and homes have no, or very restricted, outdoor areas. It may be necessary to rearrange furniture to create enough space indoors to provide physical activity. Sometimes it is possible to provide a sheltered outdoor play area where children can still benefit from fresh air.

Equipment is also often limited. Some nurseries and pre-school groups have to share their premises with other organizations, so there is no room to store large-scale equipment, such as pedal cars, indoor slides etc.

You can help in the following ways:

* Change the activities on a regular basis; children like to try new challenges
* Choose equipment that has multiple uses: e.g. hoops, which can be bowled, jumped into, used as a target for throwing and climbed through
* Arrange visits to parks and playgrounds so that children can enjoy the freedom of running in open spaces and using large-scale equipment, such as rope ladders and swings
* Borrow equipment from a toy library.

Note: Ideas for promoting physical development at each stage of development can be found on pages 97–98.

How to avoid non-stereotypical exercise and play

Boys often seem to dominate outside play and the use of equipment. As children become more aware of their gender, and of other people's expectations of their behaviour, they might reject activities they once liked and choose instead more 'gender-appropriate' activities; for example, girls might choose skipping games, while boys may prefer a game of football.

In order to challenge these **stereotypes** and to ensure **equal opportunities** are offered to every child, follow the guidelines below.

Equal opportunities for every child

* Avoid having expectations of children's physical abilities based on **stereotypes**:
  Example: 'You're a big strong boy, Tom, please carry that chair inside for me.'
* Ensure that the provision of play does not reinforce stereotypes:

  Example: Allow only the girls to use the wheeled toys and bikes for one session.
* Be a good role model. You should be fully involved in children's physical play, rather than passively supervising. Show children that you are enjoying the session.
* Be observant. Take note of the child who seems reluctant to try new equipment and offer gentle encouragement.
* Be aware of the use of gender-specific terminology:

  Example: fireman; instead use 'fire-fighter'.
* Be sensitive to requests for privacy when changing for school PE lessons.

✱ Respect dress code based on religious beliefs, ensuring safety guidelines are still followed.

✱ **Children with special needs** may need different equipment – according to the special need they have – or they may need it to be adapted; for example, by fitting Velcro straps to bike pedals. Other ideas include:

✱ Providing soft foam-filled blocks, soft balls, bean-bags and plastic bats; these can often be obtained from a charity or from a toy library

✱ Planning activities to encourage exercise and movement of all body parts – an occupational therapist or play specialist can offer valuable advice.

For more information on stereotypes and promoting equal opportunity, see pages 265–270.

Child protection policies and procedures

- signs and symptoms of child abuse
- observing children for signs of injuries
- policies and procedures in the work setting

Although child abuse is not common, it is important to recognise that there are, and will always be, children who are victims of abuse in one way or another. The categories of child abuse are:

- **Physical abuse**
- **Emotional abuse**
- **Neglect**
- **Sexual abuse**

Physical abuse

Non-Accidental Injury (NAI) involves someone deliberately harming a child. This may take the from of:

❑ **Bruising:** from being slapped, punched, shaken or squeezed

❑ **Cuts:** scratches, bite marks, a torn frenulum (the web of skin inside the upper lip)

❑ **Fractures:** skull and limb fractures from being thrown against hard objects

❑ **Burns and scalds:** cigarettes, irons, baths and kettles

Often the particular injuries can be easily explained, but you should always be suspicious if a child has any bruise or mark which shows the particular pattern of an object, e.g. a belt strap mark, teeth marks or the imprint of an iron. Also look out for behavioural disturbances in the child, such as aggressiveness towards others or a withdrawn attitude.

Emotional abuse

Emotional abuse occurs when a child consistently faces threatening ill treatment from an adult. This can take the form of verbal abuse, ridiculing, mocking and insulting the child. It is difficult to find out how common this form of abuse is, because it is hard to detect. Signs of emotional abuse include:

- withdrawn behaviour; child may not join in with others or appear to be having fun;

- attention-seeking behaviour;
- self-esteem and confidence is low;
- stammering and stuttering;
- tantrums beyond the expected age;
- telling lies and even stealing;
- tearfulness.

Emotional neglect means that children do not receive love and affection from the adult. They may often be left alone without the company and support of someone who loves them.

Neglect

Physical neglect occurs when the adult fails to give their child what they need to develop physically. They often leave children alone and unattended. Signs of physical neglect include:

- being underweight for their age and not thriving;
- unwashed clothes which are often dirty and smelly;
- child may have poor skin tone, dull matted hair and bad breath; a baby may have a persistent rash from infrequent nappy changing;
- being constantly tired, hungry and listless or lacking in energy;
- frequent health problems, and prone to accidents;
- low self-esteem and poor social relationships: delay in all areas of development is likely because of lack of stimulation.

Sexual abuse

There is much more awareness today about the existence of sexual abuse. Sexual abuse means that the adult uses the child to gratify their sexual needs. This could involve sexual intercourse or anal intercourse. It may involve watching pornographic material with the child. Sexual abuse might also mean children being encouraged in sexually explicit behaviour or oral sex, masturbation or the fondling of sexual parts. Signs of sexual abuse include the following:

- bruises or scratches as in a Non-Accidental Injury or physical injury;
- itching or pain in the genital area;
- wetting or soiling themselves;
- discharge from the penis or vagina;
- poor self-esteem and lack of confidence;
- may regress and want to be treated like a baby;
- poor sleeping and eating patterns;
- withdrawn and solitary behaviour.

Your role in reporting suspected abuse

You need to be aware of the indicators of child abuse as outlined above. However, it is important not to jump to conclusions. If you have any cause for concern, you should always talk to your immediate superior or to the head of the nursery or school. Every child care setting has a policy for dealing with suspected child abuse.

If you suspect child abuse in the home setting, then you should contact your local Social Services or the NSPCC (The National Society for the Protection of Children).

If a child tells you he or she has been abused

You should:

- Reassure the child, saying that you are glad that they have told you about this.
- Believe the child. Tell the child that you will do your best to protect them, but don't promise that you can do that.
- Remember that the child is not to blame, and that it is important that you make the child understand this.
- Do a lot of listening; don't ask questions.
- Report your conversation with the child to your immediate superior.
- Write down what was said by the child as soon as possible after the conversation.

The role of the adult

Although child abuse is not common, it is important to recognise that there are, and will always be, children who are victims of abuse in one way or another. You have a responsibility to children and their families to learn as much as possible about the signs and symptoms of all kinds of child abuse. If you have any concerns about a child, you should discuss them with the person in charge at the nursery or school. If you have concerns about a child within the home setting, then you should take your worries to your school or college tutor in the first instance.

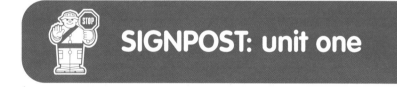

SIGNPOST: unit one

1   Looking back through the information provided in this chapter and using **at least one other book or article**, complete the chart (see Appendix for Unit 1) to show the stage of physical development children of the ages shown are likely to have reached:

Age/Aspect	Growth	Gross motor skills	Fine motor skills	Sensory skills
1 year	Wt: Ht:			
2 years	Wt: Ht:			
3 years	Wt: Ht:			
4 years	Wt: Ht:			
5 years	Wt: Ht:			
6 years	Wt: Ht:			
7 years	Wt: Ht:			

2   This group activity will help you to gather information for your assignment. A Family Centre has decided to provide a range of leaflets to help and support young families. There will be a leaflet for each 'age' of child, i.e. 'Your one-year-old', 'Your two-year-old', etc.

Your group task is to produce one of the leaflets. Each group should work on a different age. The following information must be in your leaflet and each student in your group should take responsibility for one topic:

- The physical care needed by a child of that age (hygiene, rest, exercise, etc.)
- The dietary needs (nutritional balance, etc.)
- How an adult can support the child's physical care (hygienic practices, regular checks, etc.)
- Explaining what is needed for a healthy and safe environment and how an adult can provide and maintain it.

In completing this exercise you are fulfilling **Key Skills** requirements for Communication level 2.2. However, you must identify your two 'extended' sources of information. Note: one of them must include an image such as a chart or picture that is relevant to your work. SO ... if you have obtained your weights and heights from a graph showing averages for children 0–8 years or percentile charts **or** gained information from a picture of a child riding a bike, sitting unsupported, etc., then you meet the requirements! Your written work, produced in the suitable format for the leaflet, can be used for one of the documents required for Key Skills Communication 2.3. Your finished assignment (which will need to contain a relevant image) will provide the extended piece of writing (the second document) needed.

When you are dealing with these topics you must remember that different cultures may have particular requirements that you must include, e.g. special diets or hair care, etc.

You will need to discuss your work and share your ideas, making sure you listen carefully to everyone's opinions – Key Skills Communication 2.1a. Part of your discussion may focus on how you will present your information (layout, font, use of images, style of language) and you will want your leaflet to appear as if one person has written it, not several!

3 A nursery chain, which also runs 'after-school' clubs, has decided that staff would benefit from some step-by-step advice sheets (to be kept in an easily accessible folder) for dealing with a range of first aid and other health and child protection procedures. The sheets need to be A4 sized with clearly sequenced steps. They can include diagrams or pictures to aid explanation and can be in the format of a numbered or bullet-pointed list or a flow diagram/'decision tree'.

Produce *three* sheets, choosing **one** topic from each of the three groups – make special reference to the ages given in brackets.

Group 1
- Bruising – particularly clusters of small bruises on both upper arms (one year old)
- Round burn marks on legs and upper body (two year old)
- A swollen and bruised eye (four year old).

Group 2
- Bumped head (three year old)
- Grazed knees (four year old)
- Nose bleed (five year old).

Group 3
- Symptoms of sickness and diarrhoea (one year old)
- An asthma attack (five year old)
- Symptoms of meningitis (seven year old).

Using your prepared sheets, choose one topic and give a short talk to the rest of your group (Key Skills Communication 2.1b). Make sure you use an image (this could be a picture of burn marks or a diagram to show how an inhaler helps during an asthma attack or a chart showing statistics relating to the growing number of asthma sufferers) to support what you are saying. To deliver your talk, you will need to plan the main points and any props (objects or diagrams, etc.) you want to use. Think about speaking at a steady pace and projecting your voice (right volume level) so everyone can hear. Try to vary your tone of voice so it remains interesting to your listeners. Stand confidently, avoid fiddling with clothing or hair and try to make eye contact with your audience'.

Working with Young Children

The sequence of sensory and intellectual development

- stages of sensory and intellectual development
- the sequence of development of children's play
- the different types of play
- how play relates to a child's learning and development
- range of play materials and equipment for indoors and outdoors

Psychologists have tried for many years to find out how children learn. The area of development connected with knowledge, understanding and reasoning is referred to as **intellectual** or **cognitive development**.

Intellectual or **cognitive development** involves:

❋ what a person knows and the ability to reason, understand and problem-solve;

❋ memory, concentration, attention and perception;

❋ imagination and creativity.

Language development is very closely linked with cognitive development and a delay in one area usually affects progress in the other.

There is an ongoing debate about how children develop and learn often referred to as the **nature/nurture** debate and centres on this question:

Is our ability to learn determined by our inherited genes and characteristics? (i.e. NATURE) – OR – Is our ability to learn determined by our upbringing? (i.e. NURTURE)

The illustration below shows features important for intellectual development:

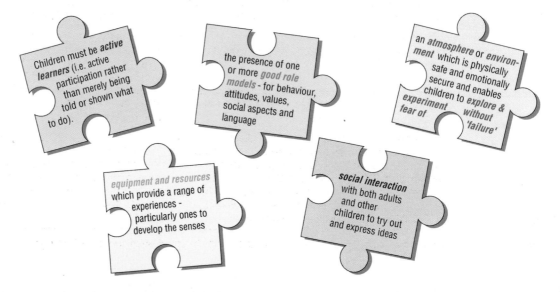

Jean Piaget (1896–1990), a Swiss psychologist, identified particular stages of cognitive development which continue to influence how we work with children. His stage theory stated that:

✱ children move through a series of stages which are loosely related to age ranges;

✱ children progress through the stages in a particular sequence (or order);

✱ no stage can be missed out or 'jumped over';

✱ basic concepts are formed early and are refined as children gain first-hand experiences;

✱ very young children are 'egocentric' – i.e. they see things from their own viewpoint and have difficulty in putting themselves in another's place.

Sensory motor stage 0–2 years

0–6 months	Babies explore objects around them using their senses – squeezing, sucking, shaking etc. They enjoy bright colours and can recognise familiar objects. They begin to differentiate familiar sounds, tastes and smells. They use their voices to produce a range of sounds. Their developing physical skills mean they can co-ordinate movements to help them explore their environment.
6–12 months	During this period babies learn that objects exist even when they cannot be seen – this is know as developing 'object permanence'. They may repeat actions to watch cause and effect. They watch and imitate adults and at this stage develop memory of events they have experienced. This helps them to understand familiar routines.
1–2 years	Increasing physical skills and mobility help children to play with a wider range of objects. They can understand the names of objects and can follow simple instructions. They continue to experiment by repeating actions and movements and are developing early concepts linked to them. They begin 'symbolic' play using toys or objects to represent things in real life e.g. a doll becomes a baby, a box becomes a car or television. They will also 'talk' to themselves and be aware of other children playing although they will not necessarily play 'with' others.

Pre-operational stage 2–7 years

2–3 years	Manipulative skills develop and children are more able to control their movements to use tools and implements e.g. hold a crayon and move it up and down, connect construction materials. They have some understanding of their own daily routine and are developing memory skills which help their understanding of basic concepts. They can often match two (sometimes three) colours – usually yellow and red – and begin to name them. They are becoming able communicators. Play may involve 'looking on' at others and, sometimes, joining in although they may still play alone or in parallel.
3–4 years	Pincer grasp is developed and helps them to use paintbrushes, pencils, beads (large) and other play materials with increasing control. Developing independence in everyday tasks – toileting, handwashing, dressing etc. Play with a wide range of materials helps to develop their understanding of concepts – colour, weight, size, number etc. and may say the number sequence up to ten but with varying degrees of accuracy. Becoming fluent speakers and beginning to use written symbols to represent an object or word ('pretend' writing). They can also recognise environmental print i.e. road name, shop signs etc. Play may now involve co-operation with others and they learn through trial and error and opportunities to solve relevant problems.
4–5 years	Physical skills help children to do up buttons, zips and other fastenings. They are becoming more independent in managing their own routines but still need adult help. They are developing concepts of: time – day and night, sequence of their day; number – know number sequence to ten and may count reliably up to ten; colour – can name some accurately and sort objects by colour; size – can identify big and small when given two appropriate objects and begin to order by size; shape – can identify and name basic 2D shapes and some 3D shapes. Can remember and talk about their own experiences. Beginning to recognise letter shapes and associated sounds. Play is often co-operative and can involve taking on identified roles.
5–7+ years	Increasing independence through developing physical skills and ability to choose and make decisions. During this period they are able to **conserve**. They are increasingly able to express their ideas and creativity in a variety of ways – through words (spoken and written), movement, music, pictures, models and other craft work. Their drawings include greater detail. Concepts are becoming more refined e.g. time – understanding of seasons, months of the year, days of the week, hours in the day etc. Are able to play more complex games and sustain interest and co-operation for longer periods of time. Beginning to develop own research skills – knowing where to find information they are interested in.

Table 2.1 Stages of sensory and intellectual development with indication of the age at which each stage is usually experienced

What is play?

Play brings together:

* ideas and creativity

* feelings

* relationships

* physical co-ordination

* spiritual development.

Play helps children to use what they know and understand about the world and people they meet.

During play children:

- get things under control so that they can face the world and deal with it

- get ready for the future

- think about things that have happened.

The role of play – understanding its importance

😊   Play is important for human beings in their development.

😊   Play is complex, and understanding play is not easy.

There are different ideas about how to develop play, but although there are wide cultural variations, all children seem to develop and learn through play, including children with severe disabilities.

Children who do not play find it difficult to learn, e.g. children in the Romanian orphanages were held back in learning about objects, ideas, feelings, relationships and people.

Your role will be important in providing opportunities which support and extend children's play.

The charter of Children's Rights (1989) says that every child in the world should have the right to play.

The role of play – why play?

Play helps children:

- deal with tragedies and setbacks (be resilient)   **Emotional development**
- have a sense of well being and good self-esteem
- have a sense of control

- make good relationships   **Social development**
- understand and care about others

• be creative and imaginative	**Cognitive (concept) development**
• think and have ideas (concepts)	
• have a go and try hard	
• develop concentration	

• be physically well co-ordinated	**Physical development**

Ideas about play are influenced by thinkers from the past and thinkers from around the world.

Ideas from the past

Friedrich Froebel (1782–1852)

Froebel was a forester and mathematician. He was the first person to write about the importance of the play in development and learning. He started a community school, where parents were welcome at any time. He trained his staff to observe and value children's play.

- He thought it was important to talk with parents and learn with them how to help children learn through their play.
- He designed a set of wooden blocks (**Gifts**) which are still used in early childhood settings today. He also designed many other kinds of play equipment (**Occupations**) and **Movement Games** (action songs and finger play rhymes and dancing) through which children learn by doing.
- He encouraged pretend play. He encouraged play with other children.
- He thought both indoor and outdoor play to be important.
- He helped children to make dens in the garden and to play with natural materials such as sand, water and wood.
- He called his schools **kindergartens** (for children 2–8 years). This means the **garden of children** in German.
- Even today there are kindergartens all over the world. His influence on early childhood education and care is deep.

Maria Montessori (1880–1952)

Montessori was an Italian doctor who worked in the poorest areas of Rome in the 1900s. She did not believe that pretend play was important. She thought children wanted to do real things, e.g. not play at being cooks but to actually do some cooking. However, she did like Froebel's play equipment, and she designed more (didactic materials) to help them learn, for example, about shapes, weight, colour, size and numbers.

Montessori thought children should be guided by a trained adult to use her equipment until they could use it confidently on their own and independently. She called her schools **Children's Houses** and these are still to be found all over the world.

Rudolf Steiner (1861–1925)

Rudolf Steiner encouraged play through natural materials, such as clay, beeswax, silk scarves for dressing up and wooden blocks which are irregularly shaped. He believed singing and dancing were important and that stories give children ideas for their play. There are schools today which carry out these ideas.

Ideas about play from around the world

In Western Europe and the USA, children are often given toys to play with. Sometimes they are very expensive to buy. In other countries, specially designed toys may not be part of the way of life, and children will play mainly with **natural materials**, such as **stones**, **twigs**, **sand**, **water** and **mud**, and make their own **pretend play**.

In some cultures, adults think it is not a good idea to play with children. They let children play together and older children play with younger children (for example Maori children in New Zealand). In other cultures, adults think adults (usually mothers) ought to play with their children and to teach them through their play.

Why do children play – learning through play

A **theory** is something which helps us to explain and answer '**why?**' It helps us to look at the **role of play** in a child's development.

The different theories of play emphasise different aspects. They all help us to learn more about children's play.

Practice play – children practise for later life

Psychoanalytic – they are learning how to deal with feelings

Theory of mind (moral development) – they are helped through play to think of others

Concepts (cognitive) – ideas and thinking

Learning through practice play

Some theories emphasise the importance of childhood play because it encourages children to practise things they need to do later on in life. It helps them with the physical co-ordination of their bodies, objects and people.

There are two sides to practice play:

1 The biological side of practice play

Studies of young animals playing show that, for example, lion cubs playing together quite naturally begin catching and chewing. This helps them to learn what they need to know later in order to hunt for their food and survive.

2 The social/cultural aspect of practice play

Even newborn babies are very aware of other people. Children imitate people who are important role models for them.

Play and feelings

Some theories emphasise the importance of children's feelings. These are psychoanalytic ideas about why children play.

The play scenarios children create deal with their feelings of happiness, sadness, anger etc. in an emotionally healthy way. Although this helps any child, therapists particularly emphasise sad and angry feelings through play for the children they work with.

Research shows that emotional health is helped through play, and leads to children developing **resilience**.

Play helps socially acceptable behaviour

Other theories show that children learn to think of others through their play. They learn to behave in ways which are socially acceptable as they play. It helps them to understand how other people feel and this helps them to develop morally (to value and respect others and to care about other people). This is called **theory of mind**.

Research shows that serial murderers have not played as children, and find it difficult to care about other people.

Play helps thinking and ideas (concepts) to develop

There are three important theories about how play helps children to have ideas and learn to think. They are all useful for adults working with young children. Two of these theories emphasise social/cultural learning.

Both these theories show that other people are important in developing a child's play.

Vygotsky was a psychologist in the 1930s who found that children do their best thinking when they play with others. This is because play helps them to feel in **control** of their ideas, and to make sense of things that have happened. Play helps children to **think ahead**.

Bruner believes that play helps children to learn how adults do things in their culture. Adults observe children as they play and break things down into easily manageable steps for them. This is called **scaffolding the learning**.

The third theory emphasises both biology and social/cultural learning. It is the most famous theory.

Piaget emphasised that children are active learners. They learn through their senses (seeing, touching, hearing, smelling, tasting) and through their own movement.

☐ Sometimes children will **play alone**.

☐ Sometimes they will **play with others** (children or adults)

☐ Children are like scientists, exploring their world and working at different levels about the world.

☐ Although each of the stages builds on the one before, they also overlap. Modern research shows some children do things earlier, and some later than others.

Play and the development of physical co-ordination

Children who can	Gross motor	Fine motor
Sit (usually 6–9 months)	• Play with feet (put them in mouth) • Cruise around furniture	• Play with objects using a pincer movement (i.e. finger and thumb) • Transfer toys from one hand to the other • Enjoy dropping objects over the side of the high chair and look to see where they have gone • Play with objects by putting them into the mouth • Enjoy 'treasure baskets' (natural objects and household objects) *Provide:* • Cups, boxes, pots of different sizes
Crawl (usually 9–12 months)	• When sitting, the baby leans forward and picks up objects • Enjoy playing by crawling upstairs or onto low furniture • Love to bounce in time to music	• Pick things up with a pincer movement (finger and thumb) • Pull objects towards themselves • Can point at toys • Clasp hands and love to copy adults' actions in play • Love to play by throwing toys on purpose • Hold toys easily in hands • Put objects in and out of pots and boxes *Provide:* • Push and pull toys
Walk (but with sudden falling into a sitting position) (12–15 months)	• Can manage stairs with adult supervision • Can stand and kneel without support	• Begin to build towers with wooden blocks • Make lines of objects on the floor • Begin using books and turn several pages at a time • Use both hands but often prefer one • Lot of pointing • Pull toys along and push buttons *Provide:* • Board books and picture books with lines • Big empty cardboard boxes • Messy play with water paints and sand (be alert for physical safety)
Walk confidently (usually 18 months)	• Can kneel, squat, climb and carry things, can climb on chairs • Can twist around to sit • Can creep downstairs on tummy going backwards	• Pick up small objects and threads • Build towers • Scribble on paper • Push and pull toys • Enjoy banging toys e.g. hammer and peg drums *Provide:* • Large crayons for drawing and paper
Jump (usually 2 years)	• Can jump on the spot and run and climb stairs two feet at a time • Kick but are not good at catching ball • Enjoy space to run and play (trips to the park) • Enjoy climbing frames (supervised)	• Draw circles • Build tall towers • Pick up tiny objects • Turn the pages of books one at a time • Enjoy toys to ride on and climb on • Enjoy messy play with water paints and sand pits *Provide:* • Duplo, jigsaws, crayons and paper, picture books, puppets, simple dressing up clothes, hats, belts and shoes
Hop (usually 3 years)	• Jump from low steps • Walk forwards, backwards and sideways • Stand and walk on tiptoe • Stand on one foot • Try to hop • Use pedals on tricycle • Climb stairs one foot at a time	• Build taller and taller towers with blocks • Begin to use pencil grip • Paint and make lines and circles in drawings • Use play dough, sand for modelling, paint • Hold objects to explore *Provide:* • Enjoy trip to the park, walks, library, swimming • Enjoy cooking, small world, gluing, pouring, cutting

Children who can	Gross motor	Fine motor
Skip (usually 4 years)	• Balance (walking on a line) • Catch a ball, kick, throw and bounce • Bend at the waist to pick up objects from the floor • Climbing trees and frames • Can run up and down stairs one foot at a time	• Build tower with blocks which are taller and taller • Draw people, houses etc • Thread beads • Enjoy exercise, swimming, climbing (climbing frames and bikes) *Provide:* • Jigsaws, construction toys, wooden blocks, small world, glue and stick, paint, sand, water, clay, play dough, dressing up clothes and home area play • Cooking (measuring, pouring and cutting)
Jump, hop, skip and run with co-ordination (usually 5 years)	• Use a variety of play equipment (slides, swings, climbing frames) • Enjoy ball games • Hop and run lightly on toes, and can move rhythmically to music • Well developed sense of balance	• Sew large stitches • Draw with people, animals and places etc • Co-ordinate paint brushes and pencils and a variety of tools • Enjoy outdoor activities (skipping ropes, football – both boys and girls enjoy these) • Make models, do jigsaws
Move with increased co-ordination and balance (usually 6–7 years)	• Can ride two wheel bicycle • Hops easily with good balance • Can jump off apparatus at • school	• Build play scenarios with wooden blocks • Draw play scenarios in drawings and paintings • Hold pencil as adults do • Enjoy ball games • Enjoy vigorous activity (riding a bike, swimming) NB children should never be forced to take part unless they want to • Enjoy board games and computer games • Often (but not always) enjoys work being displayed on interest tables and walls NB Children should never be forced to display their work

Piaget's stages of development in play

Babyhood and beginning to be a toddler	**0–18 months** The senses and movement play	Learning through play: through the senses and through their movement to co-ordinate their bodies; to crawl and play with objects – rattles; to play with people (peek a boo). They love to repeat their play over and over again.
Toddler times and early childhood years	**18 months–5 years** Symbolic (pretend) play	A symbol is something which stands for something else. Symbolic play might mean carrying a bag and saying 'I am pretending to be mum going shopping'; a stone might stand for a pretend potato; children begin to use language (or signs) as they play; the word dog stands for a dog; the sign for a dog stands for a dog; words and signs are symbols.
The years of Early Childhood Education	**4–8 years** Learning about rules through games and through play	Children take part in games with rules: Games – other people make the rules of a game e.g snakes and ladders or snap; Play – children make the rules up as they go e.g. 'I am driving a car'.
Middle childhood	**8–11 years**	Children develop more games with rules e.g. football, dance routines that they learn to perform exactly.

Table 2.2 Play helps children to use symbols

Play and development

Knowing the way that play progresses as children grow older, helps adults to plan appropriate play materials and play opportunities for different children according to their stage of development.

This is called knowing about **progression** in the development of play.

Play and the development of physical co-ordination

Children vary and develop at different rates. This depends partly on their biological stage. It also depends on where they grow up and what play opportunities and materials they are given. A child who has played with wooden blocks since toddler times might well be building towers that are castles by the age of 4 years. A child who has not had these experiences is unlikely to do this.

This shows that what children learn is influenced by how adults help their development. This is why observing children as they play is important, especially if they have disabilities.

Play and the development of feelings and social play (social/emotional development)

It used to be thought that there were four stages of social play:

☐ solitary play

☐ parallel play

☐ associative play

☐ co-operative play

Modern research shows that children do not develop as if they are climbing up a ladder. Instead, brain studies show that their play develops like a network. Sometimes they will play alone (solitary play). Sometimes with others (parallel, associatively or co-operatively).

It will partly depend on their age, but it will also depend on their mood, who they are with, where they are, whether they are tired, hungry or comfortable.

It is certainly easier for toddlers and young children to play together in parallel, associatively or co-operatively if they are in a pair (two children). Larger groups are more of a challenge for young children. Gradually three or four children might play co-operatively together. This tends to develop from 3 or 4 years of age.

A child might play alone – solitary play

A child might play alone, for example with a dolls house, because they want to play out a story that they have in their head. Having other children join the play would stop them being able to do this.

Children might play together

A pair – in parallel play

Two children might both put dolls to bed in the home area. They don't take much notice of each other.

Pairs – in associative play

Two children might play so that one is the cook in the cafe and the other is the waitress. They don't take much notice of each other. They don't seem to care that they have no customers.

Pairs – in co-operative play

One child might be the baby and the other might be the parent, as they play going to the shops. They talk about their play ideas: "you say 'mum' and I say 'yes, darling'."

Progression in play development

A group – children involved in co-operative play

A group of children 3–5 years old have been on an outing in the local market. When they return, the adult sets up a market stall. Some children become customers and buy things. Others sell things.

John has a hearing impairment and uses sign language. Jack understands his sign to give him three oranges. Other children talk as they play: 'You come and bag these apples.'

Play and the development of thinking (concepts)

Look at the chart on Piaget's stages of cognitive development in play on page 109.

Play and learning

The terms structured play and free play are rather old fashioned ways of describing the way children learn through play. Research is showing that we need to think about these in a modern way.

Free play

Children lead their own play, and adults leave them to it. They might make a play scenario with toy cars and pretend they are playing garages.

Adults provide:

- play materials
- play opportunities, both indoors and outdoors.

Children choose what to do and are given plenty of free time to develop their play.

Structured play

Research is showing that there are two kinds of structured play:

Directly structured play

Adults guide and lead the play. The adult might set up a shop and show the children how to play in it, introducing shop vocabulary (words about shopping) and guiding the play story that develops.

Indirectly structured play

The adult structures the environment indoors and outdoors. The materials offered to the children are carefully chosen and organised. Children have plenty of time for play. The adult observes the children as they play, and joins in following the children's play scenario ideas. The adult does not take over but follows the children's ideas.

This is a bit like the way a conversation between people goes along. One person speaks, and the other listens. Then the other person replies.

Indirectly structured play means that adults have to be sensitive to the child's play ideas. The adult is very important because they add ideas to help the child's play develop.

Learning through play – pleasure and pain

There is a popular idea that learning through play means always having fun. Certainly, children will have plenty of fun as they learn through play. However, children also learn about sad and angry feelings. They are challenged to learn about difficult things such as:

* death

* being separated from people they love

* being hurt.

Learning through play is not just about having fun. Play is about learning for life.

How adults can help children play

* Adults need to choose play materials carefully and to create:
  * play opportunities
  * time to play
  * space for play indoors and outdoors
  * places for dens, physical play, manipulative play and creative play
  * play props and clothes for dressing up and role play
  * an adapted play environment for children with disabilities

* Adults who provide open ended materials create more play possibilities for children
  * recycled junk materials (string, boxes, wood)
  * natural materials (clay, woodwork, sand, water, twigs, leaves, feathers)
  * traditional areas (home area, wooden blocks, work shop area with scissors, glue etc)

Tidy up time

The role of the adult is important at tidy up time. This can be enjoyable if adults think of tidying up as part of the child's learning through play. Children love to sweep with dustpans and brooms with shortened handles, which can be made safe for the children to use. They enjoy wiping tables. If boxes have labels, pictures and words, they take pride in putting things away in the right box. If children have choices about taking things off shelves to use play materials, they know where to put them back when they have finished using them. Children will willingly help to water plants.

It is important to encourage both boys and girls to join in with tidying up. Knowing a child's interests helps adults to find something the child will enjoy tidying away. Children are eager to help put away large equipment in an outside shed. They will work as a team if encouraged.

Children with visual impairment

A child with a visual impairment might enjoy creative play with paper and paint. A flat table is better than an easel:

✳ The child will need to be able to reach out in space and easily find the paint pots. A row of paint pots can be placed in a plant window box. This means the paint pots won't fall over or move about. This would be frustrating for the child.

✳ You can encourage the child to experiment with painting. Does the child prefer to paint with the lids on the pots of paint or without the lids? It is important to see what the child finds easiest.

✳ Thick paints full of texture are best.

✳ The child should face the window to get the most light possible on to the table. However, if it is sunny, this might be painful if the sunlight dances about and causes glare. An overhead light might help the child to use any residual sight.

✳ Make sure the child's glasses are clean, or that will also reduce vision.

✳ Let children express their ideas and feelings with the paint in their creative play. They might enjoy talking with you as they do so.

This way of presenting paint for a child with a visual impairment might also be suitable for a child who is only just beginning to learn about paint. It suits several children. This is the advantage of an **inclusive** approach to working with young children.

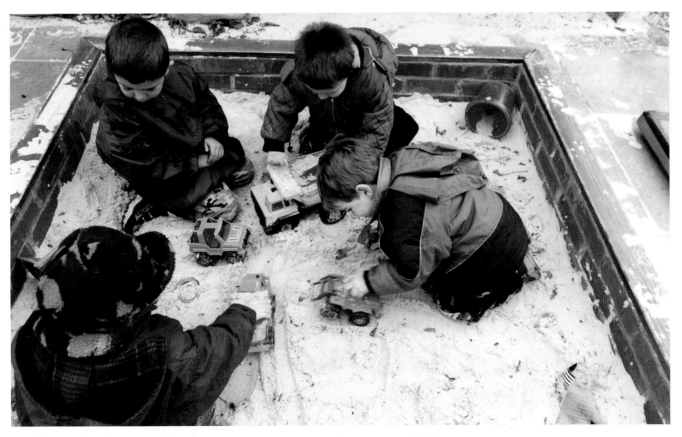

Keeping children safe as they learn through play

Physical safety

Children who play in a physically safe environment are more likely to develop confidence, self esteem and self reliance. They are in a can-do situation.

In modern life it is often dangerous for children to play outside in the street. It is therefore very important that when they attend group settings they can be physically safe.

Children with disabilities may find it more challenging to play, and will need careful help from others.

Safety should always be in mind when working with young children so that accidents are prevented. This is called **risk assessment** because adults are thinking ahead about possible physical danger to children. It is important to check materials such as pens, crayons, and felt pens for the safety mark. Remember, children put objects into their mouths as part of the way they learn.

✓ Worn equipment should be mended or replaced.

✓ Equipment should be checked for splinters, sharp edges or peeling paint.

✓ At the end of each day all aprons should be checked and wiped clean.

✓ Tables need to be disinfected.

✓ Floors need sweeping and washing once the rooms have been tidied.

✓ Carpets need to be cleaned with a vacuum.

Setting up materials and equipment

- Check large apparatus such as climbing frames and trucks for safety catches and safety surfaces. Do the children have enough space to move about safely?

- Heavy objects should not be on shelves in case they fall on children.

- All fire exits must be kept free at all times.

- Doors must not be left half open, especially if there are children with visual impairments as they bump into them.

- Objects on shelves should not stick out at a child's head height in case they bump their heads.

Emotional safety

☐ Children need to feel emotionally safe or they will not be confident enough to play.

☐ They need to play with or near an adult, especially if they are just settling in or they have been upset.

☐ They may need to have a special friend with them in order to feel secure enough to play confidently.

Social safety

When children quarrel they often begin to shout at each other and even fight. Shouting means they are trying to put their feelings into words. Adults can help them by saying something like 'I think you are angry. What shall we do about it? Do you want the bike? When Mary has finished with it she will give you a turn'.

If children become very quiet they might be blocking the drains or something adults don't want them to do. Children need to be supervised carefully. It is important for adults never to sit with their back to the group, either indoors or outdoors.

If children rush about and become over excited, it is sometimes best to join their play and help them to develop a story line. Sometimes they may have lost their play ideas in the excitement.

Violence and play	Dealing with sad and frightening events in play	Promoting anti-discriminatory play
In some settings, both war play and guns are banned. The thinking here is that this discourages children from becoming violent. Some adults think that children need to learn about the terribleness of violence in ways that are emotionally safe. Some adults think that children learn how to stop violence through play about violence.	Children will see things on television and in videos which show wars, starvation etc. They might want to use these ideas in their play scenarios as a way of helping them to understand these events.	Children need to be helped not to develop ideas which are discriminatory or which stereotype people (think of other people in narrow ways).

In some settings, both war play and guns are banned. The thinking here is that this discourages children from becoming violent. Some adults think that children need to learn about the terribleness of violence in ways that are emotionally safe. Some adults think that children learn how to stop violence through play about violence.

In this approach, adults usually allow war play as long as these emotional safety rules are kept.

- Children can only play war with children who have agreed to join this play scenario;
- they cannot pretend to shoot at or pretend to kill children or adults who are not playing this war scenario;
- they must stop if children decide they want to leave the play, or they don't like it;
- adults usually join the play to help children think about pain, hurting people and the sadness of losing people they love, not having food to eat, being tired, being rough.

Children will see things on television and in videos which show wars, starvation etc. They might want to use these ideas in their play scenarios as a way of helping them to understand these events.

Children often think about monster, giants, witches, ghosts, people from outer space. It is best if adults do not introduce these ideas into children's play. Children are usually emotionally safe if they do this for themselves. This is because if they create the monster, then the monster is under *their* control. They can decide how the monster behaves and when to stop the play.

Feeling in control is important for children's emotional safety when they play with danger and fear. This is why hospital play is often important for children before and after a visit.

A new baby in the family also brings fears, such as 'am I still loved?' and play scenarios help children to deal with this fear.

Children need to be helped not to develop ideas which are discriminatory or which stereotype people (think of other people in narrow ways).

- Play scenarios, for example where Eskimos (now called Inuits) are stereotyped as still living in igloos, might lead children to think that is how people live nowadays.
- Children see gender stereotypes on television and in videos. This often leads to superhero play;
  - Boys will be macho-men.
  - Girls will be glamorous sex symbols.

This can be dealt with by helping children to decide as they play, what does Superman eat for breakfast? When does he shop for his food? Who irons his shirts?

Types of play

Physical play

Physical play promotes a child's health. Physical play links with all other areas of a child's development.

The brain works better if children have plenty of fresh air and exercise. This is why both indoor and outdoor play are important.

Through physical play children learn to challenge gender stereotypes.

Boys and girls can enjoy playing ball games e.g. football play scenarios, running and climbing. Children need to be encouraged in these activities. It helps if children wear clothes and shoes which allow freedom of movement.

They also:

- learn through their **senses**
- co-ordinate their **movements**
- develop their **muscles**
- learn about pace and keeping going (**stamina**)
- learn how to use space in a **co-ordinated way**
- learn to challenge **gender stereotypes**

Running in a wide space

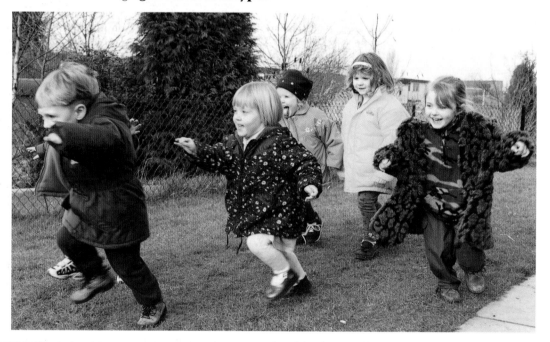

Physical Development
Co-ordinates movements (fine motor and gross motor)
Develops muscles
Develops stamina
Helps children to use space in a co-ordinated way
Learn through the senses
Learn through movement

Language development
There are endless opportunities e.g adults need to give children words they need (vocabulary) e.g fast, slow, up, down, nearly, a good landing.

Relationships (social development)
Children who play physically learn to be sensitive and aware of others, to give them enough space, take turns and share.
They co-operate with each other so that they can all have fun together.
During rough and tumble play, they bond with each other emotionally.
This physical play is usually for short periods and can often end quickly and sometimes in tears!

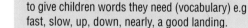

Physical play

Ideas (cognitive development)
e.g children develop understanding of:
- timing
- awareness of space
- reasons why things happen, e.g if I jump from the second step I need to push off harder and to bend my knees when I land. Otherwise I will fall.

Feelings (emotional development)
When a child falls over but gets back on the climbing frame, they are becoming resilient.
When children shout "look at me I am high up", as they climb, it builds their confidence and gives them high self esteem.
Children who have plenty of time for free movement in a safe physical environment, have opportunities to become adventurous.

Co-operative play at the sand tray

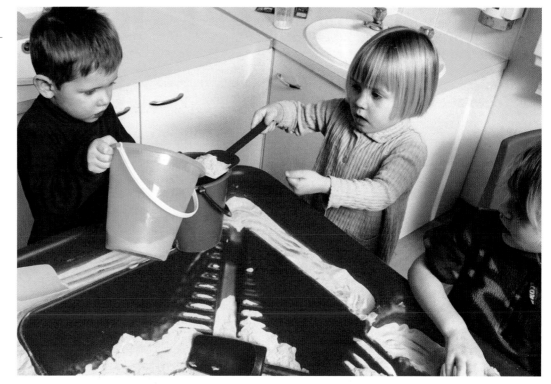

Manipulative play

Children need plenty of opportunities to play using manipulative skills. This particularly encourages children to use their hands, which are very important in human development.

☐ Boys and girls can enjoy manipulative play.

☐ Manipulative play links with the Foundation Stage Curriculum Framework, with the area of learning called physical development.

Relationships (social development)
Children talking about what they are doing with each other and passing each other materials they need – sharing and co-operating.
Children learn to challenge gender stereotypes.

Physical development
Using fingers and thumbs (pincer movements)
Hand/Eye Co-ordination
Develops hand muscles

Manipulative play

Language development
Adults and children talk together as they use materials. Does it fit? Do you have enough? It's too big, will you pass me the scissors please?

Ideas (cognitive development)
Children solve problems as they make models, paint, draw etc. They think ahead, estimate sizes, use shapes, and make choices. They develop ideas of their own.

Feelings (emotional development)
Helps resilience
Builds confidence and high self-esteem
Helps children to persevere (keep going)

Pretend Play

Children make play scenarios, for example about a shop or a boat, a garage, an office, a swimming pool.

The important thing to remember about pretend play is that there will be nothing left to show anyone when the play finishes. Pretend play scenarios do not last. This is why it is difficult to explain to parents the importance of pretend play.

Some adults take video or photographs of children during their play, to try and capture it on film. They want to value pretend play as they do all the other learning that children do.

Bathing dolls in the home corner

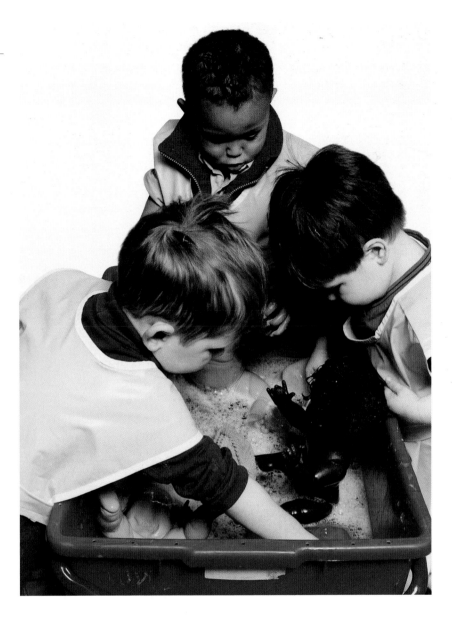

What to look out for in pretend play

☐ They use **play props**; for example, they pretend a box is a fridge, or a stick is a spoon, or a daisy is a fried egg;

☐ they **role play** and pretend that they are someone else, e.g. the shopkeeper;

☐ when they pretend play together, co-operatively, this is called **socio-dramatic play**;

☐ young children pretend play **everyday situations**, getting up, going to sleep, eating (just as the Teletubbies do);

☐ gradually children develop their pretend play scenarios to include situations that are not everyday events and which they may only have heard about but not experienced. This is called **fantasy play**. They might pretend to go to the moon or go on an aeroplane. It is not impossible that these things will happen to them;

☐ **superhero play** develops when they use unreal situations, like Superman or Power Rangers or cartoon characters;

❏ they use **imaginative play** to act out situations that they have definitely experienced, like going to the supermarket.

A group of children made a swimming pool out of wooden blocks. One of them pretended to be the lifeguard and rescued someone drowning. All the children had visited a swimming pool so this pretend play was based on a real experience.

Pretend play links with the Foundation Stage Curriculum Framework and is part of all six areas of learning. Pretend play also links with all areas of a child's development:

- emotional development
- social development
- language development
- cognitive (thinking) development
- physical development.

Creative play

Children must not be expected to 'make something'. Creative play is about experimenting with materials and music. It is not about producing things to go on displays, or to be taken home; for example, when children are involved with messy finger play with paint, nothing is left at the end of the session once it has been cleared away.

Adults can encourage creative play by offering children a **range of materials** and **play opportunities** in dance, music, drawing, collage, paintings, model making and woodwork, sand (small world scenarios), water (small world scenarios) miniature garden scenarios.

Creative play helps children to express their feelings and ideas about people and objects and events. It helps children to:

✱ be physically co-ordinated

✱ develop language

✱ develop ideas (concepts)

✱ develop relationships with people

✱ be more confident and it boosts their self-esteem.

Messy finger play with paint

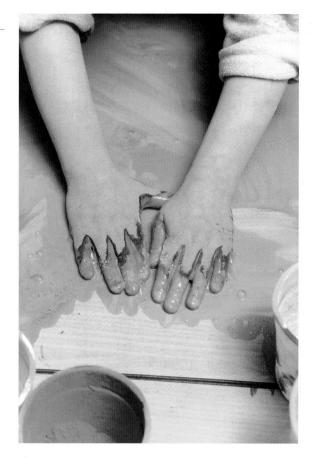

The Foundation Stage Curriculum Framework

During the Foundation Stage, children might be attending a play group, pre-school, nursery school, nursery class, day care setting, reception class, private nursery or be with a childminder or nanny.

The Foundation Stage applies to children from 3 years of age until they enter Year 1, Key Stage 1.

The National Curriculum

When children enter Year 1, Key Stage 1, they begin to follow the National Curriculum until the time they leave school. Children must attend school from the term after they are 5 years old until they are 16 years old.

What is in the Foundation Stage Curriculum Framework?

Well-planned play, both indoors and outdoors, is an important part of the Foundation Stage Curriculum Framework. Well planned play helps children to reach the early learning goals by the time they enter Year 1, Key Stage 1 of the National Curriculum.

There are six areas of learning.

* personal, social and emotional development
* communication, language and literacy
* mathematics

* knowledge and understanding of the world
* physical development
* creative development

Personal, social and emotional development

This encourages play which develops co-operation, playing together, sharing, taking turns, having a go at things.

Communication, language and literacy

This encourages play which develops non-verbal communication (eye contact, body gestures) talking and listening, being listened to, play scenarios with stories, books and rhymes, vocabulary building (learning new words).

Mathematics

This encourages children to play and enjoy numbers, patterns, shapes, space awareness and to solve problems with puzzles etc.

Knowledge and understanding of the world

This encourages play which helps children to learn about different materials through their senses and movements, and to ask questions about how things are made and what they are for. It helps children to explore nature, things from the past, and other cultures.

Physical development

This encourages children to move confidently and safely as they play, to co-ordinate their movements, and to be aware of space and others.

Children should be helped to be healthy with plenty of exercise to help the brain work well, and opportunities to develop fine and gross motor skills.

Creative development

Children should be encouraged to express their ideas and feelings, through creative play in drawings, paintings, models, music, dance and play scenarios.

The **Foundation Stage guidelines** show adults what to look out for in play, and how to promote it through the six areas of learning. It is very important to look at everything in the curriculum document before looking at the early learning goals. Children do not have to achieve these until they leave the Foundation Stage. It is important that they do all the other things which are part of good early years practice. It would be very wrong only to teach children the goals. Children need to learn through a rich play environment and make their own individual learning journeys using the stepping stones which are right for them towards each goal.

Well-planned play

The best planning comes from knowing the children really well. This develops from using the observations adults make of children to plan the next step in their play. For example, Andrew enjoyed playing at making a waterfall in the water tray by pouring water out of a bottle from as high as he could reach up. Other children joined in.

Adults can develop this play by setting up more bottles and having two water trays. Then the activity won't become too crowded. They can set up the paddling pool outside to use as a big water tray, and let children use the hosepipe to fill it. Put guttering in the paddling pool to act as a water chute and jugs to pour water down the chutes. Spare clothes are needed in case children get wet.

It is important to keep floors indoors safe from becoming slippery with too much water. Always keep a mop and bucket near a water activity.

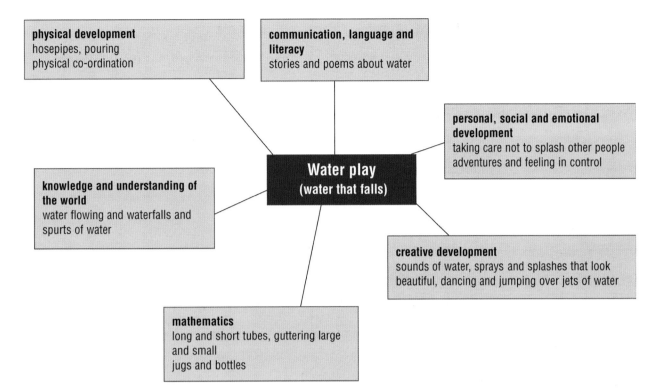

physical development
hosepipes, pouring
physical co-ordination

communication, language and literacy
stories and poems about water

personal, social and emotional development
taking care not to splash other people
adventures and feeling in control

Water play
(water that falls)

knowledge and understanding of the world
water flowing and waterfalls and spurts of water

creative development
sounds of water, sprays and splashes that look beautiful, dancing and jumping over jets of water

mathematics
long and short tubes, guttering large and small
jugs and bottles

Choosing materials and equipment to give children play opportunities

Children learn about play from natural and recycled materials as well as specially designed toys and equipment. They need a balance, for example wooden hollow blocks and cardboard boxes.

Child playing in a cardboard box

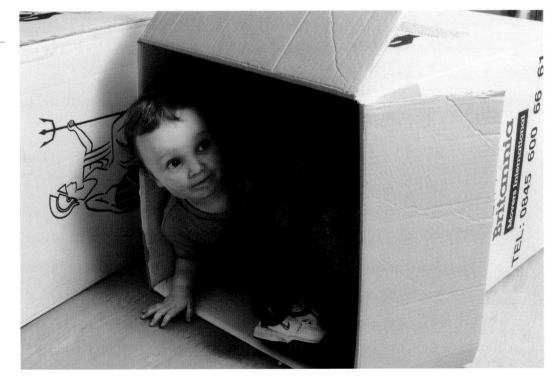

Natural materials

These should be attractively presented. They are important for children living in a modern world. Plastic is everywhere. Natural materials help children to learn about sand, water, wood and clay. These show children how they can find materials for themselves. They are cheap to provide.

Recycled materials

These cost nothing to provide. Margarine tubs, bottle corks and plastic bottles, for example, need to be set out in attractive containers, easy to reach and use. Children need enough space and table room for creative play with these materials.

Commercially made equipment

These can be expensive. They need to be carefully chosen. Look at Unit 1 which emphasises safety of equipment, non-toxic materials and cleanliness. They are often pre-structured which means that children can only use them in a narrow way. Open-ended equipment which can be used in a variety of ways is better value for money e.g. wooden blocks, Lego™, Duplo™.

Children gain if there are plenty of these so that they can build exciting models. It is best to have all the same brand of wooden blocks, or Lego™ or Duplo™, then these can be added to over the years.

✻ Check equipment for safety marks

✻ Can it be cleaned easily?

✻ Can it be mended easily or are there replacement parts?

✻ Is it open-ended so that it can be used in many different ways e.g. dolls house, farm, home area equipment, wooden blocks.

The indoor and outdoor areas

It is best not to change the room around too often because children take some time to find out where things are, both indoors and outdoors. Adults need to know about the **child's development in play** so that they, in their curriculum, can provide what is needed for play in their **curriculum plan**. Important points to consider when providing for children's play are:

- Things should be **set out so that they are interesting**, with enough variety to **keep stimulating the play**.

- The **layout of the room** should take account of different children's cultural experiences and heritage.

- There should be specially adapted equipment for **children with disabilities**.

- Adults should think carefully about what materials to set out, and **how to present them in order to encourage play**.

Planning the indoor and outdoor area

The materials that adults set up **indoors** should (whenever possible) be available **outdoors** in any group setting (see the Foundation Stage Guidance document). Examples include:

Indoors	**Outdoors**
❏ Sand tray	❏ Covered sand pit
❏ Water tray	❏ Watering cans to water plants and buckets of water

This means that children can learn as much outdoors as they do indoors. See also layout plans on page 145.

Climbing frames. These need to be carefully designed to offer children plenty of challenges as safely as possible. One side of the frame might have evenly spaced rungs for children who are less experienced in climbing. The other side might have unevenly spaced rungs, which need more thinking by the child.

Tarmac. An outdoor area needs some tarmac or tiled area so that in wet weather it is possible to run or walk about without muddy feet tramping back indoors.

Wild area. Many gardens now have an old wild area, which has plants that encourage butterflies, moths and birds. A bird table is also a source of great interest.

Grass. Outdoor areas also need grass where children can find worms, make daisy chains and blow dandelion clocks. A grassy slope can also provide rough and tumble play and roly-poly possibilities on a fine day.

Paddling pools. These are suitable for fine days. When providing a pool, remember:

- the pool must be constantly supervised; there should always be towels near it so that children do not become cold;
- to protect children's skin from **sunburn** – follow your setting's policy;
- that there are **cultural sensitivities** with regard to children taking off their clothes when using a pool. This needs to be carefully discussed between staff and parents before introducing children to a paddling pool;
- some children do not like to be splashed and this needs to be respected; perhaps there can be 10 minutes at the end of a session for **'splashy times'** so that children who enjoy this can stay on in the pool and other children can get out if they want to. In this way children learn to respect each other's feelings.

Digging patches. Some outdoor areas provide digging patches and a vegetable planting area. Younger children tend to dig, carry earth about, find worms and tip water into holes. (Often 2- to 3-year-olds.) Older children (often aged 3–5 years) begin to understand the process of digging, planting, watering and growing. This shows in their play; they want to play farmers or gardeners, and a sandpit is often where they will choose to do this.

Bikes, carts and other wheeled equipment. Bikes are often the source of conflict among children. Some children *always* want to ride them. For this reason many settings now provide carts and different types of bikes and trikes, which two or three children can ride on and on which they can pull each other around. These are very useful in encouraging children to help each other so that they become a team. Adults often make special zones in the outdoor area where children can use bikes without knocking other people over.

Providing well-planned play for the Foundation Stage

The following pages look more closely at seven different types of **play provision** and at the way they link to the six areas of the Foundation Stage Curriculum. These areas are:

- **Wooden block play**
- **Sand and water play**
- **Home area**
- **Dressing up clothes**
- **Small world play**
- **Clay, dough and mud patches**
- **Painting and drawing.**

Wooden block play

Personal, emotional & social development

- Interested, excited, motivated to learn
- Try out new ideas & activities
- Select blocks they want to use without help and feel valued
- Sensitive to others; share and take turns
- Make good relationships with other children and adults

Communication, language & literacy

- Talk as they build
- Listen to each other
- Make up play scenarios with stories
- Make comments and ask questions
- Increase vocabulary about blocks (It's taller, could you pass me the cylinder, please?)

Mathematics

- Use number ideas
- Use maths language: talk about shapes & sizes of blocks
- Solve practical problems – Is this too tall?
- Space awareness about blocks

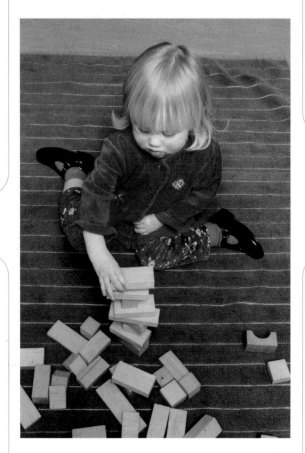

Knowledge & understanding of the world

- Find out about materials – wooden blocks, foam blocks
- Ask questions about how to do things with blocks
- Think about how wooden blocks are made from trees
- Building and constructung with blocks

Physical development

- Use blocks with confidence and safety
- Use a range of wooden blocks, hollow and unit blocks to develop fine and gross motor skills
- Balance blocks with increasing control
- Aware of space and of others using the block play area

Creative development

- Explore shape, form, texture and space of wooden blocks
- Use senses and movement to explore blocks
- Use imagination to make play scenarios
- Design and make constructions (children use their own ideas)

Indoors

Wooden blocks are best if they are free standing. They never wear out and can easily be reconditioned (sanded). There are three kinds of blocks:

☐ Unit blocks

☐ Mini hollow bricks

☐ Large hollow bricks.

All of these link with each other. To use wooden blocks, children need:

✓ Enough space to build

✓ To play with the blocks away from 'traffic' of people walking through the area

✓ To have the blocks set out on shelves with outlines of shapes showing each type of block, so that children know where different types of blocks should be stored – children need to see them and to choose which they will use

✓ A complete set of blocks (and not to lose any!); they should be easily tidied away

✓ To have blocks available each day

Outdoors

Blocks could also be milk crates or wooden boxes, which can be stored outside along the wall and used each day. Children make stepping-stones and build with them.

Safety

Children must not build too high unless supervised (except when using soft foam blocks), in case blocks fall on them.

Look at the section on general safety on pages 27–32 to see whether you have missed things you need to remember when you are working with wooden blocks with the children.

Progression in block play

- **At 1 to 2 years:** children mainly build towers and put blocks in rows.

- **At 2 to 3 years:** children make enclosures, towers get taller and they put blocks in rows. Balance is important now. They sometimes call their models something, e.g. a house.

- **At 3 to 5 years:** children begin to put together a variety of patterns. They begin to create play scenarios with more complicated stories. They make many patterns and quite difficult balancing is achieved. They are interested in how to balance and build blocks.

- **At 5 to 7 years:** the stories and buildings become very complex and are highly co-ordinated.

Construction

Construction is similar to block play except that all the pieces connect with each other, whereas blocks balance. Ideally, a variety of construction sets should be available – e.g. Lego™, Duplo™, Stickle Bricks™, Construct-O-Straws™, etc. However it is important that whatever sets you have should contain enough pieces to interest a group of children. Younger children find Duplo™ easier than Lego™ because the pieces are larger and easier to hold as they develop muscle control in their hands. By then they have developed their pincer movement and enjoy practising using it.

Sand and water play

Personal, emotional & social development

- Interested, excited, motivated to learn
- Confidently play, try out new ideas
- Concentrate, aware of what they need
- Take turns & share
- Choose sand & water on their own – no help
- Make good relationships with other children and adults

Communication, language & literacy

- Enjoy listening to others
- Use action words – filling, pouring, spilling etc
- Talk to others as they play
- Explore sounds of water – splash, drip etc
- Learn words about sand & water – dry, wet, cold, warm etc

Mathematics

- Use maths language: capacity – e.g. how many cups to fill this jug?
- Solve practical problems, e.g. pouring water through a funnel
- Make patterns and shapes in the sand

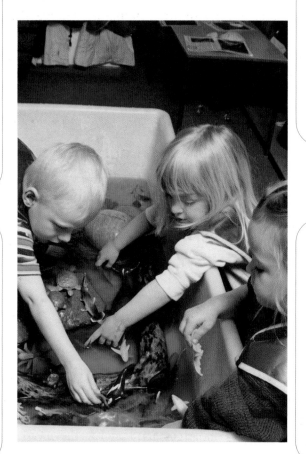

Knowledge & understanding of the world

- Use the senses to investigate – differences between wet & dry sand
- Ask questions about what is happening
- Choose tools – watering can for plants, spade for digging
- Find out about the environment – water pipes for sinks, sand found on beaches

Physical development

- Use sand & water with confidence, safely
- Move with control & co-ordination, aware of space, how many can use area easily
- Use large sandpits & paddling pools, supervised
- Swimming (gross motor skills)
- Small trays with sand (fine motor skills)

Creative development

- Ask questions – how does water fill a space?
- Pour water and dry sand, using senses to feel the texture of sand & water
- See, smell, listen to sounds of water
- Make play scenarios, express ideas, feelings & thoughts

Sand and water play

Indoors

Sand can be offered in a commercial sand tray, in seed boxes from a garden shop or in washing up bowls on tables. It can be poured on to a plastic mat and used as a 'beach' experience with shells, buckets, spades and pebbles. The mat can be rolled up at the end of the session and the sand poured into a sand tray to use again.

* There should always be both wet and dry sand on offer, e.g. dry sand in bowls on tables, or wet sand in a sand tray.

* Provide jugs, scoops, funnels, sponges, small world scenarios, farms, tubes, spades, small buckets and rakes.

* Miniature gardens can be made adding twigs, moss, and leaves.

Outdoors

Sand and water play outside is similar to indoors. However, the following equipment can also be used outdoors:

* Hoses

* Watering cans

* Water washable paint for use on the tarmac (using buckets of water and giant brushes)

* Large, covered sand pit where several children can play.

Safety

Make sure that sand and water play is carefully supervised:

* Be alert as children can drown in very shallow water, get sand in their eyes or slip on wet floors

* Outdoor sand pits need covers to keep animals and insects out

* Place the indoor water tray near to the sink (because it's heavy and in case people slip)

* Change the water every day

* Always sweep the floor after sand play

* Use a mop to ensure floors are not slippery after water play.

Progression in sand and water play

* **At 1 to 2 years:** children begin by pouring and carrying water and sand and by putting these materials in and out of containers.

* **At 3 to 5 years:** children begin to enjoy practical problems, and to solve them as they develop their learning, e.g. how to make a strong jet of water, how to make sand keep its shape.

* **At 5 to 7 years:** children's play scenarios have more of a story than before. They use a variety of play people and co-operate more with other children.

Home area

Personal, emotional & social development

- Interested, excited, motivated to learn
- Cofidently play, try out new ideas
- Concentrate, have play scenarios of their own
- Take turns & sharing
- Aware of which cups and pots to use for cooking
- Make good relationships with others

Communication, language & literacy

- Enjoy talking and listening to other children as they play
- Enjoy making stories and acting out ones they know
- Think about ideas, feelings, events
- Learn new words about the home area, e.g. saucepan, cooker, wok

Mathematics

- Use numbers ideas, e.g. No. 5 on the gas cooker, four places at the table, three beds
- Use shapes: a plate is a circle

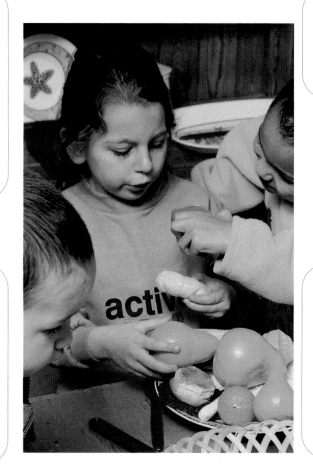

Knowledge & understanding of the world

- Find out about materials – e.g. how plastic snaps or bends, metal gets hot and cold
- Ask questions about what is happening
- Choose utensils – pan for frying, pram for pushing etc

Physical development

- Use equipment with more co-ordination and control
- Stir the pot, turn the knobs, lift the dishes – manipulative skills
- Use a range of materials – cutlery, crockery, bedclothes, dressing & undressing dolls

Creative development

- Express and communicate ideas, thoughts and feelings
- Use a range of objects in the home area – e.g. putting dolls to bed, preparing food
- Role play with families

Indoors

The home area is one of the most important areas in early childhood settings. The home area should ideally have:

- ☐ Some things in it that are like those in the child's home, e.g. cups, cooking pots
- ☐ Some things that are from other cultures, e.g. a wok, chopsticks
- ☐ A proper place for everything, and children should be encouraged to tidy up carefully
- ☐ A large dresser – with hooks for cups and cupboards to store dishes and saucepans
- ☐ Big, middle-sized and small dolls, representing children of different cultures
- ☐ A cooker (this can be homemade – e.g. from a cardboard box)
- ☐ Wooden boxes, which can be used as beds, tables, chairs
- ☐ Food can be pre-structured (plastic fruit), transformable (dough), real food (a salad) or pretend food
- ☐ Clothes can be kept in a chest of drawers, labelled with pictures and words
- ☐ Magazines, notepads and writing implements which can be put by the telephone, and perhaps a bookcase with books
- ☐ Adaptations for children with disabilities – e.g. a child who is a wheelchair user will need a low table so that they can use the bowls and plates, etc.

Outdoors

The home area outside is a **den**. Children at home enjoy playing in outside dens.

- Old furniture can be used outside to make a home area. An old airer (clothes horse) with a sheet or blanket over it makes good walls.
- Children can make pretend food using sand, water and messy materials.
- A rug can be put in the den and furniture can be made by collecting spare cardboard boxes; e.g. they can become tables or beds for dolls.
- Cushions can make seats or beds.
- A box on its side can become a cupboard with flaps as the cupboard doors.
- Cups and saucers can be made out of old yoghurt pots and margarine containers.

Safety

- ☐ Wooden equipment should be checked regularly for rough edges and splinters.
- ☐ Cutlery must be carefully introduced. Ask your supervisor for advice.
- ☐ Glass and china break easily and should not be used in the home area.

Progression in home area play

- ☐ **At 1 to 2 years:** children carry materials – pots, pans, dolls etc. – about; put them in and out of boxes, prams; puts them in rows.
- ☐ **At 2 to 3 years:** they begin to make play scenarios, often about food.
- ☐ **At 3 to 5 years:** more of the story develops about a wider range of events and people.

Dressing up clothes

Personal, emotional & social development

- Dress and undress
- Choose clothes to wear
- Show a range of feelings
- Make a good relationship with other children and adults
- Respect their own and other cultures

Communication, language & literacy

- Enjoy listening to and telling stories in role play
- Talk to others as they play
- Make up play stories and act out some already known
- Take turns and share with others

Mathematics

- Use number ideas – four buttons, two shoes, one hat

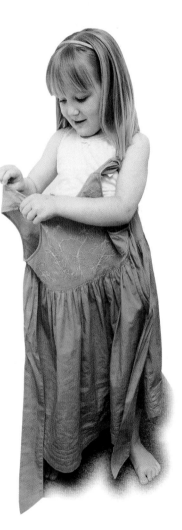

Knowledge & understanding of the world

- Choose clothes suitable for their role play

Physical development

- Use different fastenings on clothes – zips, buttons, velcro etc – development of manipulative skills
- Move with confidence and control

Creative development

- Choose colours and textures – wool, nylon, glitter
- Make play scenarios, express ideas, feelings, relationships and thoughts through role play

Dressing up clothes

Indoors and outdoors

Children wear dressing up clothes indoors, but enjoy wearing them outdoors too.

- The clothes need to be simple and flexible in use.
- A basic cape, some basic hats – including 'uniform' hats such as a fire-fighter's helmet, scarves and drapes, sari, tunic, shoes and baggy trousers help children in role playing. They need to reflect different cultures.
- Fastenings should be varied to give children different experiences of connecting clothes together, e.g. zips, buttons, tying bows, buckles and Velcro.
- The clothes need to be hanging on a rack, with separate boxes for shoes and hats. A large safety mirror at child height is useful.

Safety

- There should be no strings, ribbons or purses on strings around the neck, which might strangle a child.
- Beware of children tripping over clothes that are too long.
- Make sure children wear suitable footwear – e.g. no high heels when playing on climbing frames or running out of doors.
- Clothes should be washed regularly.

Progression in dressing up clothes play

- **At 1 to 2 years:** children wear hats and shoes.
- **At 2 to 3 years:** children wear hats, shoes, capes and scarves.
- **At 3 to 5 years:** children are more adventurous – they begin to wear whole outfits and want more accuracy to look right for the role they play.

🧸 Small world play

Personal, emotional & social development

- Interested, excited, motivated to learn
- Concentrate & try out new ideas
- Know which equipment they might need to use
- Take turns, share & play with others
- Show a range of feelings as they create their play scenarios
- Show they understand how other people feel through the people in their play stories

Mathematics

- Show an interest in shape & space by making arrangements with objects (e.g. a square field to make a farm)
- Use size language such as "big" and "little"
- Use words about position in space ('the cow is next to the sheep')
- Solve practical problems (e.g. the house falls over so prop it up against a wall)

Communication, language & literacy

- Enjoy listening to and talking with their friends as they play
- Make up their own stories and re-tell some they know as they play with small world materials
- Extend vocabulary, especially by grouping and naming

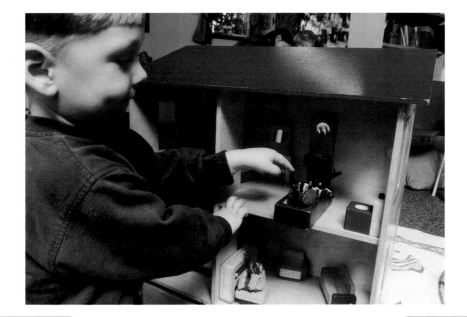

Knowledge & understanding of the world

- Observe, find out about and identify features in the place they live and the natural world
- Find out about small world materials & see how things work and can be changed
- Show curiosity, observe and manipulate objects

Creative development

- Make play scenarios, express ideas, feelings & thoughts
- Engage in imaginative and role play based on own first-hand experiences
- Play alongside other children who are engaged in the same theme
- Think about the countryside (farm) and wildlife (elephants, zebras etc)

Physical development

- Manipulate materials and objects by picking up, releasing, arranging, threading and posting them
- Use small world materials in a co-ordinated way with fine motor skills and a range of play scenarios

Garages, farms, zoos, space scenes, domestic, hospitals, boats and castles all feature in small world play.

Indoors

Children can easily create play scenarios with pretend people and make up imaginative stories using small world materials to help them. These are best set out on a floormat or carpet, or in a sand tray (see sand and water play).

�֍ Miniature gardens make a good play scene; these can be made in seed trays from garden centres and put on tables.

✖ Children can make their own gardens and make up stories using them – pots of moss, gravel, twigs, pebbles and feathers.

✖ They can also make paths, trees, grass and hills.

✖ Older children begin to use dolls houses, garages and castles.

Outdoors

Small world materials are easily lost outside.

Safety

Check that the pieces are not so small that a younger child might choke.

Progression in play

● **At 1 to 2 years:** children mainly put toys in rows and make constructions.

● **At 2 to 4 years:** they make more complex constructions, e.g. a house; simple everyday stories.

● **At 4 to 6 years:** children use play scenarios, e.g. going shopping, and having a story with different people, e.g. hospital scenes, outer space, garage scenes.

Clay, dough and mud patches

Personal, emotional & social development

- Interested, excited, motivated to learn
- Confidently try out new ideas with clay
- Concentrate, aware of what they need – e.g. rolling pins or hands
- Think of others by taking turns & sharing
- Make good relationships with other children and adults
- Understand other people will respect them

Communication, language & literacy

- Enjoy listening & talking to each other
- Learn new words – soft, hard, rolling pin
- Make play scenarios with stories
- Make comments and ask questions

Mathematics

- Use number ideas – 'I am making six cakes' or 'I have got more than you'
- Concepts of size and weight
- Make patterns and shapes

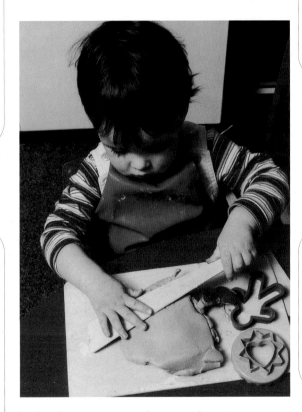

Knowledge & understanding of the world

- Use the senses to find out about dough, clay and plasticine
- Look at the differences between materials
- Ask questions and make models
- Choose tools – rollers, containers
- Find out about the environment

Physical development

- Use the clay with co-ordination
- Use the tools with confidence
- Develop manipulative skills – punching, pinching, pulling, rolling, squashing etc

Creative development

- Explore (through the senses) texture, shape and form of clay and dough
- Make designs – which do not have to be a product to keep or to display

Indoors

Types of clay and dough	
Clay, dough and plasticine are best used on a table. Plasticine can be tough when it is cold	Provide rolling pins, spatulas, smooth sticks for making patterns on the surface
Clay can be very messy when too much water is added. Some children dislike the feel of the clay on their hands, so be prepared to wash their hands when needed	Children need aprons or old clothes
Adults can show children how to pinch the clay to make it flat, or roll into coils	A shelf nearby can display children's models/work
Self-hardening clay: can be used instead of traditional clay. This is supplied in moist form and is stored in its own plastic bucket. When dry (1–3 days) models can be painted with acrylic paints	
Play dough: use different recipes and make it with the children so that they see how it is made. Children love to have plain dough that is not coloured (pastry) to play with in the home area	

Children often do not make anything in particular because this is **creative play**. There is no need to have any sort of result or finished product. It is important not to force children into this.

Storing clay

Clay can be brown or grey. It is stored by rolling it into a ball, the size of a large orange, pressing a thumb into it, pouring water into the hole, and covering the hole full of water with clay. It should then be stored in a bin with a well-fitting lid.

Outdoors

A mud patch for digging is a popular area outdoors. Spades and rakes with short handles are useful. Children love to bury things and fill holes with water. They enjoy planting flowers and vegetables.

Safety

☐ Dough must be made using salt and cream of tartar if it is to be stored and used more than once.

☐ Deter children from putting the dough in their mouths. Be extra vigilant with children who have coeliac disease as they must not consume any gluten (present in ordinary flour).

Progression in play

- **At 1 to 3 years:** children bash and bang clay.

- **At 3 to 5 years:** they learn to pinch, pull and roll it as well:
  > They can make shapes
  > They choose their tools or use their hands more carefully
  > They begin to design and make models, which they sometimes like to keep and display, but not often.

Painting and drawing

Personal, emotional & social development

- Interested, excited, motivated to learn
- Find out how to use different pens, chalks, crayons – with new ideas as they do so
- Concentrate, knowing which colours or materials they need
- Take turns & share; respect what other children draw or paint
- Choose what to draw, when to draw and how to draw

Communication, language & literacy

- Enjoy talking about their drawings and paintings
- Organise materials & ideas, feelings & events
- Learn new words about drawing & painting
- Show interest in having their name written on their drawings – may have a go at doing this themselves – or ask an adult to do this for them
- Hold a pencil, however they like and how it feels comfortable
- By Key Stage I learn to hold pencil correctly

Mathematics

- Use number ideas in their drawings – i.e. two legs, two eyes, three bears, four sides on the house
- Make patterns and learn new words to define them – e.g. round, square, zig-zag etc

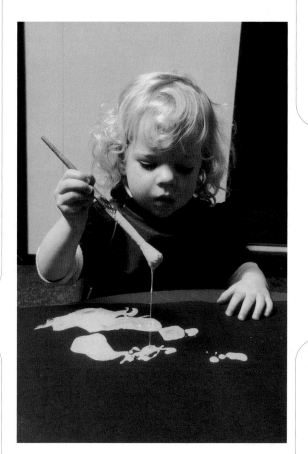

Knowledge & understanding of the world

- Investigate paint & different drawing pencils, chalks, felt pens, crayons
- Observe living things, objects and events they decide they will draw
- Decide which tools to paint or draw with
- Know about their own culture and draw their experiences

Physical development

- Use crayons, paints etc. confidently and safely
- Aware of the space they need when drawing – e.g. not jogging each other
- Use a wide range of drawing tools and a wide choice of paints (different colours and thicknesses)
- Handle pencils & paint brushes with increasing control

Creative development

- Explore colour, texture, shape, form and space in paintings & drawings
- Respond to how paint feels – (e.g. finger painting) or chalks
- Use their imagination as they make patterns, pictures and scribbles of their choice

Indoors

For **drawing:** children need a variety of materials to draw with (fat and thin felt pens, chubby crayons, pastels, chalks, charcoal and pencils).

☐ Different size, texture, shape and colour of paper; paper should be attractively set out and stored on shelves or in boxes or trays

For **painting**, provide a variety of paints – freshly mixed every day – and brushes, clean water, non-spillable paint containers, and pots to mix colours.

☐ Children need a range of paint brushes (thick, middle and thin) ideally made from good quality hog's hair. Poor quality brushes lead to poor quality paintings and are frustrating to use

☐ Flat tables are easier for younger children to use than easels

☐ Children should choose which paper and tools to use

☐ A well-designed paint dryer which stacks paintings while allowing them to dry is ideal, but you can spread paintings out on the floor under a radiator – or hang with pegs to dry from a washing line

☐ **Mixing colours:** It is best only to provide primary colours (red, blue and yellow paints) and to make shades by adding white or black to lighten or darken the colours
> Red + blue = purple
> Red + yellow = orange
> Blue + yellow = green
> Red + white = pink
> All colours mixed together = brown

☐ Children can mix their own colours if these are presented in large tins in the middle of the table, with a spoon in each tin. Patty pan pallets can be used for mixing, and water can be scooped with a small ladle from a large bowl in the centre into small, easily manageable jugs. In this way, children can pour small amounts and learn to mix the colours and shades of paint they need with a paint brush

☐ Children need encouragement to wear aprons. Those they step into using their arms first are the most popular, as aprons over the head can be frightening for very young children

☐ If children want to keep their paintings or drawings they need to be kept in a safe place. They might like to see them displayed on the wall. They must have the right to say if they do not want this

☐ Painting is a messy activity, which is probably why it is not always done in the home. Protect the floor, easels and tables with newspaper

☐ Young children should always be given the opportunity to express themselves through painting, undisturbed by adults. Adults should never interrupt, ask questions about the child's painting or make their own suggestions; these actions will discourage creativity and may stop the children from valuing their own work

☐ Many children are not interested in the product of their paintings. At this stage they are interested in the process

Safety

- Children should be discouraged from walking around with pencils or brushes in their mouths – in case they fall and injure themselves or someone else.

- Mop up any major water spills quickly to avoid floors becoming slippery.

Recycled materials

Indoors

✱ Children used recycled materials such as cardboard boxes, scraps of material, string, buttons to make models and collages, pipe cleaners.

✱ Children often make small world props to put in miniature gardens etc if they are encouraged.

Safety

✱ Use of scissors must be supervised.

✱ Glue and felt pens must be non toxic.

✱ Children can be taught how to use a sellotape dispenser but ask your supervisor if it is appropriate in your setting.

Planning the layout of materials and equipment both indoors and outdoors

Children 1–2 years

Children need both outdoor and indoor play from an early age. Many of the materials can be set out both indoors and outdoors.

✱ Children need personal spaces e.g. toddlers can sit on a mat with objects with heuristic play (play with objects made up of everyday bits and bobs e.g. paper plate, bath sponge, nail brush, spoon). Check these for safety.

✱ They need toys which are good to hold, shake and bang.

✱ They need interesting sounds (sturdy musical instruments).

✱ They need books which can be chewed and sucked.

✱ They need comfortable flooring to crawl over which is a mixture of carpets and other surfaces.

✱ They need outdoors exploring grass to fall on and fall over on for beginning walkers.

✱ They need stable furniture to pull themselves up and cruise between.

✱ They need push and pull toys.

✱ They need messy play with paints, water, sand, dough.

✱ They need wooden building blocks.

✱ They need large foam building blocks.

See diagrams (p. 147) of the layout plans for the indoor and outdoor areas for two early years settings. These are used for children 2–5 years of age.

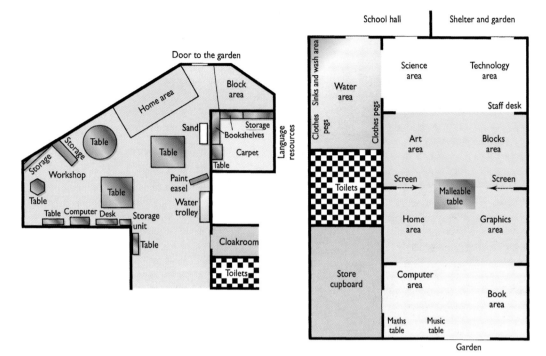

a) James Lee Nursery School

b) Eastwood Nursery School

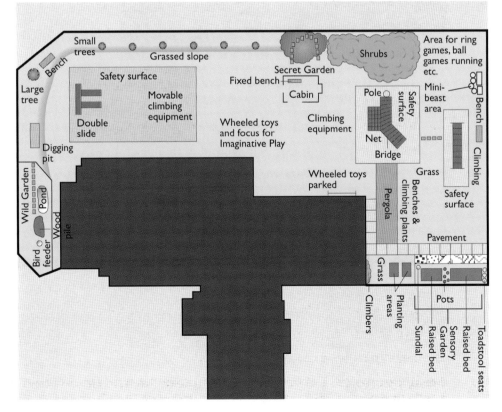

c) the garden at Eastwood

Heuristic play with natural objects

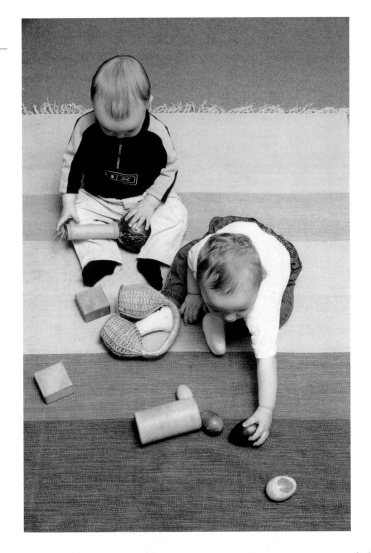

Most 2 year olds will enjoy being in these areas most of the time. However, they will need specially alert adults to support their play so that they feel secure and have a sense of well-being and remain confident. It is important to have a range of provisions. In this way the adult can find something to suit younger, or less experienced children, or can help a child with a disability to use the areas.

This is called an **inclusive** approach. It means the general play environment is planned to be suitable for a variety of play needs, ages and stages, as well as children with disabilities.

For example:

- at to 2 to 3 years wheeled trucks to sit in and be pulled along and wheeled trucks to sit on and scoot with feet on the ground;
- at 3 to 5 years tricycles with pedals;
- a few children may manage to use two wheeled bicycles;
- a child who is a wheelchair user can join in wheeled play in the zone where children have space to go fast and feel freedom of movement together;
- it is important to think about progression in play, so that you challenge children to learn through their play;

Shop play scenario

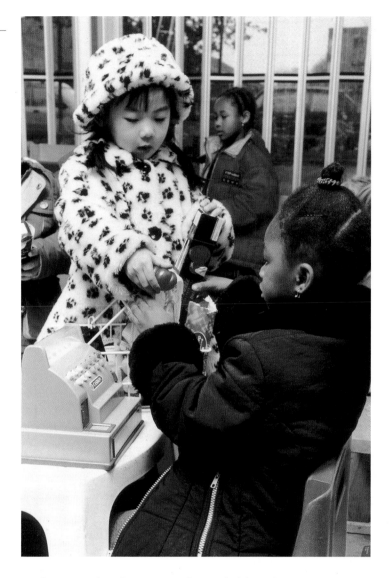

- there need to be zones where children have enough space to use wheeled toys safely;

- other areas need to be available where children can play without these so that they don't have to worry about being knocked over. This means dividing the outdoor area into wheeled truck zones and other areas where children are not allowed to take wheeled trucks or bikes;

- children aged 2 to 3 years are easily frustrated;

- they concentrate well if they are allowed to make choices and decide what they do. Otherwise, their concentration will only last for a few minutes;

- they will not share easily with other children, so there need to be enough boxes, hats, toy cars, teaset pieces, wooden blocks etc. or there will be fights;

- children from 3 to 5 years will use the area without so much adult support. Even so, adults will need to make sure that children feel confident as they move about indoors and outdoors.

Progression in the way children use indoor and outdoor areas

☐ 2 to 3 year olds need to stay near their special adults. Some early years settings make sure that each child has an adult who especially stays alert to their needs.

☐ Children 3 to 5 years are beginning to have friends who they enjoy playing with. If their special friend is away, they may not be so confident about playing as they are when their friend is there.

In most of Europe children's play is supported, encouraged and extended with the help of adults throughout the first eight years of life. This is because play is an important and central way in which children learn.

From 0 to 2 years the foundations of imaginative play are being laid.

From 2 to 4 years imaginative play develops. Children in most parts of the world use the theme of food preparation in their play. They begin to pretend to be other people (role play) and they make up stories which they act out. Their play stories are often about everyday living, although monsters do appear quite often. Their play has simple themes, and children find it hard to play these out in large groups. They find it easier in pairs, or when playing alone with small world (for instance, dolls-house, farm, garage, or zoo).

From 5 to 8 years play will blossom if it is encouraged to do so. The characters children pretend to be go beyond everyday life, and are often from story books or TV programmes. So are the storylines (narratives) the children develop. They begin to be able to play out their themes in a larger group (often 3 or 4 children) with lots of chasing about, leading and following each other about. Play shows increasingly elaborate themes which are about very important areas, such as evil.

They love to play goodies and baddies, kind or cruel people, and monsters which invade, or ghosts which haunt. This is because by this stage of development in their play, they can begin to move from the here and now (the present time) and go beyond to thinking about time in the past or future.

'Here and now' play themes cover settings from hospitals, clinics, libraries, outings on boats, to parks, stories in books, shopping, and markets.

Beyond the here and now in time and space, themes include 'old-fashioned days' such as King Arthur, Captain Hook, Princesses and Princes, exploring outer space or rain forests, or deserts, ship wrecks on islands, and so on.

Physical play also develops so that children become more co-ordinated and can play on two wheeler bikes, roller blades, or with skipping ropes. Because they have more control of their bodies, they can play on more elaborate bits of equipment. This is why they introduce writing and cards into their play; for example in offices, shops or hairdresser salons. Children at this age need to feel in control of the equipment they use when they play.

Time to go home

Look around the room.

● Is it clean and tidy?

● Is it attractively set out for tomorrow?

● Can children reach materials? (check this by going around on your knees, to see if you can reach things at a child's height)

● Is it a safe environment?

- Are all the basic materials ready for children to use?
- Do you know what you need to do when you arrive the next morning?
- What do you need to remember to bring tomorrow?
- What did the children teach you today about what they need in their play?

Different play activities for children

2

- cooking activities
- playing different types of games with young children
- creative play with natural and other materials
- pretend play
- physical play

Cooking activities

Almost all children have some experience of cooking, or at the very least, food preparation, in their own homes. This experience can range from watching tins being opened and the contents heated, seeing fruit being peeled and cut, or bread being put in a toaster and then spread, to a full-scale three- (or more) course meal being cooked. All cultures have their own food traditions and cooking activities with young children provide an ideal opportunity to introduce and celebrate their diversity and richness.

Mealtimes are, for most of us, social occasions which involve sharing, turn-taking and an understanding of acceptable behaviour – manners! Apart from allowing children to develop these social skills, cooking activities are valuable in promoting scientific understanding in terms of materials and their properties and processes of change – both physical and chemical. Physical changes are those which can be reversed e.g. water, when frozen, becomes ice but, when allowed to thaw, returns to its original state – water. Chemical changes are those which have brought about a change in the substance which cannot be reversed e.g. a piece of bread once toasted will not return to its original state when left to cool or cheese which has been heated and become melted will not return to its original form or texture even if it retains its essential flavour. Most importantly children are learning these fascinating facts in the context of an everyday activity.

Safety and hygiene are paramount considerations when planning and implementing such activities. As you will have read in **Unit 1** some people have **food allergies** which must be taken into account when planning what foodstuffs will be used. Less obvious may be **skin conditions** (e.g. **eczema**) which may be painful particularly if in contact with fruit juices or, sometimes, soaps and washing-up liquids. Some thought at the planning stage should enable you to check with parents and take the necessary steps (e.g. thin disposable gloves) to involve all the children.

A cooking activity

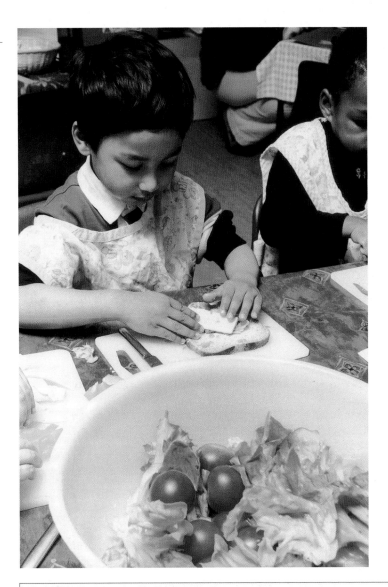

Guidelines for cooking with children

✓ Always prepare surfaces with anti-bacterial spray and clean cloths

✓ Always ensure children have washed their hands and scrubbed their fingernails

✓ Always provide protective clothing and, if necessary, roll up long sleeves

✓ Always tie back long hair

✓ Always check equipment for damage

✓ Always follow safety procedures and policies of the work setting

✓ Always ensure adequate supervision

✓ Always remind children not to cough over food or put their fingers or utensils in their mouths when handling food

✓ Always check sell-by dates of food items and store them correctly

✓ Always check for 'E' numbers and artificial ingredients in bought food items

As you make these preparations for the activity you can use them to develop children's understanding and awareness of hygiene. Whenever possible you should provide a set of equipment, appropriately sized, for each child and ensure that the finished product is given to the child who made it.

Strangely enough cooking activities do not always need to involve using a cooker or even a microwave oven! The diagram below shows a wide range of processes which offer opportunities to use food with children. For some you need only the food and basic utensils (e.g. for spreading, decorating biscuits, preparing fruit salad etc.) and for others the use of a kettle or access to hot water may be sufficient. Use of a refrigerator will be needed for others.

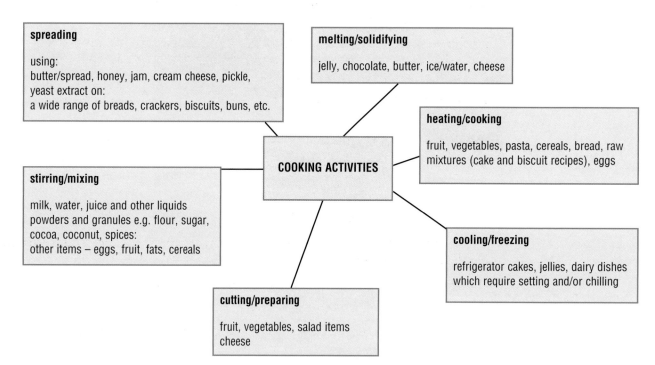

spreading

using:
butter/spread, honey, jam, cream cheese, pickle, yeast extract on:
a wide range of breads, crackers, biscuits, buns, etc.

melting/solidifying

jelly, chocolate, butter, ice/water, cheese

heating/cooking

fruit, vegetables, pasta, cereals, bread, raw mixtures (cake and biscuit recipes), eggs

COOKING ACTIVITIES

stirring/mixing

milk, water, juice and other liquids
powders and granules e.g. flour, sugar, cocoa, coconut, spices:
other items – eggs, fruit, fats, cereals

cooling/freezing

refrigerator cakes, jellies, dairy dishes which require setting and/or chilling

cutting/preparing

fruit, vegetables, salad items
cheese

Important skills in science are those of observation and prediction. Through cooking activities children will be able to observe changes in appearance – colour, shape, texture – during all the processes. It is beneficial to encourage children to look closely at the ingredients before they are cut, sliced, combined and/or cooked (or whatever process is being used) and, perhaps to guess (or predict) what they think will happen. Even a disaster can provide learning opportunities by discussing what went wrong! Children can extend their vocabulary to include not only words which describe the look and taste of food but also those instructions which are commonplace in recipes such as 'beating', 'creaming', 'sieving', 'grating'.

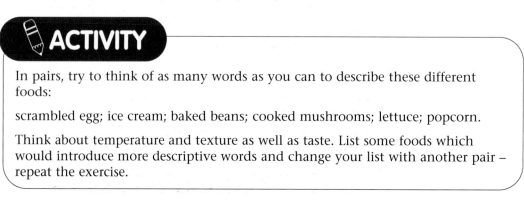

ACTIVITY

In pairs, try to think of as many words as you can to describe these different foods:

scrambled egg; ice cream; baked beans; cooked mushrooms; lettuce; popcorn.

Think about temperature and texture as well as taste. List some foods which would introduce more descriptive words and change your list with another pair – repeat the exercise.

These activities are also valuable in raising children's awareness of healthy and nutritious foods, educating them about diet and choice. By discussing the need for an ingredient to sweeten food children can be introduced to the variety available and be made aware of healthy options – for example using honey instead of sugar.

As stated at the beginning of this chapter, children learn through active involvement so any cooking activity must be chosen carefully to ensure that children can participate. There is very limited value in them watching an adult carry out the instructions and occasionally letting them have a stir!

Other learning outcomes include:

- development of physical skills through using the equipment – pouring, beating, whisking, stirring etc.;
- aspects of counting, sorting, measuring – size and quantity – sharing, fractions, ordinal number (i.e. first, second), sequencing and memory through following and recalling the recipe instructions;
- independence skills through preparation, controlling their own food and equipment, tidying up;
- expressing their ideas, opinions, likes and dislikes;
- understanding how to present food attractively through arrangement and decoration.

Multi-cultural ideas for cooking and preparing food

The following recipes are for different foods from around the world. When selecting a cooking activity, remember:

- that parental wishes must always be respected
- to check that *all* children can eat the food to be cooked
- to check that there are no problems regarding **allergies** or religious dietary restrictions
- to follow the basic food safety and hygiene guidelines on pages 74–76.

If possible, invite parents from different ethnic and cultural backgrounds to join in the planning of cooking activities, so that their child's culture is represented in the setting, and so that the food provided is authentic, rather than based on our (often stereotyped) ideas of what a child might eat at home. Not everyone feels comfortable actually undertaking the cooking with the children, but anyone could help by providing recipes and any special utensils.

Sweets for Diwali

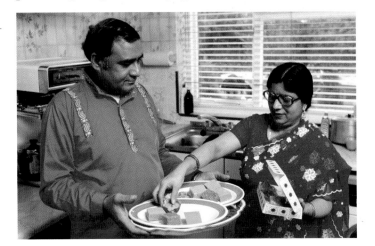

Sweets for Diwali

These sweets involve no cooking; they are traditionally eaten at **Diwali, the Hindu Festival of Lights**.

  1 large tin of condensed milk
  1 packet of desiccated coconut
  100 g ground almonds
  500 g icing sugar
  55 g chopped nuts
  Pinch of ground cardamom
  Pinch of nutmeg
  1 or 2 strands of saffron

1   Mix all the ingredients together.

2   Either spread the mixture in trays and cut into pieces, or roll into small balls.

3   Place in paper cases and sprinkle with icing sugar and nutmeg.

Chinese Moon cakes

These little cakes are often eaten during the **Chinese Festival of the Autumn Moon**, which falls in September. During this festival of lights there is a procession during which animal-shaped lanterns, each containing a small candle, are carried before the main feast.

  125 g slightly salted butter
  2 egg yolks
  60 g sugar
  140 g flour
  Small jar of jam (or red bean paste)

1   In a large mixing bowl combine the butter, sugar and 1 egg yolk. Stir until creamy.

2   Add the flour and mix thoroughly. Form the dough into one large ball and wrap it in cling film or foil. Put this in the fridge for 30 minutes.

3   Preheat the oven to 190°C or Gas Mark 5. Unwrap the chilled dough and, with clean hands, form small balls in the palms of your hand. (These are the moon cakes.)

4   Make a hole with your thumb gently in the centre of each moon cake and fill with about half a teaspoon of the jam or red bean paste.

5   Brush each cake with the other egg yolk, beaten.

6   Bake the moon cakes for about 20 minutes or until the outside edges are just slightly brown. Makes about 24 moon cakes.

Potato Latkes

These savoury 'pancakes' are often eaten during **Hanukkah, the Jewish Feast of lights**. Hanukkah usually begins in December and lasts for about 8 days. Each day is celebrated with songs, games, food, and the lighting of the Hanukkah candles. (Adults will need to fry the pancakes.)

  For 12 children under 6 years old, you will need:
  60 g self-raising flour or fine matzo meal
  6 medium-sized potatoes
  half a medium onion
  3 eggs

salt and pepper to taste
oil for frying

1   Using a cheese grater or food processor, grate the potatoes. Drain off the extra liquid.

2   Grate the onion. Mix the grated potatoes and onion with the eggs and flour.

3   Mix all the ingredients to a thick batter.

4   Heat the oil and drop in tablespoons of the mixture to make pancakes of about 8 cm (3 inches) diameter. Fry on both sides until golden-brown and serve warm.

Hummus

Hummus

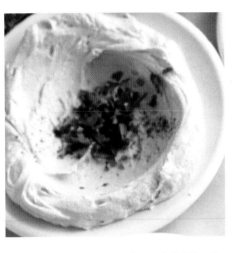

Hummus originates from Middle Eastern and Mediterranean countries. It is a savoury dip or spread that requires no cooking.

400 g can of chick peas
2 tablespoons of tahini (sesame seed paste)
3 tablespoons of lemon juice
1 large garlic clove crushed
quarter teaspoon ground cumin
salt

● Drain the chick peas and save the liquid for later.

● Put the chick peas in a blender and add the tahini, lemon juice, garlic, cumin and 4 tablespoons of the chick pea liquid.

● Blend until it is really smooth. Hummus can be eaten on toast, with pitta bread or with crunchy vegetables like carrots and sweet peppers.

Adapting cooking activities for children with particular needs

All children should have the opportunity to enjoy cooking and food preparation. The most important aspect of helping children with particular needs is to have knowledge and understanding of the difficulties facing each child. You may have to adapt some recipes, provide special gadgets or offer an extra pair of hands to enable children with particular needs to join in. The best people to ask are the child's parents or primary carer. Ideas for adapting cooking activities fall into the following categories.

● **Problems with mobility or co-ordination:** work with parents to find comfortable ways for a child to sit, e.g. a corner with two walls for support, a chair with a seat belt, or a wheelchair with a large tray across the arms. Children might need adult help with stirring, whisking and pouring. Provide a non-stick mat placed under the mixing bowl and utensils with easy-to-grip handles.

- **Visual impairment:** children might need to have their hands guided to handle objects. They may need to sit where there is good light and have the use of magnifying glasses.
- **Hearing impairment:** remember to use touch, gesture and facial expression to help these children to participate. Use pictures to illustrate the steps of a recipe during cooking activities.
- **Learning disability:** allow more time to complete a task. It often helps to break each task down into more stages. Other children might need pictures of food to help them make choices. Encourage them to 'have a go' and praise their efforts.
- **Special dietary needs:** always find out about each child's special dietary needs; e.g. vegetarian, vegan, diabetic diet, diet for coeliac disease, lactose intolerance, obesity. For more information on special diets, visit the website: www.waitrose.com/nutrition/special
- **Food allergies:** the most common – and dangerous – food allergy is **peanut allergy**. Always check with parents before giving peanut butter to a child for the first time. Some children are more likely than others to develop an allergy to food **additives**, especially colourings, flavour enhancers and preservatives. Children with food-related problems such as asthma, eczema, and skin rashes are often advised to avoid additives. For more information on food additives, visit the website: www.nutrition.org

Playing games with children

The term 'game' covers a wide range of activity – from simple 'round-and-round-the-garden' played with babies to complex games with special equipment and rules. Most games offer an enjoyable way of developing knowledge and/or understanding and/or practical skills. Babies and very young children enjoy one-to-one games which adults initiate. At this early stage they are not socially ready to join with other children and still spend much of their time exploring their world and objects in it.

Playing games with rules

As children develop intellectually they can begin to cope with games involving colour matching and recognition, shape matching and recognition, counting, sequencing and memory. Their increasing ability to copy those around them means that they can follow simple rules although taking turns and waiting patiently often causes problems!

Games which actively involve them can promote development in all areas. Ring and action games can help co-ordination, decision-making, language, rhythm and social skills of turn-taking and sharing. Where some children are chosen and others are not (e.g. 'The Farmer's in his den') they learn an important lesson of consideration for others and discover that they, themselves, cannot always be first but will get a turn at some point.

Table-top games

Earlier sections of this chapter have given many ideas for speaking, listening and musical games. Table-top games introduce children to rules and special equipment and can be used to teach and consolidate basic concepts. The best games available are those which offer versatility – the possibility of adaptation for differing abilities and stages of development.

✳ Ages 3–5 years – in these early stages children cope well with games that have a definite ending – with or without a 'winner'. This can be when a picture has been completed or a playing board has been filled. In most instances, although the first player to complete may be the 'winner', games are usually continued until all players have finished. It is the skill of the adult to maintain everyone's interest and involve children in each other's success.

Lotto games are among the most versatile as they:

✳ can be based on a wide range of topics e.g. number (numerals, patterns, objects), shapes, colours, words, seasons, weather, transport etc.

✳ have individual baseboards appropriate to young children

✳ can be adapted to suit needs of individual children

✳ can be for two to four (sometimes six) players

✳ can easily be made

✳ may have different versions (see below)

To create versatility a single baseboard may have two, or three, sets of cards. For example a lotto game to promote number may have baseboards with pictures of objects – one apple, two boots, three fish etc. One set of cards could have exactly the same set of pictures for direct matching, another set could have the numerals, or number symbols – 1, 2, 3 etc and yet a third might have the number words – one, two, three etc. The cards can be used for simple snap or pairs-type games or for labelling sets of objects that children have sorted. Other lotto-type games may include baseboards with a single picture which require pieces to be collected e.g. body parts/coloured balloons etc.

Other popular games are **dominoes** and **pairs**. For both these games adult supervision is important as for dominoes children need to be constantly reminded of the choices which can change at each turn, and for pairs young children tend to move the cards from their original places and the 'memory' element is lost. These games can last too long and result in children losing their concentration and enthusiasm.

✳ **Age 5–8 years** – at this stage children are able to share a playing board or area and games involving throwing a die or dice, counting on or back with the winner being the first to the finish are popular. There is a wide range available, some will develop reading skills as there are instructions to be followed on the board. Be aware of the needs of the children you are working with, think carefully before you introduce a 100 square board for snakes and ladders – it will be too long a game for the younger end of this age range and the direction changes – left to right and then back again – are confusing.

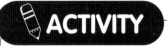

ACTIVITY

Design and make a table-top game for use with an individual child or small group of children of your chosen age from the range 3–8 years. In designing and making your game consider the following factors:

- age/stage of development

- clear objectives or purpose

- subject matter or content

- safety

- number of players

- rules

- attractiveness and appeal

- presentation

- storage/packaging

Remember to make your pieces an appropriate size, durable (laminate or cover with sticky-back plastic), colourful and attractive. If your game involves **visual matching** then make sure your pictures are **identical** (use wrapping paper or photocopied images) rather than 'nearly the same'. Try to think about children's interests e.g. book or television characters. You should state the age for which you consider the game to be suitable, provide storage and attractive packaging. Rules should be clearly presented so that any adult wishing to use the game would understand what the main aim was – e.g. to develop children's memory/counting/shape recognition etc. – and step-by-step playing instructions should be included. Explain how to play alternative versions, if applicable. When you have made the game you should try it out with the correct age children in your work setting. **Evaluate it** by identifying whether: it achieved your stated objectives; the children enjoyed it; they understood what they had to do; it maintained everyone's interest; there were any difficulties; there are any changes which could improve it.

Competitive games

Apart from the games described already, children in this age range are beginning to become involved in team games – perhaps in PE lessons – and the element of competition increases. However, many still find it difficult to 'lose' and need sensitive handling. Success and failure are facts of life and everybody experiences both at some time or another. Children can be helped to deal with their feelings through games in a safe and reassuring context.

Competitive games can:

- encourage children to try harder, concentrate more, foster determination;

- help children understand that 'luck' often plays a part in success and failure;

- promote positive attitudes towards co-operative and collaborative working;

- help children recognise their own particular talents and those of others;

- enable children to experience success and a sense of achievement;

- enable children to experience 'losing' and to recognise the talents of others;

- teach children the importance of rules and 'fair play';
- help children accept that there may be the ultimate decision of an umpire or referee against which there is no appeal.

Drawbacks can be that children:

- who seem never to win may lose confidence and self-esteem;
- may believe that winning is the most important thing;
- may not be given opportunities to express their feelings of disappointment e.g. being told to be a 'good loser';
- blame other team members for failure.

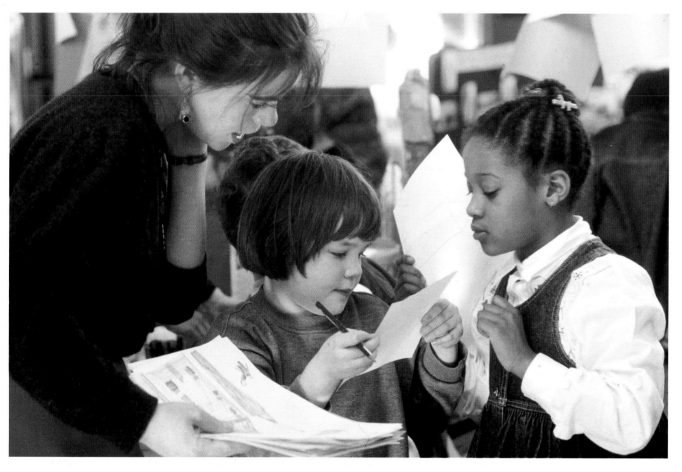

3

Communication and language experiences

- talking and listening to young children
- common communication difficulties in children
- where to obtain books, poems and rhymes from different sources
- setting up a book area
- children's reactions to different types of story
- choosing and using visual aids
- songs, rhymes, finger play and musical activities/experiences

Communicating effectively with young children

It is important to remember that there is more to communication than the words being spoken. It also involves:

☐ facial expressions;

☐ body language (posture and actions or gestures) which help to convey meaning;

☐ tone of voice which can, in itself, alter the meaning of what has been said e.g. the tone used to say our name instantly tells us whether we are in trouble, being appealed to or just having our attention drawn – particularly if it is our parent!

☐ pauses;

☐ turn taking.

It is thought that more than 70% of messages are conveyed through non-verbal means.

When talking to babies and young children most adults will naturally adopt a slightly higher-pitched voice than normal and may also emphasise and repeat important words.

To make communication effective:

- Make eye contact and show that you are listening – it is very difficult to have a conversation with someone who never looks at you!

- Listen carefully to the child's own spoken language and use it as a basis for conversation – very young children tend to use one or two words to mean any of a number of things e.g. 'drink' can mean 'this is my drink', 'I want a drink', 'Where is my drink?' or 'You have got a drink'.

- Repeat the child's words in a correct form, or a complete sentence. This checks understanding and provides the child with an accurate model for the future. For example, young children often use speech such as 'feeded' instead of 'fed', 'runned' instead of 'ran' – in checking what they mean the adult must use the correct term – Child: 'I feeded carrots to my rabbit' Adult: 'Oh, you fed your rabbit some carrots.'

> As you may expect, young children understand more than they can express themselves. They may be able to follow simple instructions (especially if they are accompanied by a gesture e.g. pointing) such as 'give daddy a kiss' or 'fetch your teddy' long before they can use sentences themselves. They learn new words – initially names of objects and important people – by listening carefully and copying. Many words which have unstressed syllables – such as important and computer – are learned as 'portant' and 'puter' because these are the sounds that they are able to hear easily.

- Be a good role model, speak clearly and use correct grammar and patterns of speech.
- Encourage children to speak by asking 'open' questions which require an answer in phrases and/or sentences rather than a simple 'yes' or 'no' – e.g. 'Tell me about your party' instead of 'Did you have a good time at your party?' This opens up opportunities for the child to talk about a range of different things or one single event of his/her own choice – you can always ask more questions as the conversation progresses to check the information, supply additional vocabulary and correct grammar.

Because intellectual and language development are so closely linked, a delay in one area will usually result in delay in the other.

Factors which particularly affect language development and/or communication are:

☐ any hearing impairments – permanent or temporary;

☐ physical impairments such as cleft palate and hare lip;

☐ stammers and stutters;

☐ other medical conditions which affect other aspects of development and, as a consequence, a child's confidence or self-esteem;

☐ disorders which affect learning such as autism;

☐ an additional language – children's home language must be valued. Adults should recognise that these children are, most likely, competent communicators at home and need support to develop an additional vocabulary which, for the very young child, may only apply in the early childhood setting;

☐ lack of language input (conversations) with an interested adult or good role model;

☐ emotional factors which can result in shyness, low self-esteem and a lack of confidence.

Speaking and listening activities

These range from individual conversations between adult and child to whole class/group 'news' times. In addition there are many games and activities which provide ideal opportunities for children to use and practise their speaking and listening skills. For very young children sharing rhymes – traditional nursery, finger and action – songs and books with an adult are both valuable and enjoyable.

As language develops and listening skills develop, older children will be able to play games which involve 'active' listening such as:

- ❑ 'What (or who) am I?' This involves the adult (or a child – perhaps with help) giving clues until the animal/person/object is identified. **I have sharp teeth. I have a long tail. I have a striped coat. I eat meat. Answer: a tiger or a tabby cat.**

- ❑ Taped sounds – these can be environmental (kettle boiling, doorbell, someone eating crisps) or related to a particular topic – farm animals, pet animals, machines – or of familiar people's voices.

- ❑ Taped voices – reception or Year 1 children tape their own voices giving clues about themselves but without saying who they are. 'I have brown eyes. I have two brothers. I have a Lion King lunchbox. I have short, dark hair. Who am I?' This activity is best done with a small group so they are not guessing from amongst the whole class! They find it difficult not to say their names but love hearing themselves and their friends. The enjoyment factor makes it valuable and ensures concentrated listening once the excitement has died down.

- ❑ Feely box – use varied objects for children to feel (without being able to see) and encourage them to describe the shape, size, texture, surface etc. This can be topic-related e.g. fruit or solid shapes. A very good activity for extending children's vocabulary.

- ❑ 'Snowball' games which involve active listening and memory – 'I went to market and I bought . . .' There are many versions of this. It can be used for number – one cabbage, 2 bananas, 3 flannels etc . . . or to reinforce the alphabet – an apple, a budgie, a crane etc . . . or topic related – food items, transport items, clothing etc.

- ❑ Chinese whispers – this is appropriate for older children who are more able to wait patiently for their turn.

- ❑ Circle activities in which children and adult/s sit in a circle and a 'special' object is held by the person who is speaking. Rules are that only the person holding the object is allowed to speak – the object is passed around in turn or to whoever wants to say something – adult supervision needed! Alternatively a large ball can be rolled across the circle and the person rolling the ball makes his/her contribution (this can be on a theme – favourite foods/colours/games etc.) and the person who receives the ball makes the next contribution.

These activities encourage children to take turns, to use language to express their thoughts, feelings and ideas and to gain confidence as communicators. The circle activities are particularly good for encouraging shy or withdrawn children who may not, otherwise, get a word in – literally!

Selecting and using books with young children

What to look for in choosing books

It is never too early to introduce children to books and it certainly helps them to have positive attitudes towards books and reading if they see familiar adults enjoying them. They can quickly learn 'reading behaviour' – how books work, turning pages, following pictures and print, flow of text from left to right and (not always, but usually) top to bottom – by sitting on an adult's lap and following a finger along the print or pointing to pictures.

Many books will have an indication of the age for which they are suitable but sometimes this is very broad. In making your selection these factors need to be considered:

- type and size of book
- illustrations
- print (size and font) and text
- content
- language
- plot or storyline
- length

Apart from thinking about individual books it is important to make sure that you have allowed for variety in your overall selection to include story (**fiction**) books, fact (**non-fiction**) books, picture books and poetry or rhyme books.

There are some general guidelines which can help you in your choice.

Age 0–1 year:

Provide **board**, **picture**, **bath**, **fabric**, **feely**, and **simple rhyme books**. Small hands which have not yet developed manipulative skills to turn thin pages will manage thicker card/board ones. Board books are also more likely to stand up to the chewing and exploring by mouth that babies do! Bath and fabric books are also good and can be washed. They should not be too large for a baby to handle. **Clear**, **simple**, **brightly-coloured illustrations** are suitable at this stage, preferably of **everyday objects** to encourage 'naming' for first words. Simple picture books without words are appropriate as adults can point to and talk about the pictures. Early picture books often have a single word for each page e.g. 'spoon' or 'a spoon', 'teddy' or 'a teddy'. Pictures of common animals and objects they are not familiar with can help to build vocabulary. The print needs to be fairly large and in a simple **lower case** script or font. Books for this age tend to have a few pages – perhaps up to ten.

Age 1–2 years:

This is a very important age for speech development and children are beginning to link two and three words to communicate their needs. Books can be of the same type as for 0–1 year but can include **a wider variety of subject matter. Fact and story books which reflect their own everyday activities** e.g. getting dressed, mealtimes, bathtime, bedtime, going to the park etc. are important to emphasise and introduce the idea of a sequence of events. There may be a **single line of text** which describes the picture e.g. 'under the bed', 'on the chair'. This can develop vocabulary and understanding of positional words. **Print needs to be large and bold. Rhyme books which encourage repetition**, perhaps with actions, are particularly good at this stage.

Age 2–3 years:

As children's spoken vocabulary grows and becomes more fluent they are ready for **slightly longer books** which may have a simple story – one which has a beginning, a middle and an end. Children can cope with only a small number of characters. At this stage they are beginning to enjoy and repeat rhymes and songs. Pictures still need to be large and colourful. **Lift-the-flap** and **pop-up books** allow children to get actively involved although care and supervision are advisable as they are not always gentle in handling them. **Print should be large** and where sentences are used, **correct use of punctuation** (full stops and question marks) **and capital letters** is important. In a work setting children of this age are likely to share story sessions with larger groups of children as well as look at books on an individual or paired basis.

Age 3/4/5 years:

At these ages children are developing fluency and can speak and understand an increasing number of words. Their first 'reading' has been signs and labels around them and they can read their own names. They can relate to a wider range of subjects and fact books help them to develop their understanding. Books which show a sequence of events are still important. Children are beginning to read whole words and identify letter shapes at around four years of age. They can use **pictures** to help them understand the text (story or factual information) as well as **noticing and appreciating** more detail. The **amount of text on a page increases** to several lines but **the print is still quite large**. Throughout this period children gradually come to understand more complex stories and enjoy **humorous situations**. Stories with more **characters** are suitable. Children will have favourite books which they will enjoy over and over again and will be able to retell the main parts of a well-known story (these are called **core texts**). They still like listening to stories but also look at books independently – younger children often 'pretend read' to themselves or a friend as they imitate adults and older children.

Age 5/6/7+ years:

It is during this period that most children become fluent readers. They will manage **smaller print, more lines of text and fewer illustrations**. Many will still enjoy their favourite picture books even if they can cope with more challenging ones. They are beginning to use books as a **source of information** about subjects that interest them. They enjoy jokes and can follow stories written in **'comic strip' style**. Stories can be **longer, more complex and have more characters**. Longer stories and short books can be listened to and enjoyed in serial form by children aged around seven. By this time their listening skills and concentration are further developed and they have less need for pictures. They can use the descriptions to imagine characters and places.

✏ ACTIVITY

Connor, aged 6, was taken to see the Walt Disney film 'Beauty and the Beast'. He loved it, could tell the story and asked for the story book as a birthday present. His grandmother bought him a beautiful version. It was a fairly thick, hardback book containing several chapters, long descriptive passages and with one lovely picture at the start of each chapter. After a few days he put the book on a shelf and left it there!

In pairs or small groups discuss why Connor behaved like this. Describe the type of book which would have been appropriate for him and explain your reasons.

More about illustrations

Some illustrators have such distinctive styles that their work is instantly recognisable – e.g. Quentin Blake, Shirley Hughes. Their books have been favourites for many years and the pictures account for much of their appeal.

Look for . . .	Avoid . . .
✓ a story or factual information which is relevant to the children – particularly if pictures are 'dated'	✗ 'dated' pictures – content e.g. type of telephone, clothing, kitchen equipment, or the style e.g. use of particular colours or techniques
✓ images which show both men and women in caring roles and participating in a variety of jobs/occupations	✗ stereotyped images of gender (e.g. girl helping mummy in the kitchen while boy helps daddy with the car or garden; girl playing with a doll and boy playing with a train etc.)
✓ positive images of different races and cultures – i.e. realistic representation, as main characters, in a variety of occupations, traditions valued and respected	✗ negative images re: race (e.g. inaccurate representation of physical features, a single black person as the main 'bad', poor, or mean character).
✓ well-produced photos which are relevant to children's experience	✗ photos that are obviously out of date
✓ positive images of disabled people – i.e. as important characters showing individual abilities and personalities	✗ disabled persons shown as needy, dependent and always on the receiving end of 'good deeds'
✓ photos showing fair representation of different races	✗ photos showing only white children

More good reasons to use books

Apart from being important for language development, stories and books can be used to promote other areas. Some emotional issues such as bullying, bereavement, illness, families and friendship can be dealt with at the right level through stories. They create an opportunity for children to talk about their feelings and fears. Similarly, factual books about hospital, dentists, impairment etc. can prepare children for life experiences. A well-chosen story or book can often be used as a starting point for a topic or theme.

Cultural diversity

Most cultures seem to be rich in traditional tales and, regardless of the country they come from, these seem to have similar themes of good/bad, strong/weak, happy/sad, rich/poor. Indeed, many of the 'fairy' stories familiar to us from childhood are also well-known in other countries with, perhaps, some slight alterations and differently named characters. Including tales from other cultures in your book selection can add to the variety and richness of children's story experiences.

Many editions of these well-known stories are now available in dual-language versions which show text in English and also in the original language in which it was written (usually, although the additional language may be any). The illustrations remain appropriate for both sets of text. Even if there are no children in the work setting with English as an additional language, these books can be used to introduce children to the idea that there are many different ways of writing and communicating.

ACTIVITY

Using books that you have seen being used with children, make a selection for each of the age ranges given on pp.165 and 166. Include one fact book, one rhyme or poetry book and, for ranges 2 years and upwards, two story books. Review each book carefully, providing information about author, title, publisher and place and date of publication. In your reviews comment on the illustrations, language, content, print, layout, storyline (if applicable), and explain what age you consider the book to be appropriate for and why. Comment on any positive and negative aspects – use the 'look for' and 'avoid' lists to help you.

Setting up a book area

Most work settings have a book 'corner' or defined area where books are displayed and made accessible. Usually it is situated away from noisier and messy activities, and is carpeted for comfort and to minimise noise. There may be children's chairs or floor cushions or bean bags which offer a relaxing and comfortable environment in which to share a book or become absorbed in one. By identifying a specific area children can be discouraged from spreading their play from other, perhaps more boisterous, activities. If possible there should be a good, natural light source or, if not, sufficient overhead lighting to cover the whole area. The books themselves are best displayed in low shelves, preferably with the front covers showing. Small children cannot cope with titles written 'sideways' on thin spines. Sturdy wooden boxes on low legs, sometimes known as 'kinderboxes' offer easy access to children and allow them to look through the whole range before making a selection. Some town libraries have books stored in boxes made into 'Thomas the Tank Engine' or other well-known book characters.

The whole idea is to make the books and the area exciting and inviting. Tidying the area and changing the books out on display regularly can stimulate the children's interest. Wall and hanging displays related to popular stories and characters can add to the area's attractiveness. It is important that children are encouraged to handle books carefully, turning pages properly and not damaging the spines. Staff should make periodic checks for damage – a missing page can cause frustration to the reader and listener!

Story activities

These can be enjoyed on an individual, small group or large group basis and a story session is often used to 'round off' the morning or afternoon in work settings. Although children are actively involved in listening it is an opportunity for a quiet, shared experience, accessible to all. Through stories children develop their listening skills, their understanding of a sequence of events, their vocabulary and their imagination. They can also try to understand the feelings and actions of different characters and relate them to themselves and their own lives.

ACTIVITY

With permission from your supervisor, observe a story session which involves a small or large group of children. Give information about where the session took place, how the children were settled, what story was told/read and how it was introduced. Try to record responses of individual children as the story progresses – how attentive they are, what they say, any actions or facial expressions you notice. When you write your conclusion comment on the children's enjoyment and understanding. How did the story teller manage to maintain interest? (See 'Delivery strategies' on the next page to help you) How did he/she manage behaviour? Was the story appropriate? Why/why not?

The choice of story is very important (see pages 164–165 for more detailed information about choosing books) and the following factors should be considered:

✱ length of story – young children have a fairly short concentration span;

✱ content of story – children should be able to follow the plot and understand the situations and events;

✱ language – it should be well-written using accurate grammar and tenses and have a rich vocabulary while being appropriate for the age range;

✱ illustrations – the younger the child, the bolder these should be and many of them – older children will be able to cope with fewer and they can be more detailed;

✱ repetition – of words and phrases such as 'Then I'll huff and I'll puff . . . etc.' or 'Not now, Bernard' are suitable features for younger children.

A skillful story teller will be able to hold children's attention and bring a story alive through a range of strategies.

Delivery strategies

Eye contact Ensure that you can see all the children's faces and that you make eye contact with all of them at some point during the session This helps to maintain interest and desired behaviour.

Position You need to have your face (and book if you are using one) in the light rather than in shadow – sitting with your back to a window with light coming from behind you makes it difficult for children to see your facial expressions.

Pace Vary the speed at which you deliver the story – speeding up at exciting moments and slowing down at others adds interest.

Behaviour Try to seat any children who may have difficulty concentrating close to you or another adult. Use eye contact and non-verbal communication to deal with unwanted behaviour without halting the story.

Volume Vary the volume – you need to project your voice a little rather than speak as in a normal conversation. Use a variety of tones – whispering, shouting etc. as the story demands.

Questioning When preparing the story look for opportunities to stop the story either to recap what has happened so far, to check children's understanding and to ask what they think may happen next.

Children with particular needs Hearing-impaired children, children with English as an additional language, or who have concentration difficulties need to be given special consideration so that they can share and enjoy the session.

Range of voices Create interest by using different voices appropriately for the characters in the story. This can be very effective and many stories such as 'The 3 Billy Goats Gruff' and 'The 3 Little Pigs' are especially suitable.

Settling children There are many ways of getting the children quiet, focused and ready to listen. One of the most effective is to recite or sing rhymes, particularly action ones or fingerplays if they are fidgety. Games like 'Simon Says' will focus attention on you, ready for the story.

Use of props Appropriate props – puppets, objects, flannelgraph figures etc. help to focus children's interest and can often add to their understanding. They are particularly useful when telling a story rather than reading it. Children can be involved in the actual telling by holding and using props at the right moment in a story.

A storytime session

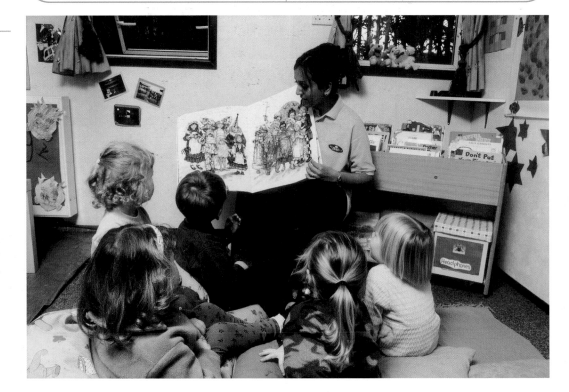

Musical activities

Although different cultures have their own traditions, music is a 'universal' language and is, therefore, accessible to everyone. Our bodies have a natural rhythm – the heartbeat and pulse and even those with hearing impairments can be aware of rhythms and vibrations caused by sound.

Nursery, finger and action rhymes are often the first songs that children participate in and each family will use its own favourites. Work settings usually introduce an even wider repertoire to children. These rhymes help to develop children's sense of rhythm as well as increasing their vocabulary and, perhaps, encouraging their number skills (counting up and down) or naming of body parts etc.

Making music

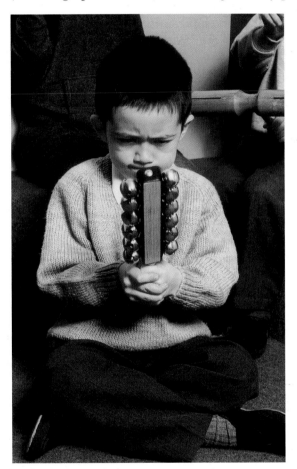

There is a range of musical activities that are appropriate.

1 **Listening to music** – live or taped.

- Try to introduce a wide range including music from different cultures – oriental, folk tunes, pan pipes from South America, unaccompanied vocal music from other continents as well as military band music and western styles. The extracts should not be too long and you can encourage **active listening** by asking them to focus on one aspect – the tempo (speed), the tune or the rhythm.

2 **Singing**

- This can be well-known rhymes or games which involve the children in imitating a short tune sung by an adult (or, with older, confident children, a child). Regular singing games develop children's **listening skills** and ability to **discriminate sound** – particularly helping them to 'pitch' a note more accurately.

3   **Playing instruments** – this involves many skills – physical, listening, social and intellectual.

- The best, and most available instruments, are our own bodies. Body percussion involves hitting, flicking, tapping, thumping etc. different parts of the body to produce a wide range of sounds – try chests, fingernails, teeth, cheeks with mouths open – in fact, anything – not forgetting the human voice! 'The Little Indian Boy' in 'This Little Puffin' (see resource list) is ideal for using body percussion. Children learn to control their movements to create loud and soft sounds, fast and slow rhythms.

- Bought instruments available should be of good quality and produce pleasing sounds – cheap ones are not sufficiently durable and often create a poor sound. Although tuned percussion (i.e. xylophone, glockenspiel, metallophone) are likely to be found in schools, individual, child-friendly instruments are better for younger children who may not be ready to share. A good range could include untuned percussion – tulip blocks, cabasa, guiro (or scraper), maracas, tambour (hand-held drum), tambourine (a tambour but with the metal discs around the side), castanets (on a hand-held stick), claves (or rhythm sticks), click-clacks, bongo drums – as well as Indian bells, triangle and beater, individual chime bars and beaters, cow bells, and hand-held bells. A group of instruments can be placed in a 'sound' corner for children to experiment with on their own or in pairs – perhaps all 'wooden' instruments on one occasion or 'ones which are struck with a beater' another time.

Large group sessions can be difficult to organise but some simple rules can make them enjoyable for all and worthwhile. Sitting in a circle and re-inforcing the names of instruments as they are given out helps to keep things under control. Even three-year-olds can understand that they must leave their instrument on the floor in front of them until asked to pick it up, although this is not easy in the first instance.

The whole point of the games is for children to **experience** music-making so there must be plenty of playing and experimenting and not too much sitting around waiting! It is usually a good idea to allow children to 'have a go' with their instruments before doing a more focused activity. Taking turns to **listen** to each child make as many different sounds on his/her instrument in as many ways as he/she can is a good way of **building their confidence** and understanding that there is no right or wrong way. They can then **choose** the sounds they liked best. Similarly work can focus on **dynamics – loud and soft** – and children can be asked to play as loudly as they can and as quietly as they can. Which instruments were difficult to do this with? Why?

Another activity involves each child having an instrument – this time make sure there are some which **resonate** (i.e. go on sounding after they have been played or struck) as well as the wooden percussion instruments. Going around the group one child plays his/her instrument and the next child cannot play until the sound has died away. Discuss which instruments had 'long' sounds and which 'short' ones.

4   **Moving to music**

- This allows children to **respond creatively** to different sounds and rhythms. A wide variety should be available as for listening. Circle singing games such as 'The farmer's in his den', 'Ring-a-ring o' roses' and 'Here we go round the mulberry bush' all encourage children to move in time with the **pulse** or beat.

5 Composing music

- Choosing sounds and putting them together in patterns around silence to create their own tunes and rhythms can develop listening and intellectual skills

There are many useful books with suggestions for games and activities – see the resource list.

Using homemade instruments adds variety and interest. The most successful of these are shakers made from 'found materials' using different containers – tins, plastic pots, boxes (these must be clean and have close fitting lids) and choosing contents which will produce interesting sounds. These could be rice grains, lentils, chick peas, black-eyed beans, runner bean seeds, dried pasta, stones, sand. Under supervision children can experiment and choose the contents, the amount and the container. If they are to be used continually it is a good idea to glue the lids on to avoid the danger of children putting small items in their mouths. They can also be decorated or covered in patterned sticky plastic.

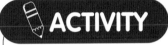 **ACTIVITY**

Choose one of the categories from the numbered list above. With permission from your supervisor, plan and carry out an activity with a small group of children aged three or over. Try to identify what musical aspects they will be learning about and how your activity can promote development in other areas. List the resources you will need including time and supervision. Explain how you will introduce any new words or experiences. After you have carried it out evaluate: whether it achieved what you had planned; whether the children enjoyed it and how they responded – give examples; how it might have been improved.

4

Encouraging young children to explore

- interesting objects for young children to explore
- the value of objects of interest in promoting development
- encouraging children to handle objects and cultural artifacts with care and respect
- enabling children with particular needs to explore
- the importance of the local environment and open spaces

Providing interest objects

Babies and young children learn about their world through their senses and by exploring objects around them. Their interaction with a wide range of objects helps them to develop the basic concepts of shape, colour, size, weight, texture, sound and many others. As mentioned in relation to displays, providing children with interesting objects in their environment is an important way to encourage curiosity, experimentation and problem-solving skills.

Playing with found materials

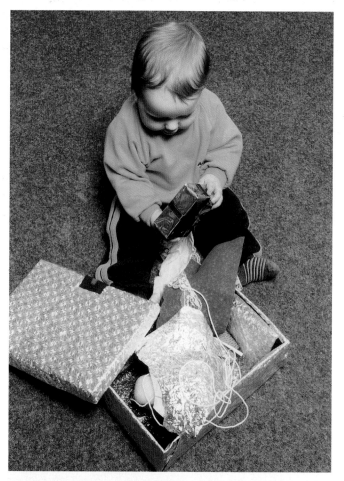

Safety must be the first consideration:

Avoid objects which:

✗ are damaged (unless they are natural objects)

✗ are made from toxic materials

✗ are too fragile to be handled

✗ are too heavy

✗ have small pieces

Choose objects which:

✓ are appropriate for the age/stage of children

✓ link to a topic/theme or concept

✓ are sufficiently robust for children to handle

✓ can be investigated through the senses

If you choose to provide objects which may be delicate e.g. a wasps' nest, pine cones or shells then it is important to set some guidelines for handling them. If they really are too fragile then allow children to use magnifying glasses to look at them or to touch the object while it is under the control of an adult. Even quite young children will understand if they are given an explanation. Using simple pictorial signs (e.g. of a hand with a tick through it or a hand with a large cross through it) to indicate whether objects may be handled or not will be clearer than a written sign saying 'Do not touch'. Objects from the past can stimulate children's interest and help them develop an understanding of history. For example collections of electrical appliances – irons, kettles, toasters, radios etc. – can be used to help them relate their grandparents' and parents' lives to their own experiences. Similarly objects which represent everyday aspects of other cultures can provide the same links. Encouraging children to bring objects from home is an ideal way of maintaining positive links with their families, raising self-esteem and valuing their home life.

Ideas for collections of objects:

* **natural objects** – leaves, nuts, seeds, flowers, twigs, pieces of bark, stones, pebbles, shells;

* **shiny objects** – safety mirrors (card), spoons, foil wrappers, 'silver' or 'gold' items;

* **different materials** – *soft* ones e.g. velvet, fur (artificial), cotton wool, velour, towelling – *rough* ones e.g. sandpaper, sacking, brick, brushes with stiff bristles;

* **items connected with a season** – e.g. clothing, related activities (buckets and spades, sunglasses or umbrellas etc.);

* **items from home connected to a theme** – baby toys, photos, favourite books etc.

Observing young children

5

- the importance of observing and planning
- policies, rules and procedures of work settings
- different types of observations and recording formats

Why observe children?

Parents, babysitters and childcare workers automatically watch the children in their care. They want to know that the children are safe, happy, healthy and developing well. Watching or observing closely can often reassure all concerned that everything is alright but may also alert them to problems or illness. Any discussion about a child usually relates to what has been seen, heard or experienced and leads to conclusions about his/her personality, likes and dislikes, difficulties etc.

Anyone who works with children needs to develop the skill of observing them (sometimes to be written/recorded) to check that a child is:

- **safe** – not in any physical danger from the environment, from itself or from others;
- **contented** – there are many reasons why a child might be miserable, some may relate to physical comfort (e.g. wet nappy, hunger, thirst) or emotional comfort (e.g. main carer is absent, comfort object is lost) or lack of attention and stimulation;
- **healthy** – eats and sleeps well and is physically active (concerns about any of these aspects may indicate that the child is unwell);
- **developing normally** – in line with general expectations for his/her age in all areas – there will be individual differences but delays in any e.g. crawling/walking or speaking, may show a need for careful monitoring and, perhaps, specialist help. Any particular strength or talent may also be identified and encouraged.

A series of observations (particularly if they are written or recorded in some way e.g. photos) can provide an ongoing record of progress which can be very useful to parents and other professionals who may be involved with a child's care and education.

Observations can provide valuable information about:

- individual children – their progress and how they behave in particular situations
- groups of children – the differences between individuals in the same situations
- adults – how they communicate with children and how they deal with behaviour
- what activities are successful and enjoyed by children

What should be recorded?

There is some information which should be included in any observation but other aspects will depend on the purpose of the observation. If it is to consider the child's fine motor skills then the detail will probably be different from one which is to find out about his/her social development – even if the same activity or situation is being observed. You should also record some introductory information – see below.

When you carry out a written observation it is usually because you want to find out something about an individual child or a group of children. This provides **an aim** which should be identified at the start of your work. For example: 'To see what gross motor skills Child R uses in a P.E. lesson and consider how confident he is on the apparatus.' A clear aim explains what you want to find out and **the activity or context** which you have decided will best show you. This is better than saying you will watch Child R in a P.E. lesson. **The aim you identify should affect what information you write in your introduction and in the actual observation.**

As well as an aim your observation should also have the following:

- [ ] date carried out
- [ ] start and finish times
- [ ] who gave permission
- [ ] where it took place (setting)
- [ ] number of children present
- [ ] number of adults present
- [ ] age of child/ages of children
- [ ] names or identification of children (remember confidentiality)
- [ ] method used (brief reason for choice)
- [ ] signature of supervisor or tutor

How should it be recorded?

Your tutors will have their own preferences for how they want you to present your work but, generally, each observation should include the following sections: Introduction: Actual Observation: Evaluation: Bibliography

- **Introduction** – In this section you must explain **where** the observation is taking place e.g. At the sand tray in a reception class, and give some information about **what is happening** e.g. the children had just returned to the classroom from assembly . . . If there is any **relevant information about the child** you might include it here e.g. Child R has been ill recently and has missed two weeks of school. Include information which is relevant to your aim – it may be important to know whether he is of average build if you are dealing with physical skills but not particularly relevant if you are dealing with imaginative play.

- **Actual observation** – There are many different methods of recording and your tutors will help you decide which one is best – perhaps a 'chart' format, a checklist, or a written record describing what you see as it happens. Remember only to write what you see and, if appropriate, hear. **Do not write your judgements, opinions, assessments etc.** Make sure you include information about other children or adults involved if it is relevant.

When recording your observation remember to maintain confidentiality by only using a child's first name or initial or some other form of identification, e.g. Child R. You may use 'T' or 'A' for 'teacher' or 'adult'.

What is an Evaluation and how might it be presented?

An **Evaluation** is an assessment of what you have observed. This section can be dealt with in two parts.

1. You need to look back at your recorded information and summarise what you have discovered e.g. *'Child R was looking around the classroom and fidgeting with his shoelaces during the story and appeared bored and uninterested. However, he was able to answer questions when asked so he must have been listening for at least part of the time.'* This is a review of what you saw.

2. You then need to consider what you have summarised and compare your findings to the 'norm' or 'average' or 'expected' for a child of this age and at this stage of development. What have you, yourself, learnt about this particular child/group of children, and how has this helped you to understand children's development more widely? Use relevant books to help you and **make reference to them or quote** directly if you can find a statement or section which relates to what you are saying or the point you are making. Your tutor or assessor wants to know what you understand *not* information s/he could read in a book, so use references carefully.

As observation of children can help carers to plan for individual needs, try to suggest what activity or caring strategy might be needed next. You may also, in this section, give your opinion as to reasons for the behaviour etc. – take care not to jump to conclusions about the role of the child's background and never make judgements about the child or the child's family.

The ***bibliography*** is a list of the books you have used when reading and researching for information relating to your observation.

Listening to a shell

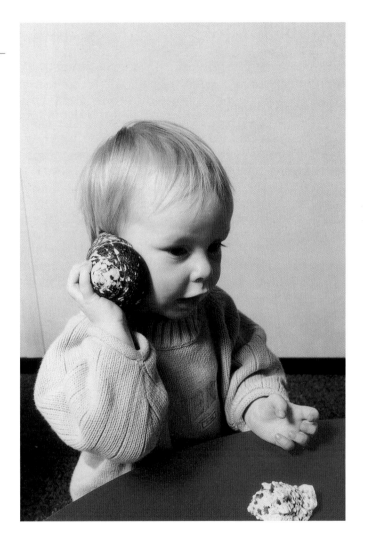

6

The role of the adult in supporting children during play and planning appropriate activities

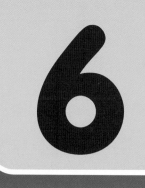

Framework for working with children

Early Years settings operate within defined guidelines. Whether the function of a work setting is to provide care and/or education it is subject to inspections by OFSTED to ensure it satisfies the legal requirements satisfactorily. Each of the UK countries has its own National Curriculum and system of testing. For more information see pages 127–128.

Adult role in supporting children

Adults can support children's learning through:

- planning activities and experiences to suit individual interests and needs of an individual child

- talking with children about the experience/activity they are involved in and extending their vocabulary

- observing and monitoring progress

- ensuring a wide range of materials and resources is available

- providing appropriate activities and experiences

- showing genuine interest in the children's activity/experience and sometimes joining in with sensitivity to the child's interests

- supervising to ensure safety

- being a good role model

- intervening when appropriate with sensitivity

- encouraging children to try new things and to express their ideas and feelings

- encouraging children to participate and experiment

Why plan activities/experiences and what factors should be considered?

Children need a variety of activities/experiences, using a range of resources, to enable them to learn and make progress in all areas of development. Planning **what** will be offered helps children to use a range of resources and materials. It encourages a 'balanced' day.

Having made decisions about **what** to provide it is then necessary to plan each activity/experience and consider the following factors:

- ☐ aim or purpose
- ☐ time needed/group size
- ☐ preparation in advance
- ☐ preparation at the time
- ☐ space/resources/safety
- ☐ suitability for age/stage of development
- ☐ supervision/adult role
- ☐ adaptation for a child with a special need
- ☐ consideration of equal opportunities issues
- ☐ opportunities for monitoring and assessing individual children

Aim or purpose

As for observations, a clear aim is preferable to one which is too wide or vague. For example:

✓ To develop fine manipulative skills through putting a straw in a carton of drink *or* To develop listening skills through a 'sound' lotto game

✗ To develop physical skills *or* To play a listening game

Almost all activities have many benefits and will help development in more than one area. It is a good idea to identify the **main purpose** and mention briefly other aspects which are also likely to be involved.

Time needed/group size

Most settings have a daily routine which fits around refreshment/food, sleep or rest, outdoor or energetic activity, perhaps assembly or group time and start and finish times (these may vary for individual children in a nursery setting). Knowing how long you are going to need to carry out an activity from start to finish for a group is very important. It helps to decide when it can be done and, if all children are to have the opportunity to do it, how many 'sessions' will be needed. Generally, the younger the children the fewer you would have in a group – perhaps for a 'messy' activity such as finger painting you may work with pairs or perhaps just one child. You need to allow time for clearing away, especially if the tables or the area is needed for another activity. Similarly, the children themselves may need to wash for lunch or get dressed for going outside/home.

Preparation/Resources

In advance:

1 The first step is to find out the setting's current topic or theme, if they have one, and **discuss with your supervisor** what activity might be appropriate.

2 You should then **plan the activity/experience**, show the plan to your supervisor and, if it is suitable, agree **when** you may **implement it**. This should avoid a similar one being carried out by someone else the day before! At this stage you can ensure that the space you need e.g. the book corner or the water tray, will be available. An activity which uses 'permanent' equipment (e.g. Lego, stickle bricks, puzzles) will need setting up – space, layout of equipment, seating if applicable. However, one which uses '**consumable materials**' i.e. ones which are used up and need replacing such as paper, paint, glue etc., requires more consideration.

3 **Make a comprehensive list** of what you need – this should be detailed. For example: not just '6 sheets of paper' but 6 sheets of A3, black, sugar paper (i.e. state size, colour, type).

4 **Check that your selected resources are available** (another staff member may have reserved the last of the gold paper for a particular display or activity so do not just go and help yourself!) and **collect them in plenty of time**. Some may need further preparation – cutting to smaller size/particular shape/arranging in pots or tubs for easy access.

5 Check that:
   - (for very young children) there are no tiny pieces
   - materials are clean
   - materials are undamaged
   - there are no toxic substances/contents

For preparation relating to food and cooking activities see pages 152–155.

At the time:

1 *Always* **allow time for preparation on the day** – arrive early if necessary. Your supervisor will have made arrangements for you to take the agreed number of children at the agreed time. If you are not ready, someone else has to supervise those children and/or find them an alternative activity.

2 Remember to **protect tables, surfaces, children and their clothing** appropriately.

3 **Prepare sufficient quantities** of paint, paper etc. for the group size identified and have them conveniently to hand – you cannot leave a group of young children to go and fetch more paper from the stock cupboard or to mix up more paint!

When planning your activity think about how you will introduce it – what will be your starting point? You might show the children the equipment and ask them about it or remind them of a previous related experience.

Suitability for age/stage of development

Although you can use books to help you understand what is the 'expected' or 'norm' ability for the age range you are working with it is more important to base your own planning on what you can see and have experienced in your particular work setting. If you have used your placement time effectively you will have helped with activities planned by other staff members and become familiar with the resources and with the children. Remember that children should be **active learners** and your plan should provide them with **'hands-on' experience**. Avoid activities which involve colouring in work sheets or 'sticking' ones which do not allow children to select their own materials and choose how to use the space.

Supervision/adult role

Your activity – perhaps a physical one involving large apparatus – may require more than one adult supervising. In this case it is important not only to check that there are sufficient adults available but also that any other adult knows your activity's aim and what is involved. If you have written a clear plan then it can be shared more easily. Try to think ahead about any aspects of your plan which may involve an adult in offering practical help to all children or an individual child.

Adaptation for a child with a special need/consideration of equal opportunities

As you will be planning for children in your work setting you will be aware of any children with special needs – whether the difficulty results from a physical condition, a sensory impairment, a learning disorder, or a behavioural or emotional problem. Notice what strategies are used by other staff members to allow access to all activities and equipment. This may be as straightforward as ensuring that you make left-handed or 'dual-handed' scissors available or more challenging in adapting space and materials for a child whose leg is in plaster. Try to think about adaptations for children with sensory impairment. Visually impaired children will depend heavily on hearing and touch so try to adapt resources or provide extra ones to support their learning e.g. samples of materials mentioned in stories like the Three Little Pigs (straw, sticks and bricks). Hearing impaired children will also benefit from learning through touch but will need visual aids too – perhaps puppets or figures to demonstrate parts of a story or clear pictures sequenced to help with a cooking or construction task. Always make sure that you have the children's attention – touching a visually impaired child on the arm so it is clear s/he needs to listen and ensuring that when talking, or giving instructions, to a hearing impaired child s/he is able to see the speaker's face (see pp. 162–164 about effective communication). Think about the equal opportunities issues dealt with in Unit 3 – e.g. gender and cultural stereotyping – and make sure that your resources promote positive images.

Opportunities for monitoring and assessing individual children

Your activity will offer opportunities for observing how children use equipment, listen to any instructions, talk about what they are doing and interact with each other. At the end of an activity make a note about any aspects that presented difficulties, caused frustration or which were not sufficiently challenging. Make a note also of those in which the children were particularly successful. This helps staff to keep **records**, report **progress** to parents and to **plan** for individual children's future needs.

Evaluating your plan

As well as recording the points mentioned above in relation to the children you need to consider your own learning. You should try to judge how suitable your activity was and how it might be improved or altered. You can also reflect on your own ability to prepare, explain, support children and maintain behaviour. Refer to all the factors you had to consider and identify which ones 'worked' (were appropriate) and which ones were less successful.

For example: Would it have been more effective with thicker paint, coloured paper, fatter brushes? Did you allow enough/too much time? Was the cutting task too fiddly for the children to manage independently? – How could it have been improved? **Do not be too dismayed if an activity seems to be a disaster BUT make sure you understand WHY and what went wrong!**

Planning activities to meet children's needs

When deciding what activities and experiences will be offered to children, staff in a work setting must consider safety, space, children's ages and stage of development, supervision and availability of resources. Most work settings plan activities around well-chosen themes or topics. These are usually relevant to the children themselves and, perhaps, the time of year – common ones are *'Ourselves'*, *'Autumn'*, *'Festivals'* (*Christmas, Diwali, Hanukkah, Chinese New Year*), *'Growth'*, *'Nursery Rhymes'*.

An opportunity for a quiet activity

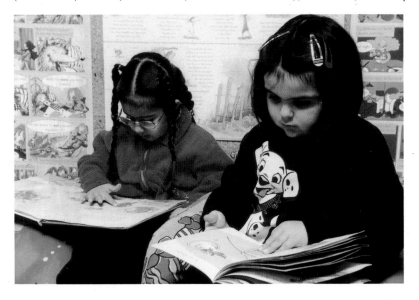

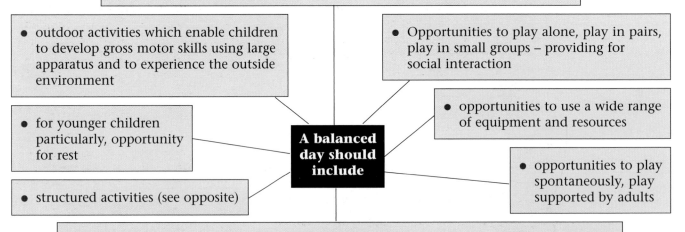

- indoor activities which enable children to – play quietly, play boisterously

- outdoor activities which enable children to develop gross motor skills using large apparatus and to experience the outside environment

- Opportunities to play alone, play in pairs, play in small groups – providing for social interaction

- opportunities to use a wide range of equipment and resources

- for younger children particularly, opportunity for rest

A balanced day should include

- opportunities to play spontaneously, play supported by adults

- structured activities (see opposite)

- some 'free-choice' activities (this usually involves the children making their own choice about which activity to do from those made available rather than their being able to choose 'anything' at all from the setting's resources. There may be some occasions when children are asked what equipment they would like to use)

Adult-led activities

These are planned, prepared and, often, initiated by adults. For example, a water activity might be planned which focuses particularly on 'force' or 'pressure'. The adult may have selected the equipment which lends itself to using water under pressure – squeezy bottles, thin plastic tubing, a water pump – and allowed children to use it in their own way, or, played alongside the children, talking about what was happening and questioning them so that they express their ideas.

Even when an activity is adult-led it should **always** involve active participation by the children. Activities which have an end-product (e.g. a model or a special occasion card) must allow for children's experimentation and creativity so that each one is different and original. There is absolutely **no value** in directing every aspect of a task. You should not aim to have all the children's work looking the same or 'perfect' (i.e. your idea of what the finished article should look like). **Ownership is very important; children need to feel that their work is their own.** What children learn from doing the activity – practical skills, understanding of materials, textures, sounds etc. is far more important than the finished article! Young children should choose whether or not to make a model, card etc.

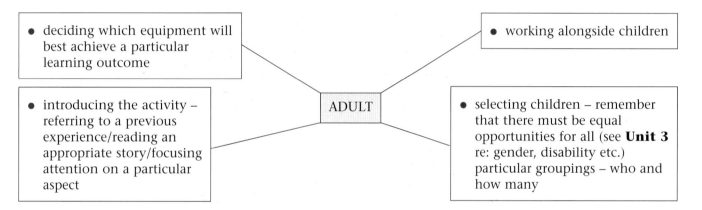

- deciding which equipment will best achieve a particular learning outcome
- introducing the activity – referring to a previous experience/reading an appropriate story/focusing attention on a particular aspect

ADULT

- working alongside children
- selecting children – remember that there must be equal opportunities for all (see **Unit 3** re: gender, disability etc.) particular groupings – who and how many

Child-initiated activities

These occur when children make their own decisions, without suggestion or guidance from adults, about the way in which they use the equipment and resources provided for them. For example, although an adult may have chosen which construction materials to set out – e.g. wooden blocks – two children may decide to work together to build a castle for 'small world' figures or 'play people'. This, then, is a child-initiated activity.

Structured activities

These should be carefully planned to develop a particular aspect of understanding or skill. They are structured in that there are resources, carefully chosen, and usually a sequence of tasks, or steps, which may lead to a desired learning outcome or objective. An adult usually leads, supervises and monitors children's responses.

Example: A simple sorting activity:

Aim – to find out if children can identify and sort all the blue objects from a selection of objects of different colours.

Ask the children individually to find something blue and put it in the sorting 'ring' with other blue things – this ensures that all children participate and enables the adult to find out if the child has understood the task and can carry it out. For this task the child has to know what 'blue' means and be able to distinguish objects of that colour from others. Some children may not realise that there are different shades of blue that are still 'blue'. Adults working with children on an activity such as this need to talk to them. Asking questions and enjoying a chat together helps adults check each child's understanding.

Spontaneous activities

These can be stimulated by natural events – a hailstorm, snow, a rainbow, puddles – or by an experience which a child has and wants to share with you – arrival of a new baby, a new pet, a birthday. The excitement generated by such occurrences makes the learning opportunities too good to let pass without capitalising on them. Planned activities can be set aside for another time in order to make the most of spontaneity. Other spontaneous activities arise when children make their own decisions about how they use the play equipment – perhaps arranging chairs to pretend they are travelling on a bus.

Offering a wide range of materials

We all need to practise skills to become competent but life would be boring and repetitive if we always had to do things in the same way. Children need to be given plenty of opportunities to practise their newly developing skills and to express their thoughts, feelings and ideas in different contexts.

A painting or drawing activity which will allow them to develop their fine manipulative skills can be varied by using:

❏ different quality paper – sugar, cartridge, 'newsprint', etc.

❏ paper of different colours

❏ different sizes of paper

❏ different **media** – pastels, wax crayons, colouring crayons, chalk etc.

❏ paint – ready-mixed, powder, thick, thin, fluorescent, pearlised etc.

❏ different techniques – finger, bubble, printing, marble-rolling, string etc.

While using such a variety the children are also learning about textures, which are appropriate materials to express an idea, colours and developing concepts about materials – how runny paint 'behaves', how chalk smudges etc. Other types of activity – construction, water, sand, small world, role play etc. – can easily be varied to broaden children's experience.

Adult role during an activity

The most obvious role is that of ensuring safety by supervising effectively. Regardless of age and setting there are always some activities which must be supervised. These include:

● cooking

● tasting

● activities involving living things

● those involving equipment which could be dangerous if wrongly used

● physical – particularly those involving climbing frames and/or gymnastic equipment

Another role is to **encourage children to try new things and to express their ideas. This involves the adult showing genuine interest in the children's activity and talking with children about the activity they are involved in.**

It is important that children experiment themselves, explore the materials and use them in creative ways rather than follow an adult's directions. Asking 'open' questions (see No.5 in 'effective communication' on page 162) encourages children to put their thoughts into words and the adult can extend their vocabulary by offering the new words in context and at the right time.

When to intervene

You **must** intervene when:

✱ children are likely to harm themselves;

✱ children could hurt others;

✱ there is a risk of damage to property or equipment;

✱ children are behaving unacceptably – e.g. showing discrimination by name-calling, physical aggression or spitefulness.

The important thing to remember is that children learn best by finding answers for themselves with encouragement and support.

The adult role is NOT to take control of the activity away from the children and 'do the difficult bits' for them.

An important aspect of the adult role is to encourage children to develop **self-reliance** and confidence in all that they do. Everyday routines help children to practise and improve **independence skills** such as dressing, eating, washing, tidying up etc.

Adults may choose to intervene when ...

- ... children become frustrated – offer support to help them through the difficult stage and move them on to the next step e.g. if they are having trouble joining two pieces of Lego assist them by calming them and then, perhaps, holding one piece firmly while they fit the other. DO NOT take both pieces and do it for them.

- ... play is becoming rough or too boisterous – sometimes just a look or a word will be enough to remind them of acceptable behaviour.

- ... children are losing interest – talk to them about the activity, ask questions which might prompt them to try something new or creative OR suggest they move to another activity.

- ... children deserve praise – for effort, acceptable behaviour, achievement.

- ... some children appear to be excluded from an activity – this may result from strong personalities 'taking over'. Just talking to the group and asking what each is doing may be enough to solve the problem.

- ... you notice the children are experimenting and you see an opportunity to develop their understanding e.g. rolling toy cars down a slope and talking about which one is fastest. Questioning – 'Why do you think the blue one reached the carpet first?' encourages them to express their ideas – they may be on the wrong track 'because it's blue' or they might think of a reason that could be tested 'because it has more wheels than the red one' or 'because its wheels are bigger'.

- ... children are experiencing difficulties – this may result in them losing concentration and not managing to persevere with what they are trying to do. A little encouragement and praise for their efforts can give them the confidence to try again.

SIGNPOST: unit two

1 (a) Write a paragraph to show your understanding of sensory development.
   (b) Write a paragraph to show your understanding of intellectual development.
   (c) Use the given list of activities to complete a table like the one below showing
       which age range they are suitable for and how they would help to promote
       sensory **and** intellectual development (remember some activities will appear in
       more than one box):

- sand play
- board game
- painting
- home play
- story telling
- water play
- listening game
- drawing

- dressing up
- poetry
- clay
- ring (or circle) game
- modelling
- drama activity/mime
- finger rhymes
- dough

- outdoor game
- music
- role-play
- songs
- natural materials play
- cooking

Age range	Activity	Aspect(s) of sensory development	Aspect(s) of intellectual development
1–2 years			
2–4 years	Cooking	Handling/smelling/tasting	Measuring; change in ingredients – mixing, heating; new words – names of tools and actions; descriptive
4–7 years			

2 (a) Choose **one** of the age ranges from the chart.
   (b) Select **3 of the listed activities** that you have identified for that age range.
   (c) For **each** of the 3 activities describe:
   - what equipment and resources you would provide;
   - the health and safety aspects you would need to consider;
   - how you would prepare your equipment and the immediate environment;
   - what the children will actually be doing and what experiences you want them
     to have;
   - what language you would want to encourage or introduce; for example, new
     vocabulary – names of objects and/or descriptive terms, such as hot/cold,
     wet/dry, etc.);
   - how you will provide for different cultural backgrounds;
   - how you will provide for children who have particular needs.

Emotional and Social Development

1   The sequence of emotional and social development
2   The development of independence, self-reliance and self-esteem
3   The effects of change and separation on children at different stages of development
4   The role of the adult in supporting children's emotional and social development
5   Children's behaviour

The sequence of emotional and social development

- factors which may affect emotional and social development
- encouraging children to recognise and deal with their strong feelings
- common stages of fear and anxiety amongst children

What is emotional and social development?

Emotional development involves:

✳ the ways in which children make sense of their feelings;

✳ the feelings children have towards other people, and

✳ the development of **self-image** and **identity**.

Social development involves:

✻ the growth of the children's relationships with other people;

✻ the development of social skills, and

✻ **socialisation**.

It is impossible to isolate emotional and social development from any other area of development: both these aspects of child development are firmly bound up with the other areas of physical, cognitive, language, spiritual and moral development.

Researchers into child development have formed theories to help us to understand the way children feel and how they interact with other people.

Theories about emotional and social development

There are two main approaches to the study of emotional and social development; these emphasise either:

Nature: this is the idea that personalities are fixed from the moment of birth. Main theories include Freud's psychodynamic theory, Erikson's stage theory and Bowlby's attachment theory.

Nurture: this is the idea that emotional and social behaviour is learnt. The main theory is Bandura's social learning theory.

Freud's psychodynamic theory of emotional development

Sigmund Freud (1856–1939) believed that there are three basic **personality** components; these he called:

- **id**: this is the primitive, impulsive part of the personality which works on what Freud described as the **pleasure principle**, that is to say, it seeks to obtain pleasure and avoid pain. The id is mainly concerned with survival and with things that give pleasure, such as food, shelter, comfort and avoidance of pain. In the newborn infant, all mental processes are **id** impulses.

- **ego**: As the child grows older, reality intervenes and the ego develops. The ego is the part of the mind which operates according to the **reality principle**, trying to balance the demands of the unconscious with what is possible or practical. The ego is rational and logical and allows the child to learn that negotiating, asking and explaining is a more effective way of satisfying demands than through the id's 'I want'. For example, the young child learns that hunger will only be satisfied when someone is available to provide food.

- **superego**: At around the age of 4 to 6 years, the child comes into contact with authority, and the **superego** emerges. This is the part of the **unconscious** mind which acts as society, or as a strict parent, and involves ideas of duty, obligation and conscience. The superego relies on the **morality principle**, acting as a censor and conscience by telling us what is right and wrong.

Freud described four stages of psychosexual development in children; he called these the oral stage, the anal stage, the phallic stage and the latency stage.

Stage	Area of physical pleasure	Influence on child care practice
Oral (0–1 year)	Mouth: Babies put things into their mouths and suck them	If babies are weaned too early from either the breast or bottle, Freud believed they would become fixated at this stage
Anal (1–3 years)	Anus: Children show pleasure in having control over their bowel movements	If there is too much emphasis on early potty training, Freud believed they would become fixated at this stage. Freud believed that children at this stage need to identify with the same gender parent
Phallic (3–6 years)	Genitals: Children develop an interest in their genitals and are aware of their own and others' gender	If children are not allowed to explore their own bodies, they may become fixated at this stage
Latency (6–12 years)	No specific area: Children tend to play with members of the same sex and often develop 'crushes' on same-sex adults	Freud saw this stage as a period of calm, when sexual energy is channelled into learning new skills. He did not believe that fixation occurred in this stage

Table 3.1 A summary of Freud's psychosexual stages

Freud believed that if children are not allowed sufficient time to experience the pleasure at each stage and move successfully on, then their personalities may become fixated.

Examples of the effect of fixation: Someone who has been rushed through the oral stage may show behaviour as an adult such as smoking, nail-biting or over-eating. If rushed through the anal stage, adult behaviour may include being anal-retentive, i.e. overly concerned with tidiness, orderliness and cleanliness.

Freud has been criticised for stating that all the main outlines of human personality are the result of experiences within the family before the age of four years.

Erikson's stage theory of psychosocial development

Erik Erikson (1902–1994) was influenced by Freud and also described definite stages that children pass through. However, he believed that children's personalities continue to develop and change right up to old age. He outlined eight stages of development, each of which is dominated by a crisis or conflict which has to be resolved. The stages relating to child development are summarised in Table 3.2 on page 191.

Stage 1: the first year of life

The psychosocial crisis at this stage is to gain a balance between trusting people and risking being let down, or being mistrustful and therefore suspicious of others. (This corresponds to Freud's oral stage.) If the mother or principal caregiver meets the baby's needs for hunger and comfort, then the baby will learn to trust. Erikson is not saying that there should be total trust, as the child needs to develop a healthy mistrust to learn about dangerous situations.

Favourable outcome: hopes for the future and trust in the environment.

Unfavourable outcome: fear of the future, insecurity and suspicion.

Stage 2: the second year of life

As children develop physically and experience wider choices, they need to assert their independence. (This stage corresponds to Freud's anal stage.) The child needs to be carefully guided by their parents and not made to feel ridiculous or a failure if their efforts towards independence are thwarted – e.g. in toilet training or in feeding themselves. Again, there needs to be a balance between **autonomy** and **doubt**, as the child needs to know which sorts of behaviour are socially acceptable and safe.

Favourable outcome: a sense of independence and self-esteem.

Unfavourable outcome: a feeling of shame, and doubt about one's own capacity for self-control.

Stage 3: 3 to 5 years

As they develop and master their physical skills, children learn to initiate their own activities and to engage in purposeful activity. (This stage relates to Freud's phallic stage.) Children begin to recognise the differences between the sexes, and will express a desire to marry the opposite-sex parent. Children will enjoy their accomplishments and try out their new intellectual and creative abilities. Parents and caregivers may perceive the child's use of initiative as aggression or forcefulness and seek to restrict and punish the child. The child will then feel guilt and will be inhibited in their creativity and use of initiative. There needs to be some sense of guilt, however, since without it there will be no conscience or self-control.

Favourable outcome: the ability to initiate activities and to enjoy carrying them out.

Unfavourable outcome: guilt about one's own feelings, and fear of being punished.

Stage 4: 6 years to puberty

This stage is centred around school and the learning of skills. (It corresponds to Freud's latency stage.) Children need to become competent in certain areas that are important within the school context and valued by adults and peers, e.g. reading and early mathematics. If they are continually rejected and criticised by their teachers, parents or peers, then they will feel **inferior** and have a sense of failure. However, if they are praised and encouraged in their achievements, they will be spurred on to further **industry**. Again, there needs to be a balance here as too much emphasis on competence leads to a 'hot-house' approach to schooling: some failure is necessary so that the child can develop some humility.

Favourable outcome: confidence in one's own ability to make and do things; a sense of achievement.

Unfavourable outcome: feelings of inferiority and inadequacy resulting from unfavourable reactions from others.

Age and stage	Effect on emotional and social development	Influence on child care practice
0–1 year **Basic trust/ mistrust**	**Optimism:** The child's main relationship is with the principal caregiver (usually the mother). Children need love and consistency of care in order to learn how to trust	Babies should not be left to cry; they need to feel loved and to know that their needs will be met
1–2 years **Autonomy/ shame**	**Independence and self-esteem:** The child's main relationship is with the parents. They need to be encouraged to be independent and to feel good about themselves	Children should be encouraged to be independent and not made to feel ridiculous if they 'fail' in their efforts
3–5 years **Initiative/guilt**	**Use of initiative:** The child's main relationship is with the family. Children need to be encouraged to explore their environment and to use their initiative	Children should be encouraged to express themselves and their sense of purpose should be fostered
6–puberty **Industry/ inferiority**	**Competence:** The child's main relationship is with the neighbourhood and school. Children need to be praised and rewarded when they achieve something and not to be rejected or criticised	Children should not be compared with other children in case they are made to feel inferior. Praise and encouragement will lead the child to try even harder

Table 3.2   A summary of Erikson's first four stages of psychosocial development

Erikson's theory when applied to child development has been criticised as not applying universally to people in different cultures and societies. For example, stage 4, industry vs. inferiority, may only be applicable to cultures such as ours, which emphasise competitiveness and which disapprove of children who do not succeed at the appropriate times.

Bowlby's theory of attachment

John Bowlby (1907–90) used many of the ideas from psychodynamics (e.g. Freud's theory) to form his basic theory. However, he also believed that the psychodynamic approach put too much emphasis on the child's fantasy world and not nearly enough on actual events.

The main principles of Bowlby's theory are that:

❏ children need a **close continuous relationship** with their mothers for successful personality development;

❏ the child must form an **attachment** by about 6 months of age; after that and until the age of 3 children strongly need to be close by their mothers;

❏ any obstacle to forming an attachment – and any disruption of the relationship constitutes **maternal deprivation**.

Secure attachment and continuous relationships are far more likely to be provided within the child's natural family than anywhere else.

Bowlby did not say that the most important attachment figure must be the natural mother. He did stress, however, that babies need one central person who is the 'mother figure'.

Bowlby's theory has been criticised for placing too much emphasis on the mother's role as primary caregiver; what is important for children is that there is familiarity, trust and continuity in their first relationships. It is now accepted that babies and young children can form several close attachments, and that it is only when such close relationships are broken that emotional damage results.

The influence of Bowlby's theory on child care practice

Bowlby's research had an enormous impact on the delivery of care both to mothers in post-natal wards and to children in institutions. Above all, his theory led to further research and highlighted the importance of meeting children's emotional needs as well as their physical and intellectual needs. Some of the changes made in response to his theory of attachment were:

- Babies are kept with their mothers after birth when at all possible.
- Parents are helped to look after their newborn babies in special care baby units.
- Children are allowed to visit their parents in hospital.
- Parents are encouraged to stay overnight when their children are in hospital, and to participate in their care.
- Parents are encouraged to stay and help to settle their children in nurseries and playgroups before leaving them.
- Children in many day nurseries and in residential care have a key worker assigned to them; this means that one person is responsible for their care when at the nursery and so becomes another attachment figure.

Social learning theory

Albert Bandura (1925–) is a social psychologist who developed the social learning theory. This theory emphasises that children learn about social behaviour by:

❏ watching other people;

❏ imitating other people.

Children are more likely to imitate people who are:

❏ warm and loving towards them;

❏ seen as powerful or competent;

❏ seen as receiving rewards for their behaviour;

❏ who are most similar to themselves e.g. the same gender.

From as early as one hour old, a baby will imitate an adult's gestures. If the baby is held in front of her mother and the mother pulls her tongue in and out, the newborn baby will almost always respond by moving her own tongue in and out.

Imitating behaviour

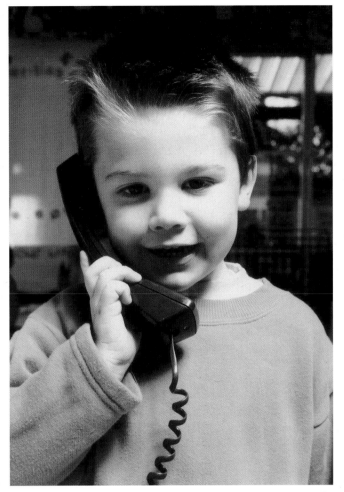

The poem on page 259 is a good example of the different ways in which children learn social behaviour. Social learning theory emphasises the important influence you will exert on the children in your care and has shaped child care practice with the following principles:

- If children are smacked by adults, they are likely to hit other children.

- If children are shouted at by adults, they are likely to shout at others.

- If children are given explanations, they will try to explain things too.

- If children are comforted when they fall, they will learn to do the same to others.

Social learning theory has been criticised for not recognising that whilst children do imitate adult behaviour, they also experiment with different ways of doing things themselves.

Stages and sequence of emotional and social development

The way in which children develop emotionally and socially is closely linked to the ways in which they develop physically and intellectually. Babies have feelings and emotions from the moment they are born. As children develop more awareness of themselves, they can be helped to become more aware of how other people feel. You need to know the stages of emotional and social development which children pass through in order to promote children's development. However these stages are only a rough guide as every child will develop in his or her own unique way.

Mother and baby smiling at each other

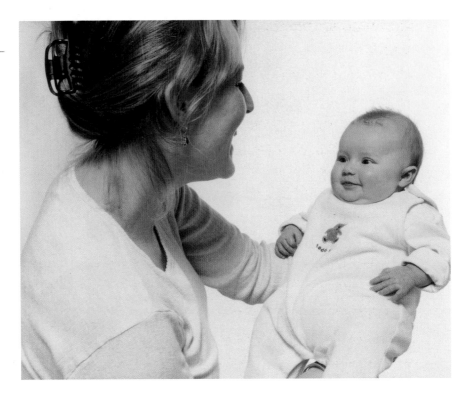

Birth to one month

Babies:

✱ use total body movements to express pleasure at bathtime or when being fed; i.e. they move their arms and legs and squirm with pleasure;

✱ enjoy feeding and cuddling;

✱ often imitate facial expressions.

At around one month old

Babies:

✳ smile in response to adult;

✳ are beginning to show a particular temperament e.g. placid or excitable;

✳ enjoy sucking;

✳ turn to regard nearby speaker's face.

At around three months

Babies:

✱ show enjoyment at caring routines such as bath-time;

✱ respond with obvious pleasure to loving attention and cuddles;

✱ fix their eyes unblinkingly on the carer's face when feeding;

✱ stay awake for longer periods of time (70% of babies sleep through the night);

✱ smile at familiar people and at strangers.

At around six months

Babies:

✷ manage to feed themselves using their fingers;

✷ offer toys to others;

✷ are more wary of strangers;

✷ show distress when their mother leaves;

✷ are more aware of other people's feelings. They cry if a sister cries, for example, and laugh with others.

At around one year

Babies:

✷ are emotionally labile; that is, they are likely to have fluctuating moods;

✷ often want a comfort object, such as a teddy or a piece of cloth;

✷ are still shy with strangers;

✷ are affectionate to familiar people;

✷ enjoy socialising at mealtimes, joining in conversations while mastering the task of self-feeding;

✷ help with daily routines, such as getting washed and dressed.

✷ play pat-a-cake and wave good-bye, both spontaneously and on request.

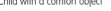

Child with a comfort object

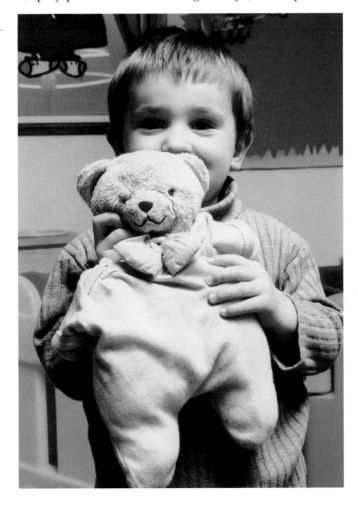

At around fifteen months

Babies:

* repeatedly throw objects to the floor in play or rejection (this is known as casting);

* watch where objects fall and seek out a hidden toy;

* carry dolls or teddies by limbs, hair or clothing.

At around eighteen months

Children:

* play contentedly alone, but prefer to be near a familiar adult or sibling;

* are eager to be independent, e.g. to dress themselves ('Me do it!');

* are aware that others are fearful or anxious for them as they climb on or off chairs, etc;

* alternate between clinging and resistance;

* may become easily frustrated, with occasional temper tantrums;

* show a marked sense of personal identity;

* can follow stories and love repetition;

At around two years

Children:

* are beginning to express how they feel;

* are impulsive and curious about their environment;

* may be clingy and dependent at times, or self-reliant and independent;

* often feel frustrated when unable to express themselves; about half of 2-year-old children have tantrums on a more or less daily basis;

* can dress themselves and go to the toilet independently; but they may need sensitive help with pulling their pants up;

* often like to help others but not when helping conflicts with their own desires;

* play alongside other children but not with them (parallel play).

At around 2½ years

Children:

* may be dry through the night, although there is wide variation;

* are emotionally still very dependent on an adult;

* play more with other children but may not share their toys with them.

At around three years

Children:

* like to do things unaided;

* can think about things from someone else's point of view;

* show affection for younger siblings;

✷ manage to use the lavatory independently, and are often dry through the night (this is very variable);

✷ enjoy helping adults e.g. tidying up;

✷ are willing to share toys with other children and are beginning to take turns when playing;

✷ often develop fears e.g. of the dark, as they become capable of pretending and imagining;

✷ are becoming aware of being male or female (developing a gender role);

✷ make friends and are interested in having friends.

At around four years

Children:

✷ wash and dry their hands and brush their teeth;

✷ can undress and dress themselves except for laces, ties and back buttons;

✷ often show sensitivity to others;

✷ show a sense of humour in both talk and activities;

✷ like to be independent and are strongly self-willed;

✷ like to be with other children.

Feeling a sense of achievement

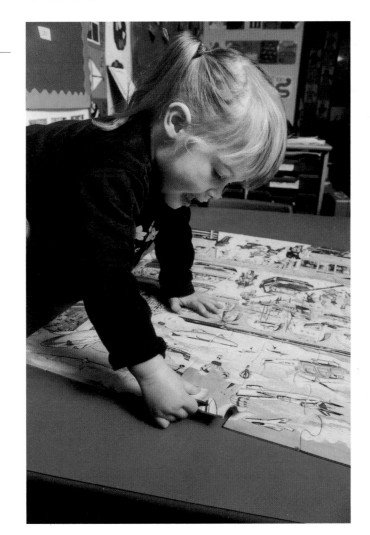

At around five years

Children:

✱ dress and undress alone, but may have difficulty with shoe laces;

✱ have very definite likes and dislikes;

✱ are able to amuse themselves for longer periods of time, looking at a book or watching a video;

✱ show sympathy and comfort friends who are hurt;

✱ enjoy caring for pets;

✱ choose their own friends.

At around six years

Children:

✱ can carry out simple tasks: e.g. peel vegetables, water plants, hang up clothes and tidy contents of drawers;

✱ choose friends mainly because of their personality and interests;

✱ begin to compare themselves with other people: e.g. 'I am like her in that way, but different in this way . . .'

✱ enjoy playing games with other children.

Showing independence

At around seven years

Children:

* learn how to control their emotions; they realise that they can keep their own thoughts private and hide their true feelings;

* begin to think in terms not only of who they are, but also of who they would like to be;

* are completely independent in washing, dressing and toileting skills;

* form friendships which are very important to them;

* form close friends mostly within their own sex;

* have a clear sense of right and wrong; for example, they realise that it is wrong to hurt other people physically.

✏ ACTIVITY

A predictable environment

In groups, discuss the ways in which your nursery or school organises the day. What regular routines are there? How do staff members ensure that children know what is expected of them – for example, before meal times and painting activities?

Children enjoying a meal together

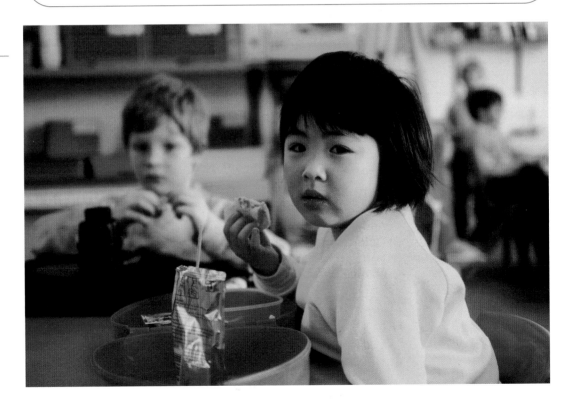

Factors affecting emotional and social development

There are many factors which affect emotional and social development in childhood. These include:

- **Genetic factors:** There are many genetic disorders which influence development. *Examples:*
  - > Children with **Down's syndrome** often have learning difficulties which can affect their understanding and their ability to communicate with others.
  - > Children with **autism** often have difficulties in forming relationships with others.

- **Physical factors:** Physical health and well-being also influences the development of self-image and socialisation. *Examples:*
  - > Poor nutrition and lack of sleep will cause a lack of energy and may result in aggressive behaviour and an inability to form relationships.
  - > Hearing impairment (even the temporary condition known as **'glue ear'**) can lead to a child lacking confidence and motivation.

- **Economic and environmental factors:** Poverty and poor housing conditions may affect children's feelings of self-esteem. *Examples:*
  - > Children who live in over-crowded homes or in temporary bed and breakfast accommodation may have fewer opportunities to play with other children and may feel isolated because they see themselves as different.
  - > Children whose family are travellers might not stay in one area long enough to form friendships.

- **Cultural and social factors:** Cultural differences may affect children's self-image and their social relationships. *Examples:*
  - > Children from a minority group may not be provided with positive role models within the wider community of nursery and school; the feelings of being different from others can lead to poor self-esteem and difficulties in making friends.
  - > Children who lack a stable relationship with their parents or primary carers will find it hard to form relationships with other adults within care and education settings.

- **Emotional factors:** Difficulties in forming attachments in early childhood and the effects of bereavement or of abuse may result in poor self-esteem and lack of confidence. *Example:*
  - > Children may experience feelings of loss when a new baby brother or sister is born. From being the only child within the family, the child has to adjust to a change in status and may feel a need to compete for parents' time and affection.

The development of independence, self-reliance and self-esteem

- why the development of independence, self-reliance and self-esteem is important
- the role of the key worker
- the role of play and other activites in developing independence, self-reliance and self-esteem
- environments which encourage the development of healthy emotional and social growth
- encouraging a positive identity for children and their families
- encouraging and supporting parents

What is self-image?

Our self-image is how we think about ourselves and involves developing a sense of identity.

Children develop a self-image (or self-concept) during their first year of life and this becomes more stable as they develop socially. Developing a sense of identity is about:

realising you exist: babies gradually begin to understand that they are separate from their parents; for example, when they explore their own bodies by grasping their hands and feet, their feelings are different from when they are being closely held by their parents;

who you are: later on during the first year of life babies learn to respond to their own name and to understand that the people around them are separate and different from them;

developing *self-esteem* (or self-worth): even before a child can understand spoken words, parents and caregivers can show approval, disappointment, anger or pleasure by the tone of voice, facial expressions and general body language;

a positive self-image: when babies begin to move about, they will keep looking at the adult who is caring for them; this is called social referencing. Developing a positive self-image depends very much on the reactions from adults towards them; children need to be encouraged to feel self-confident, by receiving unconditional love and encouragement;

learning to like and respect yourself: children need to feel valued and respected in order to develop these feelings about themselves;

developing skills of caring for and looking after yourself: between the age of 2 and 3 years, children develop independence; with their increasing physical skills, they are able to dress themselves, to wash their hands and to take care of their own toileting. These skills enhance their feelings of self-worth and confidence.

Self-image and children with special needs

People are often embarrassed when they meet a disabled person, mainly because they are 'different', but also because they feel they don't know enough about the particular disability. They are afraid that they might do or say the wrong thing. Because of this embarrassment and ignorance, disabled children have to come to terms with:

☐ their disability, and

☐ the way other people react to it.

Children with special needs need **positive role models**. You can help to improve their self-image by:

- involving disabled adults in the early childhood setting;

- carefully selecting books and activities that promote a positive self-image for disabled children – in the same way that using multicultural resources promotes a positive self-image for minority ethnic groups;

- improving your communication skills and being a good role model.

Developing self-esteem

The way we feel about ourselves leads to good or poor **self-esteem**. Our self-esteem is greatly influenced by how other people make us feel. Good self-esteem leads to a good self-image, increased self-confidence and a strong sense of identity.

The development of social and self-help skills

As early as 6 months of age, babies enjoy each other's company. When they are together, they look at each other, smile and touch each other's faces. As their social circle widens they learn how to co-operate with each other when they play and they begin to make friends.

Children need to develop certain social skills (or ways of behaving) in order to fit in – and to get on well – with the people around them. These social skills include:

✱ being able to understand how others feel;

✱ knowing how to share and to take turns;

✱ accepting rules and social codes of politeness;

✱ behaving in a way that is appropriate to the people they are with.

Children also need to learn **self-help skills**. These skills include:

✱ being able to wash their hands;

✱ being able to dress themselves;

✱ being able to brush their hair;

✱ being able to pour drinks and to feed themselves.

3

The effects of change and separation on children at different stages of development

- the child's need to feel secure
- effect of separation or change on behaviour
- recognising signs of distress in a child and how to reassure them
- supporting parents and ensuring good communication
- the 'settling-in' policy of the work setting and the reasons for it
- preparing children and adults in the setting to receive newcomers

Separation from primary carers and moving on

So many of the times that are difficult for children have to do with separation. Going to bed is separation and is often a source of anxiety in children. Some young children can be terrified as a parent walks out of the room. How children react to separation is as varied as children are themselves. For some children each new situation will bring questions and new feelings of anxiety. Other children love the challenge of meeting new friends and seeing new things.

The effects of multiple transitions

Children who have had to make many moves or changes may feel a sense of loss and grief. These changes may have a profound effect on their emotional and social development. Reasons for transitions include:

✽ Children whose parents have separated or divorced; children may have to live and get along with several 'new' people, e.g. stepfathers, stepmothers, half-brothers and sisters etc.

✽ Children who experience many different child care arrangements; e.g. frequent changes from one nanny or childminder to another.

✽ Children who are in local authority care – either in residential children's homes or in foster care.

✽ Children whose families have moved several times, e.g. for employment reasons, or as travellers.

Children who have experienced multiple transitions need to feel supported each time they enter a new setting. They may feel:

- **Disorientated:** no sooner have they settled in one place and got to know a carer, they may be uprooted and have to face the same process again.

- **A sense of loss:** Each time they make a move they lose the friends they have made and also the attachments they have formed with their carers.

- **Withdrawn:** Children may withdraw from new relationships with other children and with carers, because they do not trust the separation not to happen again.

How you can help children to settle in

The first few days at a nursery or playgroup can be very daunting for some children. They may not have been left by their parents or primary carers ever before and some children will show real distress. You need to be able to recognise their distress and to find ways of dealing with it. Children show their distress at being separated from their carer by crying and refusing to join in with activities. Parents too can feel distressed when leaving their children in the care of others; they may feel guilty because they have to return to work, or they may be upset because they have never before been separated from their child.

You can help by:

☐ **Trying to plan for the separation:** Nursery staff can help by visiting the child and their parents at home. This gives both parents and children the opportunity to talk about their fears and help them to cope with them. When children know in advance what's going to happen and not happen they can think about and get used to their feelings about it. Parents can be encouraged to prepare their child for the change by:
  > visiting the nursery with their child so that they can meet the staff;
  > reading books about starting at a nursery or going to hospital, and
  > involving their child in any preparation, such as buying clothing or packing a 'nursery bag'.

☐ **Encouraging parents to stay with their child until the child asks them to leave.** This does not mean that the parents should cling to their child. Children can always sense a parent's uncertainty. Although young children do not have a very good sense of time, parents and carers should make it very clear when they will be back, e.g. saying 'I'll be back in one hour.'

☐ **Allowing the child to bring a comforter**, e.g. a blanket or a teddy bear, to the nursery. If it is a blanket, sometimes the parent can cut a little piece and put it in the child's pocket if they think there will be any embarrassment. Then the child can handle the blanket and feel comforted when feeling lonely.

☐ **Having just one person to settle the child:** hold and cuddle the child and try to involve him or her in a quiet activity with you, e.g. reading a story. Most child care settings now employ a key worker who will be responsible for one or two children during the settling-in period.

☐ **Contacting the parent or primary carer** if the child does not settle within 20 minutes or so. Sometimes it is not possible to do this, and you will need to devise strategies for comforting and reassuring the child. Always be honest with parents regarding the time it took to settle their child.

✏ ACTIVITY

Helping children to settle in

This activity will help a child who is new to the setting to realize that he or she is not alone, and that other children also feel shy and alone at times.

- **Introduction:** Choose a teddy and introduce him to the group, saying something like: 'Teddy is rather shy and a little bit lonely. How can we help him to feel better?'

- **Discussion and display:** Take photos of teddy – using a digital camera if possible – with different groups of children, and in different places in the nursery, e.g. playing in the sand, reading a book, doing a puzzle, etc., and use later for discussion and display.

- **Circle time:** In circle time, pass teddy round, and encourage each child to say something to him: 'Hello Teddy, my name is Lara' or 'Hello Teddy, I like chocolate . . .',etc.

- **Taking teddy home:** Each child takes it in turns to take teddy home. Include a notebook and encourage parents to write a few sentences about what teddy did at their house that evening. The children can draw a picture.

- **Story time:** Read and act out the story of Goldilocks and the Three Bears, with the different sized bowls, beds, and chairs.

- **Cooking:** Use a shaped cutter to make teddy-shaped biscuits or dough teddies.

- **Teddy bears picnic:** Arrange a teddy bears picnic where each child brings in a favourite bear.

What does your teddy like to eat? Are there enough plates, biscuits and cups for all the bears?

You can probably think of many more teddy-related ideas that will help children to gain a sense of belonging.

Separating from a parent at a nursery

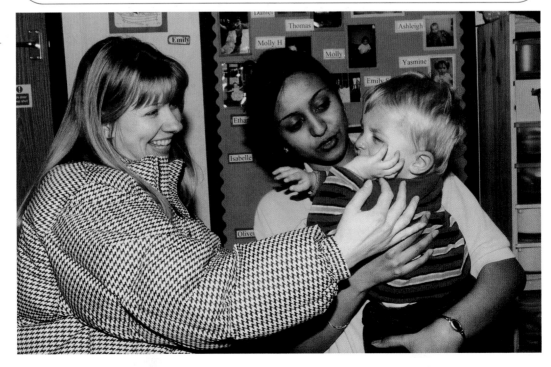

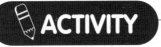

ACTIVITY

In your work placement, plan to observe an individual child's social needs during a whole session. Make a checklist which includes the following needs:

- Interaction with other children: observe how the child plays, e.g. does he or she play alone (solitary play), alongside others but not with them (parallel play) or actively with other children.

- Attention from adults: does the child seek attention from one particular adult, or from any adult? Note the number of occasions a child seeks adult attention and describe the interaction.

- Self-help skills and independence: observe the child using self-help skills, e.g. putting on coat to go outside, washing hands and going to the lavatory.

Identify the stage of social development the child is passing through and list the ways in which you can ensure that their social needs are met within the setting.

Solitary play

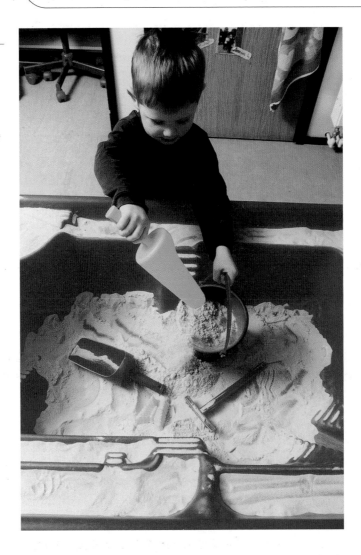

4

The role of the adult in supporting children's emotional and social development

- your role and that of others
- confidentiality in the work setting
- having respect for the individual child
- involving parents
- the importance of remaining calm when dealing with children who are upset

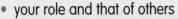 Your role and that of others

Encouraging children to recognise and deal with their strong feelings

Children feel things deeply. Feelings are hard to manage, even when we are adults. Feelings can quickly overwhelm the child and may lead to:

- sobbing and sadness;
- temper tantrums that are full of anger and rage;
- jealousy that makes a child want to hit out and hurt someone else;
- a joy that makes a child actually jump and leap with a wildness that is unnerving to many adults.

Anger

Some children become aggressive when they feel angry. They tend to be noisy and disrupt other children in their play. To help children cope with feelings of anger, you could:

☐ move the child away from the situation if necessary;

☐ try to distract the child by offering another activity;

☐ give word to the feelings; try to put into words what you think the child may be feeling, e.g. 'I know you are angry because Petra took your truck, but pinching hurts and Petra is very upset now';

☐ stay calm: don't lose your temper with the child;

☐ when the child has succeeded in overcoming feelings of anger, offer a few words of praise, which shows you understood effort made;

provide activities which will help children to express their feelings. These include:
> using malleable materials, such as dough, clay and play dough
> reading books and stories which feature children who have strong feelings of jealousy or fear;
> providing music sessions using instruments such as drums, tambourines and bells;
> encouraging children to express their feelings through drawing and painting;
> using role play in the home corner to help children to act out their feelings of frustration.

Helping children with feelings of loss and grief

When someone whom a child loves is no longer around, it may seem to the child that the person has died. This can happen when a family experiences:

☐ a mother leaving home and going to hospital to have a new baby;

☐ divorce or separation – when one parent no longer sees the child;

☐ a parent being in hospital and unable to see the child, for example, after a serious accident;

☐ a loved one who has been sent to prison;

☐ a loved one who goes abroad;

☐ the death of a loved one.

Children will go through a process of **grieving**. This process involves:

☐ feeling disbelief, numbness, shock and panic;

☐ despair and anger, and yearning for the lost person;

☐ more interest in life again eventually – but this takes time.

You can help children who are experiencing feelings of loss and grief by:

✓ explaining things in simple terms; children need to understand the reality of the situation;

✓ making sure that children do not feel that what has happened is their fault;

✓ reassuring children that it is alright to feel this way; that these feelings are normal and will eventually be less painful;

✓ being especially warm and loving – cuddle children and just be there for them;

✓ not demanding too much of children; be prepared for them to regress in their behaviour. Gently encourage children when they begin to show an interest in things once more;

✓ finding out about **play therapy** and arranging for help of this kind;

✓ making sure that children are not excluded from the rituals surrounding death; for example, let children attend the funeral, visit the grave and share the sadness;

✓ using photographs to evoke memories of the loved person.

As well as helping children in their expression of grief, we need to remember that parents also need our support.

✏ ACTIVITY

Plan and implement an activity which will allow children to express their feelings. One idea is to make some play dough and encourage them to pummel and roll the dough on a board or table. Try making the play dough recipe below as it lasts well when stored in a plastic bag or box in the fridge and it is a good texture for young children to handle.

Play dough recipe

- 1 cup of water
- 1 tablespoon of oil
- 1 heaped cup of plain flour
- 1 cup of salt
- 2 teaspoons of cream of tartar
- food colouring as required

1 Mix the water, oil and a few drops of food colouring into a pan and gently heat.

2 Add the rest of the ingredients and stir.

3 The dough will start to form and lift away from the pan.

4 Remove it from the pan and leave it to cool.

(Let children help with the measuring but take extreme care to keep the hot saucepan away from their reach.)

Allow children to handle the dough freely at first to explore the possibilities and to express their feelings. Then you could provide a variety of tools for play cooking, for example: shape cutters, a rolling pin, plastic knives, a spatula, and some small plastic bowls and plates.

Evaluate the activity in terms of how effective it was in allowing children to express their feelings.

How you can encourage children to have good self-esteem

Value children for who they are, not what they do or what they look like, or what you want them to be. Children need love, security and a feeling of trust. There is no one best way to give these feelings to children, as each child is unique and is strongly influenced by family and cultural background.

- Provide children with positive images about themselves – in terms of skin colour, language, disability, principal features, culture, economic background. Make sure that the book area and displays on the walls provide positive images for all children.

- Welcome parents and other family members to the nursery. Children need to feel that they belong and that their family background is valued.

- Provide children with positive role models. Adults who have a positive self-image help to encourage a child's self-esteem; visitors to the nursery or school can widen children's experiences of the roles adults occupy, e.g. men working in child care or women mending pieces of equipment.

- Show that you appreciate the efforts that children make. Children do not have to achieve perfect results – the effort is more important. Avoid having unrealistic expectations about what children can manage, for example, dressing, eating, going to the lavatory.

- Encourage children. When children make mistakes, don't tell them they are silly or stupid, but instead say something like 'Never mind, let's pick up the pieces and put them in the bin. Next time, if you hold it with two hands it will be easier to work with', and so on.

- Offer children the opportunity to make choices and decisions about what they do, keeping in mind the need for safety and consideration for others.

- Provide clear, consistent boundaries. Children need to know what is expected of them and what is not allowed; otherwise they become confused and begin to test out the boundaries to see what is consistent about them.

- Provide children with a predictable environment so that they can feel that there is a shape to the day. There is no need to stick rigidly to routines, but children gain in confidence if they are able to take part in routine activities, such as helping to set the table or to go to the lavatory before washing their hands.

- Always talk politely and respectfully to children, to their parents and to other members of staff. Children need first to be given respect before they can feel self-respect.

- Provide a stable environment in which there is consistency of care. Many nurseries have now introduced a **key worker** or family worker system which helps the child to be cared for by someone they know. (See page 350 for role of the key worker)

- Show interest in what children do. Develop the skill of being a good listener so that children feel encouraged to express themselves.

- Children who do not form a strong attachment with their parents are known to have poor self-esteem and may have difficulties relating to others. This could be because:
  > the parents have not themselves experienced strong attachments
  > of separation or bereavement.

✏️ ACTIVITY

Plan and implement an activity which encourages a child's self-reliance and self-esteem. One idea would be to use a 'fastenings' activity. Before starting the activity with a child or with a small group of children in a nursery setting, talk to them about how we fasten our clothes. Encourage them to talk about popper studs, zips, laces and velcro fastenings. Ask them which they find easiest and most difficult etc.? Then explain the idea of the fastenings board and encourage them to continue talking about clothes as they take it in turns to have a go.

1   Provide the child with a fabric board on which there is a variety of fastenings: popper studs, zips, laces, velcro tabs etc.

2   Encourage the child to try to fasten the various objects, offering praise for effort as well as for achievement.

3   Evaluate the activity in terms of how it met the needs of the child, and how enjoyable it was.

How to encourage the development of social and self-help skills

Many of the skills outlined above are learnt through children copying adult behaviour. You could use the following guidelines to help to encourage these skills in the nursery or school.

✓ **Encourage children to work and to play together:** Some children will need a lot of support in learning how to join in with others. You can help children to join in with others by suggesting that they copy what the other children are doing. A child asking to join in may meet with a firm 'No', but by simply starting to do the same thing, they will often be allowed to join in.

✓ **Give children choices:** Children should not always feel that they have to do what an adult suggests. Let children choose who they want to be with and what they want to do for the greater part of the day.

✓ **Make sure that children have one-to-one individual attention:** Some children feel pressure from always being in a group setting. It is important they feel that they have enough attention and time to talk without this pressure. You could try reading them a one-to-one story, for example.

✓ **Allow children personal space:** They need to be able to do things on their own without interruptions or pressure from anyone else.

✓ **Deal sensitively with any difficulties:** Children need to feel that they can talk to you, and that you will listen to them when they are experiencing difficulties.

✓ **Keep good observations of all children's social relationships:** You are in an ideal position to observe and make note of any changes in a child's social behaviour. For example, if a child who is normally outgoing and sociable suddenly becomes quiet and withdrawn, you need to report this change to the team and the parents will need to be involved in any further discussion.

✓ **Provide activities that are appropriate to the children's stage of social development:** Children in a nursery setting are still learning to share and take turns when playing together; they may enjoy activities such as playing with dough, water or sand. Older children usually enjoy being involved in group activities – such as story time and circle time. Group time is an opportunity for children to share their experiences and feelings with other children in a controlled group setting.

✓ **Be guided by a child's personality:** remember that each child is unique; what helps one child might not help another. You can help children to express and deal with their feelings positively by showing that you value them for who they are, not what you would like them to be.

✓ **Be a team member:** Discuss the policies within your workplace. Find out what is considered acceptable behaviour and always be willing to discuss any concerns you have about an individual child's behaviour.

✓ **Always appreciate and praise children for their efforts, not just for their achievements:** Children need to feel that you appreciate their efforts and that you value them for who they are. You can help them to feel valued by displaying any items they have made. You should also praise them when they have been helpful, kind or generous towards others.

✓ **Help children to develop self-help skills:** If you notice that children are having difficulty with, for example, washing and drying their hands, you could devise a way of helping them to accomplish the task by going with them to the basin and demonstrating how it is done. Remember that children learn quickly when they see an action for themselves.

Activity	How it promotes emotional and social development
Play dough, soft clay Pummelling, kneading, squeezing, shaping and punching	Children are encouraged to express their feelings and to feel a sense of control; for example, frustration can be expressed through punching and squeezing the dough
Role play Games of make-believe, pretending to be a doctor, parent or superhero	Children start to form their own identity. They can express their feelings freely and display caring and social skills in a safe environment
Dressing up	Choosing which clothes to wear promotes independence, and respect for their own and other cultures
Sand play and gardening Digging, shaping, sharing toys; planting, raking and watering	Children gain a sense of control by making towers, castles and 'building sites' and learn how to play co-operatively with others
Water play Pouring, measuring; swimming	Children feel in control and can express their imagination; swimming gives a sense of freedom and mastery of a new skill
Drawing and painting	Choosing what to draw, what colours to use, etc., gives children a sense of control. Children often express their feelings by, for example, painting an angry or a sad face
Music Drums, bells, rattles, tambourines and songs	Children can release feelings of tension or frustration. They also learn how to share and to take turns in musical games instruments
Reading stories and making books Individual or group activities	Children enjoy stories that reflect their feelings; you can tailor these to an individual child, but use the story in a group story-telling session; for example: a visit to a hospital, fear of the dark, feelings of jealousy (e.g. when a new sibling arrives), etc. They will benefit by realising that their fears are normal and they can share experiences with others. Making simple scrapbooks for each child, with photos and drawings, can increase a child's self-esteem
Games with rules Board games, e.g. Lotto, pairs; circle time; party games, e.g. musical statues, pass the parcel	Children learn how to be part of a group, to take turns and to share with others. Some games are competitive and children need to learn how to lose gracefully

Confidentiality in the work setting

Anyone working with young children, whether in a nursery setting, a school or in the family home, will need to practise confidentiality. Confidentiality is respect for the privacy of any information about a child and his or her family. Children and their parents and carers need to feel confident that:

✱ you will not interfere in their private lives and that any information you are privileged to hold will not become a source of gossip. Breaches of confidentiality can occur when you are travelling on public transport, for example, and discussing the events of your day; always remember that using the names of children in your care can cause a serious breach of confidentiality if overheard by a friend or relative of the family;

✽ you will ensure that any child or family's personal information is restricted to those who have a real **need to know**, for example, when a child's family or health circumstances are affecting their development;

✽ you will not write anything down about a child that you would feel concerned about showing their parents or carers;

✽ you understand when the safety or health needs of the child override the need for confidentiality; parents need to be reassured that you will always put the safety and well being of each child before any other considerations.

Having respect for the individual child

You need to be aware of a child's personal rights, dignity and privacy and must show this at all times; every child is unique and so your approach will need to take account of each child's individual needs. Every person deserves and needs respect from those around them. It is important to listen to children and to try to understand the world from their point of view; this is called empathy. Differences in background, upbringing and culture should all be respected too. Read also the poem on p. 259 in Unit 4.

Involving parents

Parents and primary carers should be made welcome in child care settings. It is important that parents are always valued as the child's first and most important educators. For useful information on how parents can feel more involved within their child's setting, read the section in Option Unit B, pages 343–350.

The importance of remaining calm when dealing with children who are upset

It is often only natural to feel upset when dealing with a distressed child, but it is important to react in a professional manner to be positive and caring. Children need to feel that they can express their feelings to someone they trust and who cares for them. You will respond appropriately if you follow these guidelines:

✽ always consider the **needs of the child** first and think how you can best help them when they are feeling upset;

✽ **listen to children** carefully; never dismiss their feelings as trivial – they are very important to them;

✽ **be ready to help them** when you notice they are feeling upset; this may mean intervening in their play, providing appropriate activities, or seeking advice from another member of staff or the child's parents.

There are many books available which help you to understand difficult events in children's lives, e.g. death or divorce. There are also books on these and other subjects, such as going to hospital or to the dentist, which you may want to read with children.

5

Children's behaviour

- appropriate behaviour for the child's stage of development
- causes of change in usual behaviour patterns
- the importance of establishing consistent boundaries
- managing the impact of racist, sexist, abusive and anti-social behaviour
- simple strategies of managing behaviour
- why child care and education workers never use physical punishment
- the need to ensure good communication and partnership with parents

Most societies have codes or standards of behaviour some of which are written as laws. Those relating to moral behaviour are to be found in many societies although the punishments for them may vary. Some codes, however, may not be written as rules but are generally understood. For example, in the UK queuing is an accepted form of behaviour which seems fair so people take their turns but this is viewed as strange by other societies and cultures. As children grow and develop they need to learn what behaviour is acceptable and desirable and what is unacceptable and unwanted in their families, communities and in their wider society.

Through watching children as they develop it is possible to see that at each stage there are types and patterns of behaviour which are common. Very early on babies and young children learn from their own experience what actions and sounds will gain attention. They also learn by watching others and their behaviour can be influenced positively or negatively by what they see as well as what they experience.

ACTIVITY

1 List some of the rules that you had to follow when you were a child. Include ones in your home, at primary school, general ones which applied when you were out in public.

2 In small groups compare your lists and identify which rules were common to everyone.

3 What rules do you have to follow now – at home, at school/college, in society? Are these rules fair? Who decides them and who benefits from them?

4 What rules would you abolish and what new ones would you make if you could?

 ## What is meant by the term 'behaviour'?

Behaviour is observable (can be seen and/or heard). It is the way we act, speak, and treat other people and our environment. It does not include our thoughts although these usually prompt what we do.

Behaviour is influenced in the following ways:

* by the customs and practices of the society or culture;
* by the rules, standards and expectations of the family;
* by copying others – with children, particularly through play;
* by receiving rewards or treats, or respect from others;
* by being punished or penalised or feeling humiliated;
* by the actions and attitudes of a peer group;
* by the desire to be useful to others and achieve satisfaction for doing something worthwhile.

Behaviour linked to stages of development

The following stages are, of course, only loosely linked to the ages shown. As with any 'norm' measurements, they only serve as a rough guide to help understand children's behaviour and how best to respond to it. Much will depend upon children's experiences and the way they have been helped to develop good relationships.

At age 1–2 years, children:

✓ have developed their own personalities and are sociable with close family and friends;

✓ can still become shy and anxious when parents or carers are out of sight;

✓ are developing their speech and can attract attention by calling out or crying;

✓ can become possessive over toys but can often be distracted to something else;

✓ are discovering that they are separate individuals;

✓ are self-centred (see things from their own point of view);

✓ are gaining mobility, improving their ability to explore their surroundings – this results in conflicts – often regarding safety;

✓ begin to understand the meaning of 'No' and firm boundaries can be set;

✓ can be frustrated by their own limitations but resist adult help (perhaps saying 'me do it').

At age 2–3 years, children:

✓ are not yet able to share easily;

✓ are developing greater awareness of their separate identities;

✓ are developing their language abilities which help them to communicate their need and wishes more clearly and to understand 'in a minute';

✓ can still be distracted from the cause of their anger;

✓ have tantrums (usually when parents or main carers are present) when frustrated – possibly caused by their efforts to become self-reliant e.g. feeding or dressing themselves – or having ideas which the adult does not want them to carry out (more about tantrums below);

✓ experience a range of feelings – being very affectionate and co-operative one minute and resistant the next;

✓ are aware of the feelings of others and can respond to them.

At age 3–4 years, children:

✓ are very aware of others and imitate them – especially in their play. With developing speaking and listening skills they are liable to repeat swear words they hear;

✓ are more able to express themselves through speech and, therefore, there is often a reduction in physical outbursts. However they are still likely to hit back if provoked;

✓ can be impulsive and will be less easily distracted;

✓ become more sociable in their play and may have favourite friends;

✓ can, sometimes, be reasoned with and are just becoming aware of the behaviour codes in different places or situations;

✓ like, and seek, adult approval and appreciation of their efforts.

Child showing distress

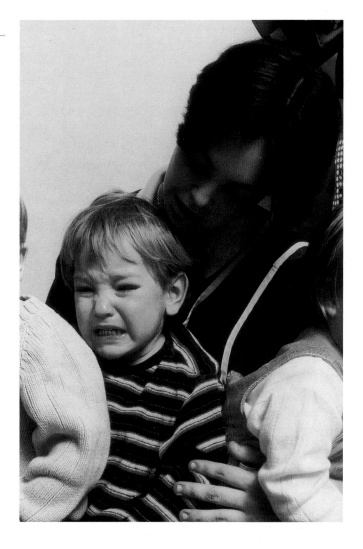

At age 4–5 years, children:

✓ can behave appropriately at mealtimes and during other 'routine' activities and may begin to understand why 'Please' and 'Thank you' (or their equivalent) are important;

✓ are able to share and take turns but often need help;

✓ are more aware of others' feelings and will be concerned if someone is hurt;

✓ are becoming more independent and self-assured but still need adult comfort when ill or tired;

✓ will respond to reason, can negotiate and be adaptable but can still be distracted;

✓ are sociable and becoming confident communicators able to make more sense of their environment. There will continue to be conflicts which they cannot resolve on their own and with which they will need adult help;

✓ can sometimes be determined, may argue and show aggression.

At age 5–6 years, children:

✓ understand that different rules apply in different places e.g. home, school, grandparents' house etc. and can adapt their behaviour accordingly;

✓ are developing control over their feelings – they argue with adults when they feel secure and need to feel there are firm boundaries in place;

✓ will respond to reason and can negotiate but are less easily distracted – anger can last longer and they need time to calm down;

✓ are able to hide their feelings in some situations;

✓ can co-operate in group play but are not yet ready for team games;

✓ may show off and boast e.g. when they celebrate an achievement;

✓ will continue to need adult support to resolve conflicts;

✓ will share and take turns and begin to have an understanding of what is 'fair' if given an explanation.

At age 6–8 years, children:

✓ can quickly adapt behaviour to suit the situation;

✓ can play games with rules;

✓ can argue their viewpoints;

✓ are growing in confidence and becoming independent;

✓ are developing some moral values and understanding of 'right' and 'wrong';

✓ can be friendly and co-operative;

✓ can control how they feel much of the time but there are still times when they want to do things their way and quarrels develop.

Children helping to unpack the family shopping

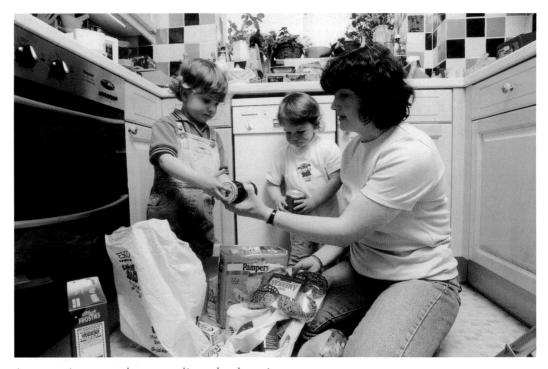

Assessing and recording behaviour

When assessing children's behaviour it is important to bear these stages in mind and to view it in the context of overall development. For example it is well known that tantrums are a common, even expected, feature of a two-year-old's behaviour. There is some cause for concern if they are a regular feature of a six-year-old's. However, some adults have unrealistic expectations of children and express surprise when unwanted behaviour occurs. *For example: A five-year-old becomes fidgety and whines during a Christmas pantomime. The adults will view the occasion as a treat and may feel resentment that their child is complaining but it is reasonable that a five-year-old should lose concentration, be unable to sit still for a lengthy period or understand all of what is going on.*

In trying to understand behaviour it is helpful to note whether there are particular incidents or situations which seem to trigger unwanted behaviour. Some of these can be avoided altogether by minor changes in routine or approach but others, such as siblings teasing each other, will occur frequently and so children need to be given some strategies and support to be able to cope with them effectively. **It is important never to reject the child but only what the child has done e.g. 'that was an unkind thing to say' rather than 'you are unkind'.**

The A-B-C of behaviour

Antecedent – what happens before, or leads up to, the observed behaviour

Behaviour – the observed behaviour – what the child says and how s/he acts (this is any behaviour, both positive and negative)

Consequence – what happens following the observed behaviour

Part of your role is to observe children's behaviour, whether or not you make a written record, so that you can contribute to discussions about a child's behaviour and develop good practice in managing unwanted aspects. In your work setting you should try to see not only how other staff and parents deal with incidents, but also which methods seem to be effective with which children.

An **event sample** is a useful way of recording negative behaviour as and when it occurs. This method involves creating a chart to note:

- the time
- the context (location, activity)
- the people involved
- actions and language of the child/ren
- actions and language of the adult
- child's response to adult/other children
- any other relevant information

This provides the **A-B-C** information and helps to identify what, or who, may have led to each incident.

You may find that:

☐ particular pairings or groupings of children present problems;

☐ some form of bullying is occurring;

☐ there is confusion about what is expected – unclear rules;

☐ large group times – register, story, assembly – are often the 'trouble' times;

☐ the child responds positively to one form of discipline or adult more readily than to another.

Time	Context/activity	Actions/behaviour	Language	Child's response
9.20 a.m.	Playing at sand tray with 2 other children	Throwing sand in face of another child. A comforts other child and takes him to basins to flush out sand	G: 'It goes everywhere doesn't it?' B: Crying and rubbing eyes A: 'Oh dear – G, you must be careful, try to keep the sand in the tray'	G looks surprised and upset, begins to cry. Goes to book corner
9.32 a.m.	In book corner just finished listening to a taped story with one other child and an adult	Putting away the book and the tape in their correct places	A: 'Well done, G, you are being helpful.'	G beams a smile and tidies other books
10.17 a.m.	Playing with the train and track with 3 other children – Adult close by at another activity	G and F are playing co-operatively when K arrives and asks if she can play	K: 'Can I play?' F: 'No, we're playing our own game' G: 'Yes she can – K, you can get those trucks' A: 'Thank you, G – we do have to share.'	K looks upset K smiles and begins to collect trucks G carries on playing with both F and K
10.45 a.m.	Outdoor play area – 11 children – bikes, prams, pushchairs to play with	G sits on a bike also holding handle of a pram which another child wants to use	R: 'Are you playing with the pram?' G: 'Yes. You can't have it' A: 'G, you can play with the bike or the pram but you can't really use both together, can you? Let R play with the pram now and you can have a turn in a minute'	G pulls pram closer to himself. G lets go of pram and rides bike away to far side of play area

Table 3.3 Specimen event table (A = adult)

Your findings can help staff to understand when unwanted behaviour is likely to occur and extra support, perhaps a talk with the child about what would be acceptable behaviour, or closer supervision can be given. They may also highlight differences in the way staff deal with it which may be confusing for children. Adults can then meet and work out how best to help the child.

A **time sample** can be even more useful and provide information, not only about the unwanted behaviour but also about the occasions when a child has behaved well.

This method involves creating a similar chart but a record of what is happening is made at regular intervals – every 30 minutes, or whatever seems appropriate and practical. This method enables you to see if the positive behaviour was noticed, appreciated and praised/rewarded. If it was overlooked the child may use unwanted behaviour to gain attention – of any kind!

Recording and sharing the information with other staff and parents helps everyone to agree on a realistic and practical course of action. Similar observations can be repeated at a later date to monitor progress and review strategies.

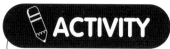 **ACTIVITY**

Ask your supervisor if you may carry out a time sample observation of a child whose behaviour is, sometimes, unacceptable. Agree the time interval you will use and the overall period (perhaps one day or two half-day sessions). Look at your information and identify the number of incidents of positive, and of negative, behaviour. Which were there more of? Is there a pattern to the situations or children present when each type occurs? Could any of the incidents of negative behaviour have been avoided? If so, how? Was the child praised on the occasions of positive behaviour? How did s/he respond?

Time	Context/activity	Actions/behaviour	Language	Other
9.00 a.m.	At the playdough table with 3 other children and an adult	Banging fist on a ball of playdough	G: 'Look, I can make it flat' A: 'You are banging hard, aren't you?'	Other children begin to copy the banging
10.00 a.m.	Playing at the water tray with 2 other children	Pouring water from a jug held high over water wheel. Water is splashing on the floor and G is 'paddling' in it. He begins to pour water directly on the floor and splash in it	W: 'Stop it, you're making me all wet' G: (excitedly) 'Look it's all up my socks' A: 'That's not very clever, G. Now we will have to clean it all up and there isn't much water left in the tray. We'll have to find you dry socks too. What do you need to remember when you're playing with the water?'	A: Notices what is happening and comes over to group. Deals with spilt water and takes G away to change socks. Tells him to choose another activity
11.00 a.m.	Playing outside – all children and adults	Taking part in a 'ring' game. Holding hands of 2 other children and walking round singing	Words of 'Here we go round the mulberry bush'	Joining in and doing appropriate actions
12. 00 a.m.	Collecting coat and pictures ready to go home	Playful pushing with another child at pegs	G: 'Hey, let me get mine' D: 'No, let me get mine'	Put on coats and start showing pictures to each other before sitting on carpet

Table 3.4 Specimen time sample

Serious incidents (for example, biting) should be recorded and reported to parents of the children involved. Parents of each child (or children) must be assured that these incidents are dealt with seriously and appropriately otherwise there is a risk that they will take issue with each other. They should be given information which explains what happened so that they:

a do not feel the need to question their child; and

b are aware of the full facts rather than their child's viewpoint.

Confidentiality is vitally important, although the children themselves will probably name names!

Ways in which adults can contribute to children's behaviour

Behaviour is very closely linked to self-esteem – children who feel bad about themselves may not behave well. The printed poem on **page 259** sums up the positive and negative ways in which adults can contribute positively and negatively to children's development and behaviour.

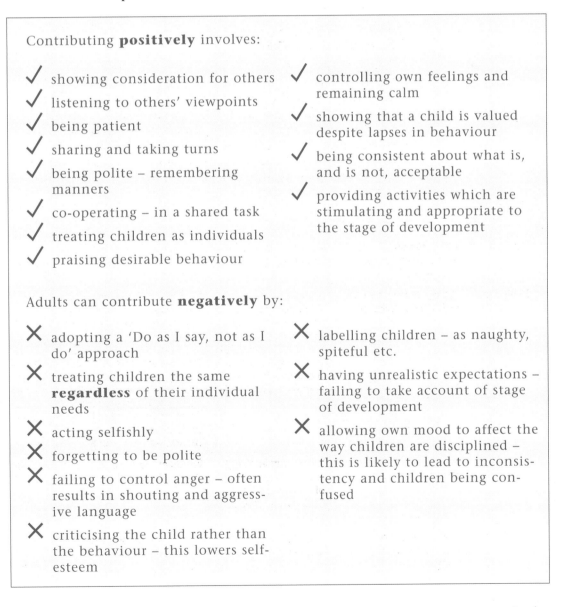

Contributing **positively** involves:

✓ showing consideration for others
✓ listening to others' viewpoints
✓ being patient
✓ sharing and taking turns
✓ being polite – remembering manners
✓ co-operating – in a shared task
✓ treating children as individuals
✓ praising desirable behaviour

✓ controlling own feelings and remaining calm
✓ showing that a child is valued despite lapses in behaviour
✓ being consistent about what is, and is not, acceptable
✓ providing activities which are stimulating and appropriate to the stage of development

Adults can contribute **negatively** by:

✗ adopting a 'Do as I say, not as I do' approach
✗ treating children the same **regardless** of their individual needs
✗ acting selfishly
✗ forgetting to be polite
✗ failing to control anger – often results in shouting and aggressive language
✗ criticising the child rather than the behaviour – this lowers self-esteem

✗ labelling children – as naughty, spiteful etc.
✗ having unrealistic expectations – failing to take account of stage of development
✗ allowing own mood to affect the way children are disciplined – this is likely to lead to inconsistency and children being confused

Factors affecting behaviour

It is well-known that behaviour is commonly affected by certain factors.

There are some factors which stem from the children themselves:

- illness
- accident and injury
- tiredness

Other factors result from their situations:

- arrival of a new baby
- moving house
- parental separation or divorce
- change of carer – either at home or in a setting
- loss or bereavement
- change of setting – e.g. transition from home to nursery or nursery to school

Individual children will respond to these situations differently but **regression** is common (usually temporary) when they revert to behaviour which is immature for them. Events which they do not understand will leave them confused, leading to frustration and aggressive outbursts, or they may blame themselves which could result in withdrawn behaviour and the development of unwanted habits through anxiety.

Generally, any factor which causes stress may result in the child:

- needing more comfort and attention;
- being less sociable;
- being unable to cope with tasks that they would normally manage;
- being subject to mood swings;
- being unable to concentrate (this includes listening to instructions) and less able to cope with challenging situations and difficulties.

A framework for behaviour – goals and boundaries

If children are to understand what is regarded as acceptable behaviour at home, in the work setting and in society, then they must be given very clear guidelines. Work settings will have a **policy** relating to behaviour and discipline which all staff should follow and which is regularly reviewed. The policy will explain the rules which are applied and how children will be helped to understand, and learn to keep, them. In most cases the rules are simple and reflect the concerns for safety and for children to be considerate of others and their environment. They should be appropriate for the age and stage of development of the children and for the particular needs of the work setting.

Goals are the forms of behaviour that are encouraged and cover physical, social and verbal aspects. They should be realistically set for the child's age and stage of development. Some examples of goals for a 4–5 year old: to say 'please' and 'thankyou'; to share play equipment; to tidy up; be quiet and listen for short periods e.g. story or register time.

Boundaries are the limits within which behaviour is acceptable – they identify what may, and may not, be done or said. Children need to understand the consequences of failing to act within those boundaries. It is important that the boundaries are appropriate for the age and stage of development. Some examples of boundaries for 4–5 year olds: that they may play outside but must not tread on the flowerbeds; that they may watch television but only until tea is ready; that they may use the dressing-up clothes if they put them away when they have finished.

It is helpful to set 'positive' rules rather than 'negative' ones. Rules which begin 'Don't' tell children what they must not do but gives them no guidance as to what they may or should do.

CASE STUDY

A boy had recently started in the reception class and displayed negative behaviour in many ways and in many situations. On arrival in the playground in the mornings, with both his parents and younger sister, he would walk around poking and kicking other children as he went. This caused anger among other parents, upset among the children and ill-feeling towards his parents who would shout at him before grabbing him, holding him by the hand and telling him off loudly. The staff discussed this with the parents and it was agreed that, in the short term, the boy should be brought to school 10 minutes later than everyone else. Every morning the father would deliver him to the classroom door with the instruction 'Behave'. The boy always said that he would. However, he did not really understand what 'behave' meant in terms of his own actions. His teacher made a point of reminding him, throughout the day, of what behaviour was expected and explained what that meant for him e.g.' sit nicely' – this means sitting still without touching any other child or anything – it was also an opportunity to reinforce the rule for other children. Improvement was very gradual. Only one aspect of behaviour was dealt with at a time. He was given one-to-one support when available and observations were recorded to monitor progress and plan future strategies.

ACTIVITY

In pairs produce some simple rules for 4–5 year olds in a reception class which give clear guidance about what they should do. For example **DO walk** instead of **DON'T run**.

Consistency in applying the boundaries is important, especially in the work setting where children need to relate to several adults. They will check that the rules have not changed and that they still apply whichever adult is present.

If you are supervising an activity the children will expect you to apply the same rules as other staff. It undermines your own position if you allow unacceptable behaviour and another staff member has to discipline the children you are working with.

Managing behaviour

First of all it needs to be agreed in a work setting what behaviour is unwanted and then some decisions made as to how staff will manage it when it does arise. These should take account of individual needs as children will respond in their own ways. For example, in a school setting, staying in at playtime is punishment for some children but, for those who have poor social skills and find the playground rather intimidating, it can be a relief. Similarly some children enjoy tidying and helping the teacher because they might get more individual attention.

Albert Bandura developed a **'social learning'** theory which states that children learn about social behaviour by watching and imitating other people, especially those they admire. Children will learn negative behaviour as well as positive behaviour so the presence of good role models is very important. **Burrhus F. Skinner** developed a **'behaviourist'** theory which states that children's behaviour is shaped by adults through positive and negative reinforcement. These two theories have influenced current practice for managing and **modifying** (shaping or reforming) behaviour.

There are three main aspects of behaviour modification:

- **identifying positive and negative behaviour** – deciding what behaviour is to be encouraged and what is to be discouraged

- **rewarding positive behaviour** – encouraging and promoting it through reward. There are different forms of reward – verbal praise, attention (this could be non-verbal e.g. smile of approval, a nod), stars or points (for older children) leading to certificates or for group/team recognition, sharing success by having other staff and parents told, own choice activity or story, tangible rewards such as stickers. These work on the principle of positive reinforcement – based on the idea that if children receive approval and/or reward for behaving acceptably they are likely to want to repeat that behaviour. *If one child is praised – e.g. for tidying up – others are often influenced to copy or join in so that they, too, will receive praise and attention.* For young children the reward must be immediate so they understand the link between it and the positive behaviour. It is of little value to promise a treat or reward in the future. Similarly, star charts and collecting points are not appropriate for children younger than five years old;

- **discouraging negative behaviour** (according to this approach) – whenever possible such behaviour should be ignored (bearing in mind safety/injury) although not if attention is drawn to it (perhaps by another child) as the message sent is that it is acceptable; giving attention and praise to another child who is behaving acceptably; distracting the child's attention (particularly appropriate with younger children) or removing him/her to another activity or group; expressing disapproval – verbally and/or non-verbally through body language, facial expression (frowning) and shaking of the head; imposing a punishment – withdrawal of a privilege e.g. watching a favourite TV programme. These work on the principle of **negative reinforcement** – based on the idea that children will avoid repeating an unpleasant experience so if they behave unacceptably and earn the disapproval of an adult or receive some sort of punishment they will be less likely to repeat that behaviour. *As they learn from watching others, older children may be deterred (put off) from behaving unacceptably by seeing someone else receive discipline.* This approach encourages the adult to act immediately so young children understand the link between the unacceptable behaviour and the adult's response to it.

Remember – **Physical, or corporal, punishment is illegal in work settings and never allowed under any circumstances – this includes pulling a child by his/her elbow or arm or grabbing him/her by the wrist. Intervention, to protect the child, others or property, should involve minimal physical restraint.**

There are problems associated with rewards in that some children may behave in a particular way purely to receive the reward rather than from an understanding of the need to consider safety, others and their environment or enjoying what they have achieved for its own sake. The type of reward also needs to be considered – is it desirable for children to be given sweets as rewards? Some parents may have strong views about this.

Rewards might work in the short term, but do not always succeed in the long term. They might even undermine lifelong learning by encouraging children to seek reward, rather than be disposed to learn because something is interesting.

CASE STUDY

In an infant school a new headteacher introduced the practice of listening to children read to her regularly. This involved children being sent individually to her office where she would reward them with a jelly bear if they read well or tried hard. One mother was surprised, when talking to her daughter about the school day, that she was upset to have read to her teacher instead of the headteacher. The girl explained that everyone was asking to read to the headteacher and she was not chosen – she missed out on a jelly bear!

The parent was alarmed that a) sweets were being given as a reward without parents knowing and b) children were not rewarded by the experience itself and the headteacher's appreciation of children's efforts.

Problem behaviour

Attention-seeking, aggression (physical and verbal) towards others, and self-destructive behaviour need to be dealt with calmly.

✱ **Attention-seeking** – This is often shown through disruptive (making noises, not responding to an instruction) or aggressive behaviour and needs managing as identified above. Sometimes children who are trying to please can be just as disruptive. Those who desperately want adults to notice them will call out, interrupt, ask questions and frequently push in front of other children to show something they have made/done. Children who seek attention challenge patience but with a bit of reminding about turn-taking, and clear expectation that they will, they can learn to wait for their turn. It is important to give attention when they have waited appropriately so that they are encouraged to do so again.

✱ **Physical aggression** – This usually results from strong feelings which are difficult to control. Whatever the cause – and it may be provocation – the adult should deal with it calmly and ensure that the needs of all the children involved are met. A child who has lost control frightens him/herself and the other children. Some work settings favour a 'time-out' approach which involves the aggressive child being taken to an identified place away from the incident – a corner or chair. This allows for a calming-down period and other children to be reassured. This method can work but needs positive follow-up by a staff member to explain that the behaviour was unacceptable, explain why and suggest how the child might have behaved otherwise – e.g. asked instead of snatched; listened to the apology for the model being broken etc. Unless this is done there is a danger that the chair or area becomes known to the children as the 'naughty chair' and staff begin to use it as a way of 'grounding' a child who is causing annoyance without addressing the issues. Many adults do not like to use this approach for this reason.

✱ **Temper tantrums** – These are usually associated with two-year-olds but can occur in older children. They may happen, particularly, when a child is ill or tired but often build from a confrontational incident when s/he is asked to do something, or not do something and a 'battle of wills' begins! They often involve shouting and crying, refusal to co-operate and mounting anger – shown through kicking, hitting, screaming, stamping – and, on occasions, self-harm. In younger children they can be over very quickly but in older ones can take longer to reach a peak and longer for the calming down afterwards.

Dealing with tantrums

1 **Try to avoid them** – if you can anticipate them try distracting the child with a game or another activity

2 **Try to ignore them** – apart from safety concerns try to give as little attention as possible during them

3 **Be consistent** – if children think, from past experience, that the adult will not keep the boundary firmly there, they will continue – clear boundaries are essential

4 **A firm hug** may help the child feel secure and under control until s/he calms down – this is useful in situations where you cannot walk away

5 **Talk about them** – this may help older children to express their feelings calmly.

6 **Provide experiences and activities** which the child finds interesting usually helps children to become involved in positive ways.

Do not give in and let the boundary go – this almost certainly leads to more rather than fewer tantrums because children are confused by inconsistency.

✱ **Self-destructive behaviour** – This includes head-banging and forms of self-mutilation (e.g. tearing out hair, excessive nailbiting causing pain and bleeding). It usually signals some emotional difficulty which needs expert intervention. Staff and parents need to discuss their concerns and agree a common approach based on the advice they are given.

✱ **Unacceptable language** – This includes swearing and name-calling which often result from children repeating what they have heard themselves. Sometimes they are unaware that it is unacceptable in one setting but not another. In these cases they need to be told firmly not to say those words 'here' – you cannot legislate for language they may use at home or criticise their families. Some children will deliberately use unacceptable language to shock or seek attention. In these cases you should state the rule calmly and firmly. Name-calling, particularly if it is discriminatory (regarding race, creed, disability, family background, appearance etc.) must always be challenged and dealt with firmly. Explain that it is hurtful and that we are all different. This behaviour is best combated through good example and through anti-discriminatory practices in the work setting which will help children to value other people as individuals. (See Unit 2 re: multi-cultural and anti-discriminatory resources.)

Sometimes the behaviour management strategies outlined above fail to be effective or are only effective for a short period of time. So when behaviour is inappropriate for the child's stage of development or is persistently challenging there are other professionals who may be called upon to help all those involved. Meetings which allow everyone to contribute information about a child will help to create an overall view of progress, development and behaviour and it is here that recorded observations will be especially useful.

Professionals who may become involved include:

- **health visitors** – who work primarily with children up to 5 years and their families checking for healthy growth and development
- **physiotherapists** – who assess children's motor skills and development and might be asked to advise on appropriate activities and equipment
- **speech therapists** – who assess mouth movement as well as speech/language itself and might suggest ways of supporting children who experience communication difficulties
- **play therapists** – who have specialist training and work with children, using play, to help them feel emotionally secure
- **paediatricians** – who specialise in the care of children up to age 16 – check for normal development and diagnose difficulties
- **educational psychologists** – who assess children who have special needs and give advice, particularly for those with emotional and behavioural difficulties
- **child psychiatrists** – who work with children and their families to help them to express their thoughts and feelings

It is important to follow correct procedures for reporting incidents. Check that you know what they are in your work setting.

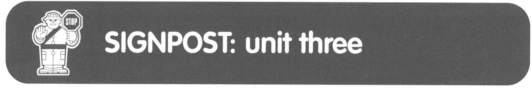

SIGNPOST: unit three

1 Write a paragraph to show your understanding of emotional development.

2 Write a paragraph to show your understanding of social development.

3 Create a flow diagram (based on the example below) which charts the sequence and stages of emotional and social development from age 1 year to age 6 years.

Age 12 months: fluctuating moods; shy with strangers; will help with daily routines; etc.
By 18 months: eager to be independent; show sense of personal identity; etc.

By 2 years: beginning to express how s/he feels; may be clingy; can be self-reliant; parallel play stage; etc.
By 2½ years: may be dry at night; play more with other children; etc.

By 3 years:

By 4 years:

By 5 years:

By 6 years

4 Taking into account what you have read about activities which promote emotional and social development, AND what you have seen during your placement experience, fill in the boxes to show which activities are appropriate for **each** age range. (See page 375 for photocopiable sheet.)

5 Choose **one** activity from each age range and explain, briefly, what is involved and **how** it can promote emotional and social development.

6 Separation from parents or main carers can have a marked effect on babies and young children.
   (a) Write a paragraph to explain how babies 'bond' with their main carers and why bonding is so important.
   (b) What is meant by 'separation anxiety'?
   (c) How are babies and young children affected by separation at various ages? Cover ages 1–6 years in your answer.

7 What is meant by the term 'behaviour'? Make a list of things that can influence a child's behaviour and factors that can affect it. Identify some of the more common types of 'problem' behaviour often displayed by young children and at what age it is most likely to occur.

8 Choose **one** of the following age ranges 1–2 years, 3–4 years, 5–6 years:
   (a) Describe the behaviour that might be expected from a child of that age.
   (b) For each type of behaviour described in 8(a), suggest how a parent might deal with it. *Remember to give guidance on responding to 'good' as well as 'problem' aspects.* NB Cultural differences mean that behaviour that is acceptable in some families and situations is not acceptable in others. Also remember that the expectations and rules for boys will be different from those for girls in some cultures and families.

Preparing for Employment with Young Children

Early years services for children and their families

- the role of statutory, voluntary and private organisations
- the range of services and facilities provided
- sources of additional information

🧸 The legal and political framework of statutory services

The Background

In the mid-1940s, the major parts of the welfare state were introduced. The thinking behind this was that everyone should be entitled to:

✱ free health care and treatment

✱ free education, and

✱ a minimum weekly income above the poverty line.

By the 1970s there was anxiety about the ever-increasing financial demands that these entitlements made on the welfare state, and in 1979, the government of the day started to move away from the welfare state approach – Margaret Thatcher, who was then Prime Minister, called it the 'Nanny State'. There was a change towards policies encouraging market forces. For example

- eye tests were no longer free to all;
- the costs of dental treatment and charges for routine dental checks were significantly increased;
- the schools meals service was decreased; many school kitchens were closed and services organised centrally;
- private pensions were encouraged.

This change was meant to enable people to have more choice in which services they used and to be more of a *safety net* than a full public service free to everyone, regardless of their income. It was also thought that if services had to compete for business, then they would become more streamlined and efficient. It coincided with a growing awareness of 'green' ecological issues, such as recycling materials and saving energy. The thinking was that there was a lot of wastage in the big public organisations, which could be remedied if more attention were given to the profit motive.

The Children Act 1989 – 'The welfare of the child is paramount'

When the welfare state was developed in the 1940s all the services for children were completely separate from each other. **The Children Act 1989** introduced a new approach which would co-ordinate the various needs of children and work in partnership with parents to meet those needs. Under The Children Act, statutory services for children are based on five linked principles:

1 **Children in need:** Children in need are:

☐ children with a **disability**;

☐ children whose health or development is:
  > likely to be significantly impaired;
  > likely to be further impaired;
  > unlikely to be maintained;

☐ children without the provision of services.

2 **Partnership with parents:** Services for children must actively seek participation, offering real choices and involving parents in decisions. For example, it should be usual for parents to join in on case conferences concerning their child.

3 **Race, culture, religion and language:** Services must link with children's experiences in relation to these areas. In work settings, staff should not discriminate, and the whole setting should reflect a multi-cultural atmosphere.

4 **The co-ordination of services:** Services are required to co-ordinate with each other in order to support a family. The idea is that families should not be passed from agency to agency. Instead, one agency (e.g. the Education Authority) should request the help of another authority (e.g. the Social Services Department).

5 **Meeting the identified needs of an individual family:** Services must be geared to meet the identified needs of a particular family. Local Authorities are therefore required to gather information and to plan services which are based on local needs.

Child Protection and The Children Act

The Children Act was drafted at a time when there was great public and professional concern about children who suffered abuse. It has led to a new approach which believes that children are better off when brought up and cared for in their own homes.

Statutory, voluntary and private services

Just as it is impossible to separate the various strands in children's development, so the way that children's needs are met within society are intricately bound up with each other. Recent changes in attitudes have meant that **health care**, **social care** and **education** are increasingly seen as essential services for children which should be provided in an integrated way. A wide range of organisations exists to provide services for young children and their families. These include:

- Statutory services
- Voluntary services
- Private services

Statutory services

Statutory services are those which are funded by Government and which have to be provided by law (or statute). Some services are provided by **central government** departments; e.g.:

- ☐ The National Health Service (NHS)
- ☐ The Department of Social Security, and
- ☐ The Department for Education and Skills (DfES)

These large departments are funded directly from taxation – income tax, VAT and National Insurance.

Other statutory services are provided by **local government**; e.g.:

- ☐ Housing Department
- ☐ Local Education Authority
- ☐ Social Services Department

These are largely funded through local taxation (Council Tax) and from grants made by central government.

Voluntary services

These are health, education and social care services which are set up by charities to provide services which Local Authorities can buy in and benefit from their expertise. Voluntary organisations are:

- Non-profit making
- Non-statutory
- Dependent on fundraising and government grants

Private services

The private sector consists of organisations set up to provide health, education and social care services 'at a price'. They are income-generating and profit-making services, which include:

- ✱ Public and independent schools
- ✱ Health insurance companies
- ✱ Some hospitals
- ✱ Childcare providers, e.g. private nurseries and crèches
- ✱ Private care homes and hostels
- ✱ Complementary and alternative medicine and therapies
- ✱ Some health screening services

🧸 Health care for young children and their families

The National Health Service

The NHS in England is the responsibility of the **Secretary of State** for Health who is a member of the government **cabinet**. The Secretary of State for Health and his or her team of Ministers set overall health policy in England, including policy for the NHS. The NHS Executive, which is a part of the **Department of Health**, acts as the HQ of the NHS in England and is responsible for translating policy into practice, setting strategic targets for the NHS and monitoring performance. The Executive has regional offices which in turn monitor the performance of the **Primary Care Trusts** in their areas. Different arrangements exist in different parts of the United Kingdom – both in Government responsibilities for the NHS and how that responsibility is discharged.

The Government decides the overall level of funding for the NHS. Currently most of this money is then allocated to Primary Care Trusts and to some GPs (called fund-holders) who decide how it should be spent to meet the health needs of their local population.

Health services for children

All services for children within the NHS structure are *free of charge*; these include:

* Hospital treatment
* Services of the Primary Health Care Team (PHCT), which includes:
    > the family doctor (GP),
    > the practice nurse
    > the health visitor
    > the community midwife
* School Health Service
* Dentist
* Optician

When children are sick, they are usually cared for in their own homes by their parents. This is known as informal care. Hospital stays are now shorter, so the care which children and their families receive in their community is very important. The Primary Health Care Team is responsible for:

* Preventative services:
    > **Routine immunisations** of children to protect them against childhood illnesses, such as diphtheria, polio, tetanus, measles, mumps, rubella etc.
    > **Developmental checks:** health visitors carry out regular health and developmental reviews of children from 6 weeks until school age
    > **Health advice:** Doctors, midwives, practice nurses and health visitors are available to advise parents on a wide range of health issues. Some practices also employ a dietician to offer advice on nutrition.
* The GP or family doctor is responsible for:
    > **Medical diagnosis and treatment**
    > The **medical care** of all the children and families within the practice
    > **Prescriptions for drugs and medicines**
    > **Referral to a specialist** doctor or other health expert when appropriate

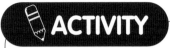

ACTIVITY

Visit your local GP surgery or health centre and find out what services are provided for young children. You could present your findings in booklet form as a word processing exercise.

Education for young children

Since 1944, schooling has been compulsory for all children between the ages of 5 and 15 (in 1972 the school-leaving age was increased to 16). The **Department for Education and Skills (DfES)** is headed by the Secretary of State for Education and is responsible for deciding the policies and the funding to the local education authorities.

A **Local Education Authority** (or **LEA**) is a type of council which has responsibility for providing education to pupils of school age in its area. LEAs vary greatly in size, from several hundred to fewer than 50 schools. The largest LEAs have responsibility for over 500 schools. The smallest LEA has responsibility for just one school.

Early Years (before compulsory education)

The **Early Years Development Plan** guarantees every four-year-old a free nursery place.

Many children under five attend:

- state nursery schools;
- nursery classes attached to primary schools;
- playgroups or pre-schools in the voluntary sector;
- privately run nurseries;
- integrated centres (including Children's Centres).

In England and Wales, many primary schools also operate an early admission policy where they admit children under five into what are called **reception classes**. Nursery provision for three-year-olds in the state sector is funded at the discretion of Local Education Authorities. Places for children under three in voluntary or private pre-school settings are paid for largely by parents.

Arrangements in Scotland and Northern Ireland are broadly similar, although there are differences of detail (for example, in Scotland, there are no reception classes and planning systems differ).

Sure Start (from birth to three years)

What is Sure Start?

The **Sure Start** programme was introduced by the Government in 1999. It is chiefly targeted at children under 4 years and their families in areas of need. The aims of **Sure Start** are as listed here.

✓ To work with parents and children to promote the physical, intellectual and social development of pre-school children, particularly those who are disadvantaged.

✓ To improve health by supporting parents in caring for their children in order to promote healthy development before and after birth.

✓ To improve social and emotional development by supporting early bonding between parents and their children.

✓ To help families to function by enabling the early identification and support of children with emotional and behavioural difficulties.

✓ To improve the ability to learn by encouraging stimulating and enjoyable play, improving language skills and through early identification and support of children with learning difficulties.

The Sure Start programme promises:	and includes:
Early education for all: Free part-time early education for 3 and 4 year olds	Helping children learn through the **Foundation Stage Curriculum** – see page 239
Outreach services and home visiting, building on existing patterns	**Support for families and parents**, including befriending and social support such as mentoring and parenting information
Services to provide good quality play, learning and childcare for children	**Primary and community healthcare** and advice about child health and development and parental health
Support for those with special needs, including support in accessing specialised services	**Establishing children's centres** where they are needed most – in disadvantaged areas – to offer families early education, childcare and health and family support with advice on employment opportunities

The Sure Start Framework: Birth to Three Matters

This framework is for all those who work with, and care for, children from birth to 3 years of age, including those with Special Educational Needs and/or disability. It shows four aspects of the development of babies and young children, each divided into four components:

❑ Inner strength
1 Me, myself and I: realisation of own individuality.
2 Being acknowledged and affirmed: experiencing and seeking closeness.
3 Developing self-assurance: becoming able to trust and rely on one's own abilities.
4 A sense of belonging: acquiring social confidence and competence.

❑ Skilful communication
1 Being together: being a sociable and effective communicator.
2 Finding a voice: being a confident and competent language user.
3 Listening and responding: listening and responding appropriately to the language of others.
4 Making meaning: understanding and being understood.

❑ Competent learning
1 Making connections: connecting ideas and understanding the world.
2 Being imaginative: responding to the world imaginatively.
3 Being creative: responding to the world creatively.
4 Representing: responding to the world with marks and symbols.

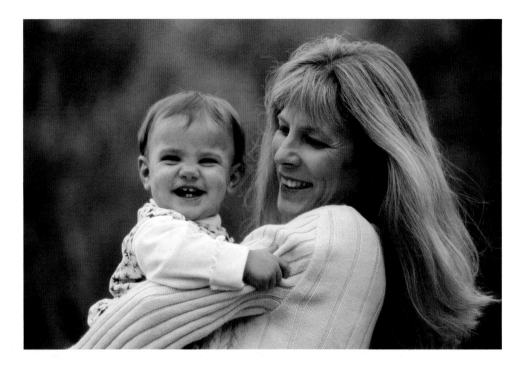

❑ Physical and mental health
1 Emotional well-being: emotional stability and resilience.
2 Growing and developing: physical well-being.
3 Keeping safe: being safe and protected.
4 Healthy choices: being able to make choices.

The key person approach

Each family is given a **key person** at nursery who gets to know them well, and this helps everyone to feel safe. A baby or young child knows that this special person and the important people at home often do the same things for them.

- They help you manage through the day

- They think about you

- They get to know you well

- They sometimes worry about you

- They get to know each other

- They talk about you

The Sure Start programme makes a distinction between the **key worker** role (described on page 350) and their **key person** role. The term 'key worker' is often used in nurseries to describe how staff work, to ensure liaison between different professionals and to enhance smooth organization and record keeping. The **key person** role is a special emotional relationship with the child and the family.

A children's commissioner

Following the tragic death of 8-year-old Victoria Climbie in 2000, after prolonged neglect and cruelty by her carers, the Government has proposed a package of child protection measures. These include:

❑ An independent **children's commissioner**, who will act as a 'champion' for young people in England (Scotland and Wales already have a children's commissioner)

☐ The creation of **'children's trusts'**, which will bring together local education authorities, health and social services

☐ A **local database** of all children within the area, showing information such as date of birth, the name of GPs and schools, and whether there had been problems, such as school exclusions, involvement with social services or trouble with the police.

State primary schools

The majority of children in the UK go to publicly funded schools, usually known as state schools. These make no charge to parents and are usually **co-educational** – that is, they take boys and girls. In 1999, four new categories of school were created: Community, Foundation, Voluntary Controlled and Voluntary Aided. Schools in all the four categories have a lot in common. They are self-managing and they do not charge fees. They work in partnership with other schools and with Local Education Authorities (LEAs), and they receive funding from LEAs.

Special schools are also provided by LEAs for certain children with **special educational needs**, though the great majority is educated in ordinary schools.

The framework of education provision for children

Children in state schools and nurseries are legally required to follow a government-controlled curriculum called the **National Curriculum**.

The **National Curriculum** is the set of guidelines that says what children should be taught in school. The aims of the National Curriculum are:

☐ to provide a balanced education for each child;

☐ to prepare the child for the opportunities, responsibilities and experiences of adult life;

☐ to develop an enterprising, adaptable and self-confident person;

☐ to give the child self-respect and encourage respect for others.

The Curriculum is divided into four stages of education, known as **Key Stages**. Each Key Stage is aimed at children between certain ages. Within each Key Stage, a number of different subjects are studied. In 1999 a new stage was introduced for children from 3 years until the end of the reception year; this **Foundation Stage Curriculum** sets goals to be reached by the time children enter **Key Stage 1** (i.e. Year 1 in a first/lower/infant/primary school) of the National Curriculum.

The Foundation Stage Curriculum

The Foundation Stage Curriculum comprises six areas of learning:

- Communication, language and literacy
- Mathematics
- Personal, social & emotional development
- Physical development
- Creative development
- Knowledge and understanding of the world

See Unit 2 pages 127–146 for more information on the Foundation Stage Curriculum and how it relates to **play**.

Key Stage 1 (5–7 years)

Children in **School Years 1 and 2 (aged 5–7 years)** work through the programme for **Key Stage 1**, which comprises the following subjects:

Key Stage 1

English
- Speaking and listening
- Reading
- Writing

Mathematics
- Using and applying mathematics
- Number
- Shape, space and measures

Science
- Experimental and investigative science
- Life processes and living things
- Materials and their properties
- Physical processes

Technology
- Designing
- Making
- Knowledge and understanding

Information technology
- Using, exploring and discussing experiences of IT
- Communicating and handling information

History
- Chronology
- Range and depth of historical knowledge
- Controlling and modelling and understanding
- Interpretations of history
- Historical enquiry
- Organisation and communication

Geography
- Geographical skills
- Places
- Thematic study

Art
- Investigating and making
- Knowledge and understanding

Music
- Performing and composing
- Listening and appraising

Physical education (PE)
- Games
- Gymnastic activities
- Dance
  (plus the option of swimming)

Religious Education *is* compulsory in schools but it is not a National Curriculum subject.

Knowledge and understanding of the world in the Early Years Curriculum

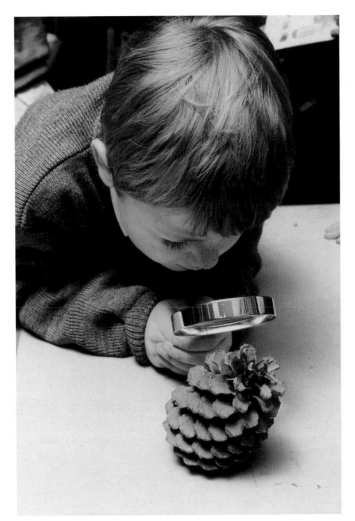

Social care provision for young children

Central government departments provide indirect social care for children:

✱ The **Department of Health** is responsible for the broad policy and central administration of welfare services, which covers both health care and social care.

✱ The **Department of Social Security (DSS)** manages the **Benefits Agency** and the **Child Support Agency**.

ACTIVITY

1 Visit your local library, Social Security office or Citizen's Advice Bureau and find out what benefits are available to families with young children, e.g. one-parent benefit.

2 Find out about the Child Support Agency.

Social Services

Local Authorities provide personal social services through their **Social Service Departments (SSDs)**. Mostly the services are statutory, i.e. they are funded by the government, but some voluntary organisations work in partnership with SSDs or services are purchased from the private sector. **Statutory social services** must be provided for children assessed as being 'in need':

Learning about balance

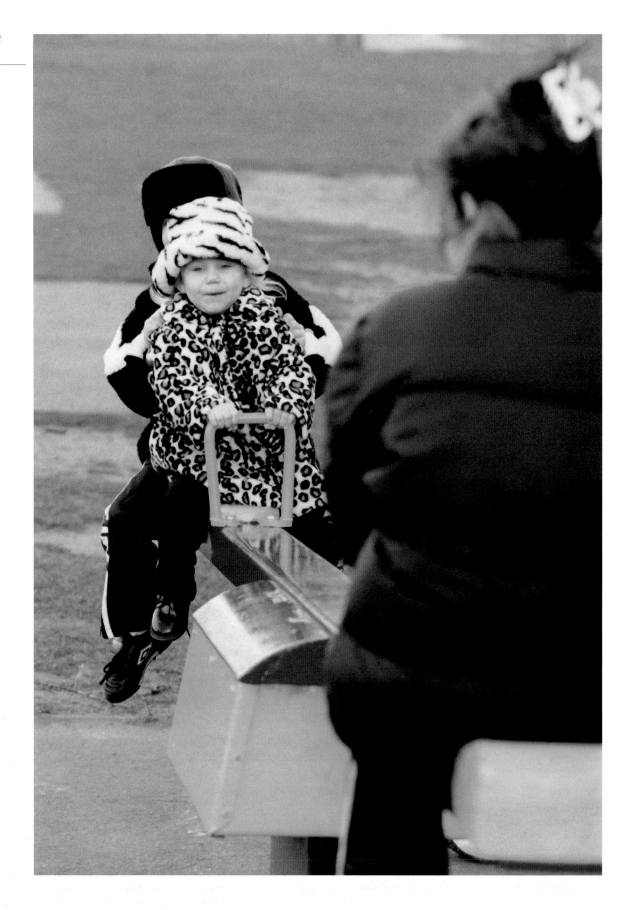

✳ assessment of needs;

✳ advice, guidance and counselling;

✳ day care services for children under 5 and not yet at school;

✳ care and supervised activities outside school hours and during school holidays;

✳ accommodation – for those children who are lost, abandoned or without carers who can provide accommodation;

✳ an emergency service 24 hours a day, 365 days a year.

Social service departments are also responsible for:

✳ **Regulating** and **registering** day care provision by voluntary and private organisations, e.g. childminders and private all-day nurseries, and

✳ Investigating the circumstances of any child believed to be at risk of harm, and taking appropriate action on their behalf.

Social Services may also provide the following caring services for children and their families:

- occupational therapy
- supplying specialist equipment
- respite care services
- training for childminders

How Local Authorities work for children and their families

Most Local Authorities have a special department to co-ordinate all the services to children within their locality. These departments are often called **Early Years Services** and deal exclusively with the needs of young children and their families. The range of services which is provided varies greatly from one Local Authority to another, but typically will include the following services (those marked with a * *must* be provided by law):

Services provided by Local Authority

- **Housing:** children and their families in need, e.g. homeless families and those seeking refuge, are a priority. Services include providing bed & breakfast accommodation or council housing.*
- **Nursery education:** most authorities are not able to offer full nursery education to all children within the borough. Nursery classes are usually attached to state primary schools. Nursery schools are separate.
- **Regulation and registration of services** such as childminders, private fostering and private or voluntary-run day care and family centres.*
- **Infant or primary education:** children must attend full-time school from the age of 5; they must follow the National Curriculum.*
- **Holiday playschemes:** these are full-day playschemes during the school holidays at various sites. A programme of activities and outings is arranged to ensure the interest and enjoyment of participating children.
- **Early Years Centres (or Family centres):** places at these nurseries are offered to children who have been identified as being 'in need of day care to assist their health or development', or to enable them to remain with their family.*

- **After school clubs:** these offer supervised play opportunities in a safe, supportive and friendly environment. They usually cater for children from five to eleven years of age, but some centres have facilities for under fives.*
- **Community places for families with low incomes:** most local authorities keep a number of full-day nursery places at Early Years Centres, specifically for the children of families with low incomes.
- **Social workers:** work with families where children are assessed as being in need, giving practical support and advice on a wide range of subjects including adoption and fostering children*
- **Residential holidays** provide opportunities for children to develop self-reliance and co-operation with others, as well as providing a break for many children who would not otherwise have the opportunity to go away.
- **Advice, information and counselling:** local authorities have a duty to provide advice, information and counselling to families where there is a child 'in need'*
- **Respite care:** families where a child has special needs may be offered a residential holiday for their child so that they can have a break from caring for them*

Recent government initiatives:

☐ Early Excellence Centres, which integrate education and care.

☐ Sure Start, which targets an area and focuses on children aged 0–3 years and their families.

🧸 Voluntary organisations

Voluntary organisations are non-profit-making organisations which usually are set up because people see a gap in provision and feel the need to provide a service. They are often staffed by a mixture of paid and volunteer workers.

Most voluntary organisations are registered charities. This means that they:

- finance their services and the running of their organisation through fund-raising;
- may also receive grants from central or local government;
- put all the money they raise back into running their services.

Within any Local Authority in the UK there are child care and education settings which come into the category of voluntary provision. Two examples are:

1 Community nurseries

Community nurseries exist to provide a service to local children and their families. They are run by local community organisations – often with financial assistance from the local authority – or by charities such as **Barnardo's** and **Save the Children**.

Most of these nurseries are open long enough to suit working parents or those at college. Many centres also provide, or act as a venue for, other services, including:

☐ parent and toddler groups;

☐ drop-in crèches;

☐ toy libraries; and

☐ after-school clubs.

Name and address of organisation	Type of support available
Action for Sick Children 85 Highbury Park London N5 1UD Tel: 020 7704 7000 www.nchafc.org.uk	Family support, information and research – campaigns by working at national and local levels to influence policy to improve the standards of health care for all children
NSPCC 42 Curtain Road London EC2A 3NH www.nspcc.org.uk	Charity specialising in child protection and the prevention of cruelty to children. The NSPCC is the only children's charity in the UK with statutory powers enabling it to act to safeguard children at risk
Gingerbread 16–17 Clerkenwell Close London EC1R 0AA Tel: 020 7336 8183 www.gingerbread.org.uk	Information and support for lone families in England and Wales
The National Children's Bureau (NCB) 8 Wakley Street London EC1V 7QE Tel: 020 7843 6000 www.ncb.org.uk	Works to identify and promote the well-being and interests of all children and young people across every aspect of their lives
Kidscape 2 Grosvenor Gardens London SW1W 0DH Tel. 020 7730 3300 www.kidscape.org.uk	Kidscape is the registered charity committed to keeping children safe from harm or abuse. Kidscape is the only national children's charity which focuses upon preventative policies – tactics to use before any abuse takes place
The Children's Society Edward Rudolf House Margery Street London WC1X 0JL Tel: 020 7841 4436 www.the-childrens-society.org.uk	Child care services for children and families in need – includes fostering and adoption services. It aims to help children to grow up in their own families and communities
Contact a Family 170 Tottenham Court Road London W1P 0HA Tel: 020 7383 3555 www.cafamily.org.uk	National charity offering information, advice and support to parents of children with special needs and disabilities. Links parents to local support groups for general support or to nationally run groups or, in the case of rare disorder, to individuals in similar circumstances.
Sure Start Level 2, Caxton House Tothill Street London SW1H 9NA www.surestart.gov.uk	Sure Start is the Government's programme to deliver the best start in life for every child by bringing together: ● early education ● childcare ● health and family support
Under5s early years education PO Box 137 Ilkley West Yorkshire LS29 7AH Tel. 07929 769493 (24hr answerphone) www.underfives.co.uk/fndtion.html	

2 Pre-School Learning Alliance Community Pre-Schools

Pre-School Learning Alliance Community Pre-Schools (**playgroups**) offer children aged between three and five years an opportunity to learn through play:

❑ They usually operate on a part-time sessional basis. Sessions are normally two and a half hours each morning or afternoon.

❑ Staff plan a varied curriculum that takes into account children's previous experiences and developing needs.

❑ The nationally set Foundation Stage curriculum framework, approved by the Department for Education and Skills (DfES), is adapted by each group to meet the needs of their own children and to allow them to make the most of a variety of learning opportunities that arise spontaneously through play.

❑ Many pre-school playgroups have received an Accreditation Certificate. This is the National Pre-school Learning Alliance kitemark of high-quality care and education.

❑ At many pre-school playgroups, parents and carers are encouraged to be involved, and there are often parent and toddler groups meeting at the same sites.

Voluntary groups tend to focus on a specific client group or issue and their publicity material reflects this focus. Some of the major voluntary organisations which provide services for young children and their families are listed in the table on p. 243.

The private sector

This sector comprises businesses making profits. It ranges from nannies looking after children in their own homes to large chains of private nurseries.

Childminders

A childminder is anyone who works at home caring for other people's children under eight years of age – usually while the parent works or is at college. Financial arrangements are a private matter to be decided between parent and childminder. Most Local Authorities recommend that parents sign a contract with their childminder, and usually provide childminders with a standard contract that can be used for this purpose.

Private nurseries

Private nurseries are set up by private individuals or organisations, but they must all be registered by the Registration and Inspection Unit of their Local Authority. All nurseries are required to display a copy of their registration certificate in their premises.

Independent schools

A small number of children under 8 years old are educated within the private sector – in independent schools, the majority of which have **charitable status**. They are not funded by the state and obtain most of their finances from fees paid by parents and income from investments. Independent schools look after their own day-to-day affairs. However, they are subject to inspection to ensure they maintain acceptable standards of premises, accommodation, instruction and staffing.

Sources of information and guidance

It is important that early years workers know how and where to obtain advice and information for families with young children. Some useful sources of information are listed below:

- **Charities Digest:** Available in Reference Library section in Public Library and most college libraries

- **Internet** www.charitynet.org.uk

- **Citizens Advice Bureau:** Trained staff provide free, impartial advice and help on legal, social and financial matters to anyone who contacts them
- **Public Library:** for information on all local voluntary groups, often on computer link
- **Yellow Pages telephone book:** Usually listed under *Charitable &Voluntary Organisations*
- **Local Authority (Council) Information Service:** Useful addresses of voluntary organisations
- **Post offices and Benefit Agency Offices (DSS):** For leaflets explaining the benefits and allowances available for families with young children

ACTIVITY

Design a booklet which you could give to a family who are new to your area to inform them about:

1   Where to find information on:

- Support groups for parents
- Mother and toddler groups
- Pre-school groups (Playgroups)
- Nursery schools and infant schools

2   How to access information on:

- Health care for their family – hospitals and Accident & Emergency Departments
- Location of health clinics, GP centres
- Community Health Councils: These are independent bodies which represent the views of patients and users of the Health Service

3   Where to find out any benefits and allowances they may be entitled to receive, for example:

- Child benefit
- Lone-parent benefit
- Housing benefit

4   List some useful general voluntary organisations which exist to support families with young children, with addresses, telephone numbers and, where possible, their internet website addresses.

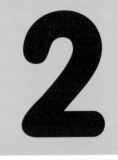
- structure, aims and routines of a range of work settings
- helping to develop good practice within the setting
- what to do if unsatisfactory practice is observed
- the work setting's equal opportunities code of practice
- the role of the multidisciplinary team and wider links

The structure, aims and routines of a range of work settings

All organisations, whatever their size, need systems in place for dealing with routine events and for communication to be effective. Many have a structure with 'tiers' or 'levels' of staff responsible to someone (a line manager) in the level above. There are more staff in the lower levels and fewer in the higher levels. The structure and organisation in Early Years work settings vary considerably depending on:

* function (what purpose or role they have)
* ownership
* size
* location
* premises
* facilities

The main **function** of nursery classes and nursery units in state and private schools is to educate although, of course, they are also caring for the children. The main function of the other settings is to care for children although, of course, in caring for them they also promote learning through the experiences and activities they provide.

Most organisations, large or small, have clear structures that enable everyone to identify the **roles** and **responsibilities** of staff members.

ACTIVITY

In pairs, try to identify the organisational structure of your study centre. Begin by listing all the staff jobs – teachers/administration staff/caretaker/cleaners/ departmental or faculty heads etc. Try to identify who reports to whom and what responsibilities or duties the jobs might entail. Who has overall responsibility?

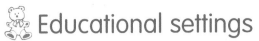 Educational settings

1 All state schools have a **Governing body** (usually comprising about 6 to 10 people) which has overall responsibility for the welfare of the pupils and staff, and educational and financial matters. Governors can be appointed (some by the Local Education Authority [LEA]) and elected. All governing bodies should have **parent governors** (the number depends on the **school roll** i.e. number of pupils who attend) who are elected by, and from, the parents of pupils.

2 The **headteacher** can be a governor too but also has the responsibility for the day-to-day running of the school and, with the teaching staff, will plan the educational programme and timetable.

3 The **deputy headteacher** stands in for the headteacher but also might have responsibility for staff meetings, staff development, administration and support staff, liaison with parents and school discipline.

4 In the next level there may be **Key Stage curriculum co-ordinators** – who oversee planning, assessment and record-keeping within the year groups –– and **subject co-ordinators** – who advise on their own subjects and order resources.

5 **Subject or class teachers** form the next level and they may have additional responsibilities (e.g. for school clubs)

6 **Nursery nurses, classroom assistants and special needs support assistants** form the next level.

Most nursery classes or units attached to schools are part of similar organisational structures but with a designated person in charge of the nursery – who is usually a **nursery trained teacher**. The nursery staff are able to work closely with reception class teachers in planning the **curriculum** for the **Foundation Stage** and ensure a smooth **transition** from nursery to school. There will also be administration and technical support staff as well as caretakers, cleaners and, possibly, catering staff.

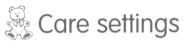 Care settings

✳ Public Sector

As detailed on p. 241, Social Services can provide care for under-fives. In this type of work setting a Nursery Manager has responsibility for the daily running but reports to the Social Services Department and Committee who deal with funding (i.e. how much money is spent on the nursery).

✳ Private Sector

Private day nurseries vary considerably in the care and facilities provided. They can be owned by companies or private individuals who employ qualified staff to organise and manage the nurseries. The size of the staff team and the level of qualifications depends largely on the number of children being cared for and their ages (there are strict regulations about staff/child ratios).

✳ Voluntary Sector

Community playgroups and nurseries run by charities belong to this category and, although qualified staff will organise and manage them, there will often be help from parents and volunteers.

The **aims** stated by work settings will vary. A playgroup may emphasise a happy, safe atmosphere in which children can experience a wide range of play experiences with other children, whereas a nursery unit in a school will focus on promoting learning opportunities through a planned curriculum. However, all now follow the Foundation Stage Curriculum guidance. Both examples will have the welfare of the children as their prime concern. **Routines** will also be different and take account of hours open, number of children, age of children, facilities (perhaps shared) etc.

Good practice – Policies and Codes of Practice

Other sections in this book have explained what methods and attitudes contribute to good practice and have given clear guidance as to what is dangerous or illegal. Following the good practice of experienced **role models** is probably the best way to develop your own confidence and ways of working.

During your practical training in different settings you will almost certainly have been:

✓ introduced to staff and children;

✓ shown where things are kept;

✓ had routines explained;

✓ told how responsibilities are shared;

✓ given documentation – Policies and Codes of Practice – to read (in some cases you will have had to sign to say that you have read and understood them).

A Code of Practice

A Code of Practice sets out a framework within which the setting will operate and must take into account legislation. For example the Health and Safety at Work Acts identify the legal responsibilities of employers and employees, so a Code of Practice must meet its requirements.

A Policy

A Policy sets out the ways in which the Code of Practice will be followed. It has an aim (e.g. to ensure that all people who use the premises are safe) and explains what steps are taken to achieve it – for example: regular checks of electrical equipment; set procedures for dealing with toxic substances and storing them; identified person given responsibility for checking etc.

In your work setting you may find Codes of Practice and Policies relating to:

✱ equal opportunities responsibilities   ✱ child protection

✱ behaviour and issues of discipline   ✱ staff development/training

✱ health and safety; first aid   ✱ food service

✱ confidentiality   ✱ record-keeping

✱ working with parents

Good practice does not, necessarily, mean that every work setting must do things in the same way. For example, there are different methods used to prevent unauthorised people entering premises; some settings have a security panel at the entrance which involves ringing a bell and announcing who you are before being admitted, others have push-button coded locks. So long as the safety and security is satisfactory then the way it is achieved is not important. Every work setting will have its own ways of achieving and ensuring good practice.

3

Working relationships and roles within the team

- your role and that of others within the team
- establishing and developing working relationships
- importance of listening to and recording information accurately
- assisting others to achieve their work priorities
- exchanging information within the work setting whilst maintaining confidentiality
- suggesting ideas and following them through

Your role and that of others within the team

To meet the needs of all the children in a setting, the staff members must work effectively together as a team.

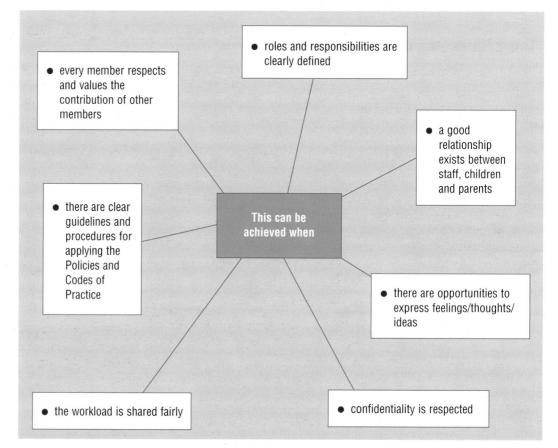

- roles and responsibilities are clearly defined
- every member respects and values the contribution of other members
- a good relationship exists between staff, children and parents
- there are clear guidelines and procedures for applying the Policies and Codes of Practice

This can be achieved when

- there are opportunities to express feelings/thoughts/ ideas
- the workload is shared fairly
- confidentiality is respected

The roles and responsibilities of team members will depend on the organisation of the work setting.

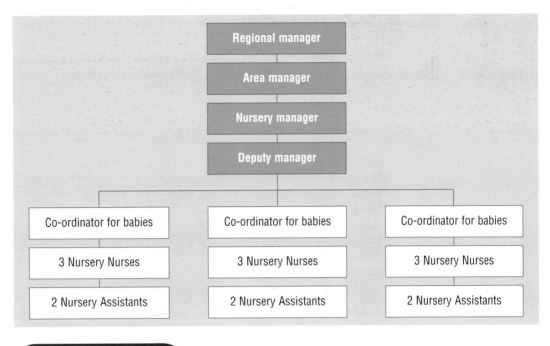

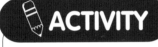**ACTIVITY**

Choose one of the following – babies, toddlers or pre-school – groups and list the duties that a Nursery Assistant may carry out. What responsibilities might the role include?

The 3 Bears Playgroup

Provides morning only care for 2–5 years

Village hall (used by other community groups) organised into play or activity areas:

- Messy area
- Indoor large apparatus
- Construction area
- Book/story area
- General activity area with tables and chairs
- Small outdoor play area.
- Toilet area. Kitchen

The **3 Bears Playgroup** is a **voluntary organisation** and employs a qualified Nursery Nurse and Nursery Assistant to organise and run the sessions. It was set up to serve the local community and has strong links with the school and other groups. Parents take turns, on a rota basis, to provide the extra help and supervision needed.

Humpty Dumpty Day Nursery

Provides all-day care for 3 months–5 years

Purpose-built with different large rooms/areas for each stage:

- babies

- toddlers

- pre-school

There are separate changing/toilet facilities for each group.

There is a kitchen area specifically for the babies and a second one which is shared by the other two groups. Each area has its own outdoor play area.

The **Humpty Dumpty Day Nursery** is one of a nation-wide chain of nurseries. The chain is owned by a large company; it employs regional and area managers to oversee the smooth operation of a number of its nurseries. All the nurseries work to the same Codes of Practice and are similarly equipped.

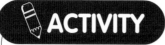

ACTIVITY

In groups, choose either the Nursery Nurse or the Nursery Assistant or a parent helper and decide what responsibilities and duties each would have in this situation. Which ones appear on all the lists? What additional roles may these staff have compared to similar positions in a private sector nursery?

In your role as a Nursery Assistant you will be supporting the work of others. You will usually work under direction, sometimes under supervision, of a Nursery Nurse or teacher, depending on the setting. There may also be professionals from other disciplines (medicine, social services, dentistry etc.) who are involved with the families and children you work with. A **special school** or nursery which cares for children with physical disabilities will have a '**multidisciplinary**' team; this may include teachers, nursery nurses and assistants, trained special care assistants, physiotherapists, paediatricians and, possibly, social workers. Effective teamwork is vital in such settings to ensure that

- all concerned know their individual roles and responsibilities and that
- parents and primary carers know which team member can deal with any specific concerns.

Forest Day Nursery

Come and work at Forest Day Nursery. We cater for babies and children aged 3 months–5 years. We have a vacancy for a Nursery Assistant to work in a friendly team of 10 staff. You should have a recognised qualification, and experience of a day nursery work setting. You should be flexible, cheerful and prepared to work hard! A shift system is operated on a rota basis. Please telephone .... or write for further details to: ....

The person we are looking for must:

✓ hold CACHE Certificate in Child Care & Education/NVQ2/SVQ2
✓ have had experience of day nursery work setting
✓ be cheerful/friendly
✓ be reliable, have a good record record for attendance and timekeeping – PDP/attendance sheets
✓ understand importance of confidentiality/evidence in PDP/references
✓ understand and practice equality of opportunity (reference/PDP)
✓ understand and practice health and safety procedures
✓ recognise and value the contribution of other staff members
✓ be willing to co-operate and be flexible in carrying out duties
✓ be able to follow instructions

Attending meetings

In most work settings being part of the staff team means participating in meetings to discuss, and to make decisions about, a wide range of issues. You are expected to attend and you must 'make your apologies' (to the person holding the meeting) if, for a genuine reason, you are unable to attend.

At any formal meeting, there is usually a set format:

1 An **agenda** (or programme): This is a list of items which will be discussed – some of which will appear at every meeting. Apologies for absence are usually received and recorded at the start of any meeting.

2 A written record, called the **minutes**. Most meetings will begin by looking at the minutes of the last one to remind everyone what was decided and to find out what has happened since. Someone will be given responsibility for 'taking the minutes'.

3 **Any other business:** most meetings will allow time for issues not included in the formal agenda to be raised and discussed; for example, a problem with discipline or damaged equipment that has arisen since the meeting was arranged.

4 **Date for the next meeting:** This is set and agreed by those attending the meeting.

After the meeting, the person who has taken the minutes will type or write them out neatly and arrange copies to be sent to all the people who attended or who were invited but were unable to attend.

Some meetings are informal and may be set up to talk about planning next month's topic or theme or to finalise arrangements for an outing. Others may be more formal, perhaps covering policy matters. There is one person who leads (or 'chairs') the meeting and makes sure the items on the agenda are being dealt with – it is very easy for people to begin their own conversations or stray from the subject in hand!

Remember that you are there to contribute your ideas and thoughts and to listen to those of others.

At a meeting try to:

☐ listen carefully to information being given;

☐ ask questions about anything you do not understand;

☐ check that you know what is expected of **you**;

☐ contribute your ideas and opinions clearly and at the appropriate time – not when everyone has started talking about the next item;

☐ make sure you bring pen and paper and any other things that will be needed – e.g. an observation of a child who is being discussed;

☐ understand that you may not share the views of others or agree with all decisions made.

Time management

There are often conflicting pressures on your time when working in early years settings. However well prepared a timetable is, something can always occur which upsets the smooth running of the day. Even when you are caring for one young baby in the parent's home, you will find it useful to follow these guidelines:

• **Prioritise** your tasks: it is a good idea to make a written list of the various tasks you have to complete in a particular session; then you can divide the tasks into essential and non-essential (but desirable) tasks.

- **Set targets:** Try to set deadlines for completing certain tasks; you may be able to fit in a simple task – such as organising the creative play area – between other tasks. Be realistic in what you hope to achieve. Be aware that you may be interrupted in what you are doing and will need to return to it later.

- **Try not to become overwhelmed:** There will be some days when you wonder if you will ever complete any one task. Take a deep breath and try to put it all into perspective. As long as you are doing your best and have the children's welfare as your primary concern, try not to panic if you are running late!

- **Share your concerns:** Your colleagues will understand the pressures (and the rewards) of working with children and about the unpredictability of such work. By sharing your worries you can learn how to manage your time and routines more effectively.

ACTIVITY

Carla has been working as a full-time nanny for just three weeks. She is in sole charge of 3-year-old Joanna and her 10-month-old brother, Liam. Her responsibilities include taking and collecting Joanna to and from a pre-school playgroup each morning and generally caring for Liam and Joanna from 8 am until their mother returns from work at 6 pm. Carla has a good relationship with the children and with their parents, but is concerned that she is not able to give as much attention as she would like to Joanna. This is because Liam cries a great deal and will only settle for a sleep if she walks him in his pram or walks around the house holding him. Even then, he tends to wake after only half an hour or so. Having completed the CCE course, Carla has a clear idea of Joanna's needs and is aware that she is failing her. Joanna is beginning to show anger and resentment towards Liam and to Carla during the long afternoons.

1 How can Carla improve daily life for (a) Joanna, (b) for Liam, and (c) for herself?

2 Discuss how you would deal with this situation.

You may find it helpful to read the section on crying babies – see Option A, page 328.

Responsibilities of an early years worker

You need to practise your skills with regard to certain responsibilities:

1 **Respect for the principles of confidentiality**

Confidentiality is about trust and sensitivity to the needs and the rights of others. You should always treat all the information you are privileged to receive within the work setting as confidential; avoid gossip and stereotyping.

2 **Commitment to meeting the needs of the children**

All children should be treated with respect and dignity and their needs must be considered as paramount. This means working within the guidelines of an equal opportunities code of practice, and not allowing any personal preferences or prejudices influence the way you treat children.

3 Responsibility and accountability in the workplace

The supervisor, line manager, teacher or parent will have certain expectations about your role, and your responsibilities should be detailed in your job contract. As a professional, you need to carry out all your duties willingly and to be answerable (or accountable) to others for your work. You need to know about the lines of reporting within a work setting and how to find out about your own particular responsibilities. If you are unsure what is expected of you – or if you do not feel confident in carrying out a particular task – then you should ask your line manager or your immediate supervisor for guidance.

4 Respect for parents and other adults

You need to respect the wishes and views of parents and other carers, even when you disagree with those views. You should also recognise that parents are usually the people who know their children best. In all your dealings with parents and other adults, you must show that you respect their cultural values and religious beliefs.

5 Communicate effectively with team members and other professionals

Being able to communicate effectively with team members, other professionals and with parents is a very important part of your role as an early years worker. You should always:

✓ be considerate of others and polite towards them;

✓ recognise the contributions made by other team members; we all like to feel we are valued for the work they do. You can help others to feel valued by being aware of their role and how it has contributed to the smooth running of the nursery;

✓ explain clearly to the relevant person any changes in routine or any actions you have taken: for example, (a) as a nanny, always informing a parent when a child you are caring for has refused a meal or been distressed in any way, or (b) reporting any behaviour problem or incident to your line manager in a nursery setting.

A team meeting at a nursery

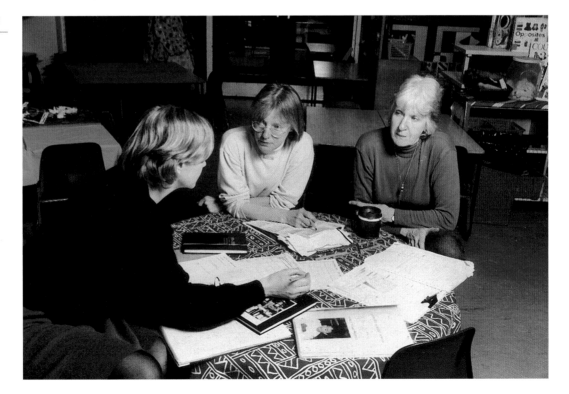

4

Values and principles

- CACHE values statement and equality of opportunity statement
- forms of discrimination
- your role in ensuring that activities, resources, equipment and relationships reflect the sector's values

CACHE Statement of Values

You must ensure that you

- Put the child first by:
  - ensuring the child's welfare and safety
  - showing compassion and sensitivity
  - respecting the child as an individual
  - upholding the child's rights and dignity
  - enabling the child to achieve their full learning potential

- Never use physical punishment

- Respect the parent as the primary carer and educator of the child

- Respect the contribution and expertise of staff in the child care and education field and other professionals with whom they may be involved

- Respect the customs, values and spiritual beliefs of the child and their family

- Uphold the Council's Equality of Opportunity policy

- Honour the confidentiality of information relating to the child and their family, unless its disclosure is required by law or is in the best interest of the child.

Values and Attitudes

Our values and attitudes towards others develop from early childhood. The way in which we are brought up and the behaviour we see around us will help us to form opinions and to make choices about every aspect of our lives. The first **values** which we absorb into our learning come from our early childhood experiences, particularly from:

☐ our parents or primary carers and our family;

☐ our friends and their families; and

☐ our early experiences in play group, nursery and school.

Children learn moral values by example and by imitation. If a child is made to feel secure and loved within their family, they will develop confidence and **self-esteem** and find it easier to make close relationships with others. Children whose early life involves unhappy or very weak relationships with others often find it difficult to make close, lasting relationships when they are older. **Attitudes** are the opinions and ways of thinking that we have towards others and their beliefs. These attitudes are shaped by our values.

Examples of moral values are:

❑ truth   ❑ right conduct

❑ love   ❑ non-violence

❑ peace

The following poem by Dorothy Law Nolte describes the effect our values have on children's development:

Children Learn What They Live

If children live with criticism, they learn to condemn.
If children live with hostility, they learn to fight.
If children live with ridicule, they learn to be shy.
If children live with shame, they learn to feel guilty.
If children live with encouragement, they learn confidence.
If children live with tolerance, they learn to be patient.
If children live with praise, they learn to appreciate.
If children live with acceptance, they learn to love.
If children live with approval, they learn to like themselves.
If children live with honesty, they learn truthfulness.
If children live with fairness, they learn justice.
If children live with kindness and consideration, they learn respect.
If children live with security, they learn to have faith in themselves and others.
If children live with friendliness, they learn the world is a nice place in which to live.

✏ ACTIVITY

Working in pairs or small groups, identify and list **five** moral values within the poem above, and for each value, discuss how this value can be promoted within the care and education setting. (One example could be the value of appreciation; by praising children every time they have achieved something, however small that thing may be, you are demonstrating your **appreciation** for them as individuals and promoting their self-concept – or feelings of self-worth.)

Attitudes

Our attitudes towards others are based on our beliefs and feelings about the world. **Negative attitudes** towards others may result from **assumptions** about people and their way of life, which may be very different from our own. Travellers, for example, have often been discriminated against within care settings because of these differences.

Positive attitudes towards children enable them:

- to feel good about themselves;
- to feel that they are valued; and
- to develop high self-esteem.

It is not our task to try to change the values and attitudes of others, but we should challenge others if their behaviour shows discrimination. What is most important is that we act as good **role models** through our work with children, so that they can learn to imitate our behaviour and express positive attitudes towards others.

ACTIVITY

Exploring your attitudes and values

Consider the following moral questions:

1   Should women go out to work when they have young children?

2   Should the armed forces accept gay men and women into their ranks?

3   Should it be against the law to smack a child? Should childminders and teachers have the right to smack a child if the parents consent?

4   Should gay couples (male *or* female) be allowed to adopt a child?

5   Should men take an equal share with women in bringing up their children?

In pairs, discuss each question in turn, making brief notes on the arguments for and against each question. Then, in the whole group, consider how each answer could affect your attitudes towards parents and children in the work setting.

Stereotypes

A stereotype is a way of thinking that assumes that all people who share one characteristic also share another set of characteristics. Examples are:

✱ **racism:** racism is the belief that some 'races' are superior to others – based on the false idea that different physical characteristics (like skin colour) or ethnic background make some people better than others;

✱ **sexism:** sexism occurs when people of one gender (or biological sex) believe that they are superior to the other;

✱ **ageism:** this occurs when negative feelings are expressed towards a person or group because of their age; in Western society it is usually directed towards older people;

✱ **disablism:** this occurs when disabled people are seen in terms of their disability, rather than as unique individuals, who happen to have special needs.

There are many other stereotypes, such as those concerning gay and lesbian groups, people from low socio-economic groups and those who practise a minority religion.

Stereotyped thinking can prevent you from seeing someone as an individual with particular life experiences and interests and so lead to negative attitudes and to **prejudice** and **discrimination**.

Scenarios – Making assumptions

1   *Sam, Jason, Laura and Fatima are playing in the home corner. The nursery teacher asks Sam and Jason to tidy away the train set and trucks and asks Laura and Fatima to put the dolls and cooking pots away, as it is nearly story-time.*

The assumption here is that dolls and cooking utensils are 'girl' playthings, whereas trains and trucks are 'boy' playthings. The teacher is reinforcing this stereotype by separating the tasks by gender.

2   *Paul's mother arrives at the school open day. She is in a wheelchair, being pushed by Paul's father. The teacher welcomes the parents and then asks Paul's father if his wife would like a drink and a biscuit.*

This is a common feature of daily life for people who use wheelchairs. They are often ignored and questions are addressed to their companion, often because the other person is embarrassed by the unusual situation and fearful of making a mistake. The assumption here is that the person in the wheelchair would not be able to understand and reply to what is said to them.

3   *Members of staff are having a tea break and discussing a new child who has just started at their school. Julie says: 'I can't stand the way these travellers think they can just turn up at school whenever they feel like it – they don't pay taxes you know and they live practically on top of rubbish dumps . . . poor little mite, he doesn't know any different.'*

An assumption has been made which is based on prejudice and stereotyped thinking; in this case, travellers are assumed to be 'scroungers' and to live in unhygienic conditions. Such attitudes will be noticed by all the children in the class and may result in the individual child being treated differently, damaging his self-esteem and leading to feelings of rejection.

4   *Harry's mother is a registered heroin addict who has been attending a drug rehabilitation programme for the last few months. Whenever Harry behaves in an aggressive way to other children or to staff, one staff member always makes a jibe about his home life: 'Harry, you may get away with that sort of thing where you come from, but it won't work here. We know all about you.'*

This is an extreme and very unkind form of stereotyping. It is assuming that, because his mother is a drug user, Harry is somehow less worthy of consideration and respect. By drawing attention to his home life, the member of staff is guilty of prejudice and discriminatory behaviour. There is also a breach of the policy of **confidentiality**.

ACTIVITY

Look at the three photographs on page 262. One of them is a student on a child care course; one is a university student studying for a degree in Law and the other is a primary school teacher. Which person do you think fits each role? (See page 264 for the correct answers.)

Different occupational roles

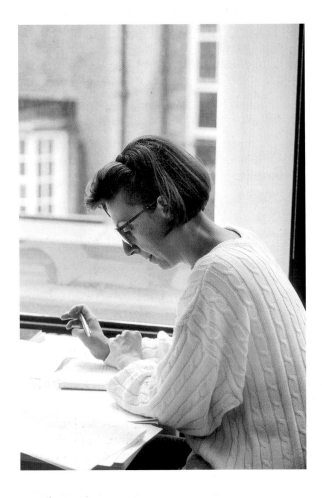

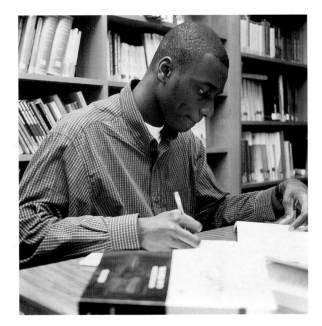

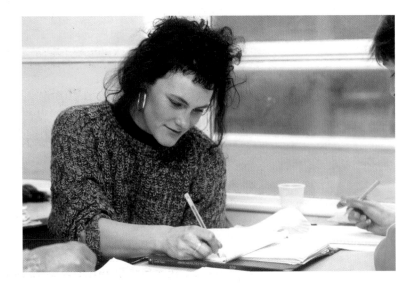

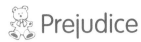 Prejudice

Prejudice literally means 'pre-judging' someone – knowing next to nothing about them but jumping to conclusions because of some characteristic, like their appearance.

It involves having pre-conceived ideas about a person based on attitudes and beliefs which often lead to **discrimination**. People have all kinds of prejudices – for example, they might not like students, people with beards or people who are fat. When such prejudices are carried into action, then it leads to discrimination; for example, if they refuse to sit next to a fat person on the bus or if they bar a group of students from a cafe.

Discrimination

What is discrimination?

Discrimination occurs when someone is treated less favourably, usually because of a negative view of some of their characteristics. This negative – or **pejorative** – view is based on stereotypical assumptions which do not have a factual basis.

Types of discrimination

The most obvious types of discrimination occur as a result of the **stereotypes** described on page 258: racism, sexism, ageism, and disablism. Children may also discriminate against other children on account of their differences. This often takes the form of name-calling and teasing and may be directed at children who are either fatter or thinner than others in the group, or who wear different clothes.

Sometimes discrimination is **institutionalised**. This means that the particular institution is not organised to meet the needs of all the people within it; in other words, the structures are not in place to prevent discrimination taking place. Examples include:

* institutional racism within the police force; many more black youths are stopped by the police than are white youths;

* children with impairments or learning difficulties are not provided with the equipment or resources to enable them to take a full part in the school or nursery curriculum;

* adults who use wheelchairs may not be allowed access to cinemas or theatres, because of lack of suitable adaptations to comply with fire regulations;

* the needs of children from minority religious or cultural groups are not recognised within the nursery or school.

Direct discrimination occurs when someone is treated less favourably on specific racial or other grounds than other people are, or would be, treated in similar circumstances.

* *Example:* If an Asian woman is turned down for a job as a shop assistant and told there are no vacancies, then a white woman with equivalent qualifications is offered the job a short while later, the Asian woman has been **directly** discriminated against.

Indirect discrimination occurs when a condition or requirement is applied equally to people of all racial or other groups, but many fewer people of a particular group are able to comply with it. Such **indirect** discrimination is against the law when it cannot be justified other than on racial or other grounds.

- *Example:* If an employer requires job applicants to have a qualification in a particular subject, but will only consider people whose degree is from a British university, this condition could amount to indirect discrimination.

Codes of practice and equal opportunities policies

At government level, laws have been passed to protect certain groups of people from discrimination. These laws cannot absolutely *prevent* discrimination from taking place, but they do make a public statement about what is acceptable in society and they also provide a framework for good practice.

Laws relating to discrimination

Sex Discrimination Act (1975 and 1986)	These Acts make it illegal to discriminate against someone on the grounds of their gender – when employing someone, when selling or renting a property to them, in their education or when providing them with goods and services. It also protects people from sexual harassment. The Equal Opportunities Commission was set up in 1975 to enforce the laws relating to sexual discrimination.
Equal Pay Act (1984)	This Act gave women the right to equal pay for equal work.
Education Reform Act (1988)	Local Education Authorities (LEAs) must provide access to the National Curriculum to all children including those with special needs and must identify and assess children's needs.
The Children Act (1989)	This Act states that the needs of children are paramount (i.e. the most important). local authorities must consider a child's race, culture, religion and languages when making decisions. Childcare services must promote self-esteem and racial identity.
Disability Discrimination Act (1995)	Disabled people are given new rights in the areas of employment, access to goods, facilities and services, and buying or renting property. A National Disability Council (NDC) advises the government on discrimination against disabled people.
The Race Relations Act 1976	This Act makes it unlawful to discriminate against anyone on grounds of race, colour, nationality (including citizenship), or ethnic or national origins. It applies to jobs, training, housing, education and the provision of goods and services. The Commission for Racial Equality (CRE) was set up to research and investigate cases of alleged racial discrimination.

Equality of opportunity

Equality of opportunity means opening up access for every child and family to full participation in early childhood services. Children and their families need to feel part of things, and a sense of belonging. Every early years setting needs:

❑ a policy on equality of opportunity

❑ a code of practice which takes the policy into action, and

❑ regular meetings to see how it is going.

> Answers to Activity on page 262:
>
> (a) Child Care course student
>
> (b) Primary school teacher
>
> (c) Law student.

All workplace policies and codes of practice must be drawn up within the framework of current legislation, in particular relating to the laws detailed above.

Equal opportunities policy

An equal opportunities policy represents a commitment by an organisation to ensuring that its activities do not lead to any individual receiving less favourable treatment on the grounds of:

- gender
- marital status
- religious belief
- race

- disability
- skin colour
- ethnic or national origin
- age

Such a policy does not mean that there will be reverse discrimination, e.g. in favour of black people. The **policy statement** should also provide information about the law on direct and indirect discrimination, and should be made available to all employees and service-users. Many local authorities demand that nurseries and playgroups have a written code of practice and policy statement before they allow them to be registered. In trying to decide how discrimination can best be prevented, the following issues could be considered:

- encouraging all staff to recognise **positively** the different racial and ethnic variations within the setting;
- promoting awareness of any discriminatory practices within the nursery or school, e.g. name-calling, teasing or aggressive behaviour – and developing strategies to deal with them;
- avoiding the use of labels – (even in private) – such as 'bully', 'thick' or 'spoiled brat';
- ensuring that all children have equal access to equipment and resources; some children may be prevented from using certain equipment because of an impairment or because other children always dominate a particular play area;
- treating all parents and carers with respect and warmth;
- promoting a sense of fair play and respect for others within the setting.

Codes of practice

A code of practice is not a legal document, but it does give direction and guidance to the organisation for which it has been designed. The code of practice covers areas of ethical (or moral) concern and good practice, such as:

- equal opportunities
- staff to children ratios
- confidentiality
- child protection
- health and safety aspects

- record-keeping
- partnerships with parents
- food provision
- first-aid responsibilities

The effects of racism, sexism and other forms of discriminatory practice on children's development

The early childhood setting – nursery, playgroup or nursery school – is often the first experience beyond their immediate family and friendship group that the child joins. When they join any wider setting, children need:

- to feel valued for themselves – as individuals;
- to feel a part of things, and a sense of belonging;
- to feel accepted by others;
- to develop a sense of self-worth, i.e. to feel that they matter to other people.

Discrimination of any kind prevents them from developing a feeling of self-worth or self-esteem. The effects of being discriminated against can last the whole of a child's life. In particular, they may:

✱ be unable to fulfil their **potential**, because they are made to feel that their efforts are not valued or recognised by others;

✱ find it hard to form **relationships** with others because of lack of self-worth or self-esteem;

✱ be so affected by the **stereotypes** or labels applied to them that they start to believe in them and so behave in accordance with others' expectations. This then becomes a **self-fulfilling prophecy**: for example, if a child is repeatedly told that he is clumsy, he may act in a clumsy way even when quite capable of acting otherwise;

✱ feel **shame** about their own cultural background;

✱ feel that they are in some way to **blame** for their unfair treatment and so withdraw into themselves;

✱ lack **confidence** in trying new activities if their attempts are always ridiculed or put down;

✱ be **aggressive** towards others; distress or anger can prevent children from playing co-operatively with other children.

Disability and discrimination

Children who are disabled (and their families) may be discriminated against in particular ways:

✱ They may face difficulty gaining access to shops. Most large stores have easy entrance arrangements, but smaller shops prevent access by wheelchair (and often by large pushchairs and prams too).

✱ Children who *look* different often face more discrimination because the **disability** is seen first rather than the *child*; for example, they may be stared at and hear remarks about themselves when out with their families. Disabled children have even been barred from cafés and restaurants because of their differences.

✱ Children who look *just like* any other child may have a 'hidden' disability, such as autism, Attention Deficit Hyperactivity Disorder (ADHD) or deafness. Their behaviour may attract disapproval when out in public and the family will feel under attack.

✴ They may have financial difficulties. There are always extra financial costs involved in bringing up a disabled child in the family; for example, mobility costs, the costs of giving full-time care, and perhaps extra laundry costs. Parents may have to rely on state benefits to enable them to give their child the care they need.

✴ Parents who are caring for a disabled child may not have the time or energy to give equivalent attention to any other children in the family. This could restrict the other child's development.

✴ Parents often have to struggle 'against the odds' to obtain the best treatment and resources for their child. Many parents find it difficult to have to ask for help all the time; others find the process very tiring. (For example, the process of **statementing** can take many months or even years).

Your role in challenging discrimination

The first step in being able to challenge discrimination is to identify when it is taking place. The most obvious and common form of indirect discrimination is when **labels** are applied to children. You may believe in private, for example, that Mark is a 'spoilt' child who gets away with the sort of behaviour that you personally think is unacceptable. It would be unnatural not to have an opinion on such matters. However, you should not initiate or join in any discussion which results in Mark being labelled as a 'difficult' or 'spoilt' child. Equally, you will find some children more likeable than others; again this is quite natural. What is important is that you are fair in your treatment of all the children in your care. You should treat them all equally and with respect.

Remember the poem on page 259 – *'Children learn what they live'* and try to develop **positive attitudes** towards all the children you meet, so that they cannot feel the effects of discrimination. It is only natural to like some children better than others, but our behaviour should always reflect the principle that all children are entitled to the same love and respect.

Valuing diversity

It is important that you recognise the differences between children and that you **value** those differences. Children should be encouraged not to feel anxious about people who are different from themselves. Many of the traditions practised within families from ethnic minorities are now adopted by Western societies, e.g. baby massage with natural oils and the carrying of babies in fabric slings. We all have a great deal to learn from one another.

Some practical ways of encouraging **cultural diversity** are by:

✱ providing a range of activities which celebrate these differences; e.g. to make children aware of what is involved in celebrations of religious festivals such as Diwali and Chinese New Year, as well as Christmas and Easter, whether or not we have children in the nursery who celebrate these occasions;

✱ promoting a multi-cultural approach to food provision; for example, parents could be invited into the setting to cook authentic national and regional dishes – Caribbean food, Yorkshire pudding as a dessert, Welsh griddle cakes, Irish Bara Brith, Asian sweets – the list is endless!

✱ encouraging self-expression in solo and in group activities; for example, by providing 'tools' for cooking and eating from other cultures – woks, chopsticks, griddles etc;

Baby being massaged

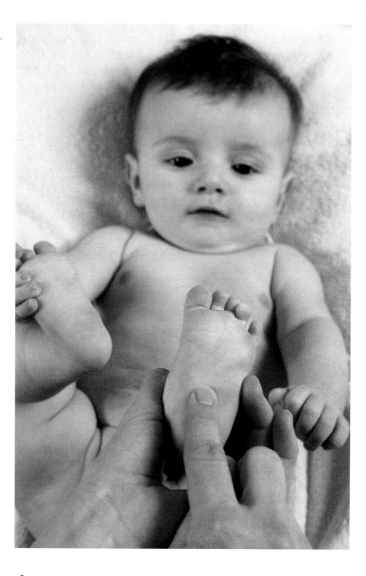

✳ celebrating the diversity of language; use body language, gesture, pictures and actions to convey messages to children whose home language is not English.

Children may feel themselves to be different in other ways too, not simply by having a different cultural heritage. Children with special needs often feel that they are the odd ones out in a group setting, for example, if a child:

- wears glasses or a hearing aid;

- has frequent bouts of asthma;

- has a mobility problem, or

- has learning difficulties.

Some practical ways of valuing and encouraging diversity are by:

✓ providing positive images: books and displays should use **positive images** of children with disabilities and from different cultures. Children also need positive images of gender roles, e.g. men caring for small children and women mending the car;

✓ arranging activities to encourage children with special needs to **participate fully** with other children: this might mean providing ramps for wheelchair users, or working with parents to find comfortable ways for a child to sit; e.g. a corner with two walls for support, a chair with a seat belt, or a wheelchair with a large tray across the arms;

✓ learning a **sign language**, such as Makaton or Signalong to help communicate with a child who has a hearing impairment or a learning difficulty.

Child and adult
communicating in Makaton

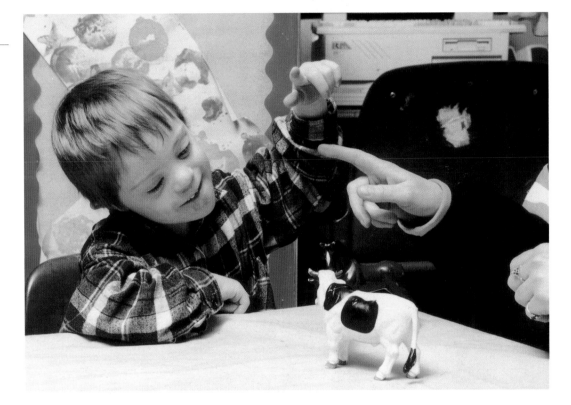

Creating a positive environment

Creating a positive environment involves attending to the needs, talents and desires of each child and encouraging them to expand their limits and broaden their horizons. Children need:

☐ **Love and security:** children need unconditional love, irrespective of who they are and how they behave; they also need the security of predictability and routines to help them understand the world around them.

☐ **Praise and recognition:** children should be praised appropriately when they have achieved something and also when they have tried hard to achieve something; recognising and praising their achievements will motivate them to greater efforts.

☐ **New experiences:** children need fresh challenges all the time; this is important in extending what they have already learned. Providing a wide range of activities and experiences within the nursery or school helps children to develop intellectual skills as well as creativity.

☐ **To form relationships** with other children and adults in an atmosphere of trust and respect; they need good role models.

Recognising achievement

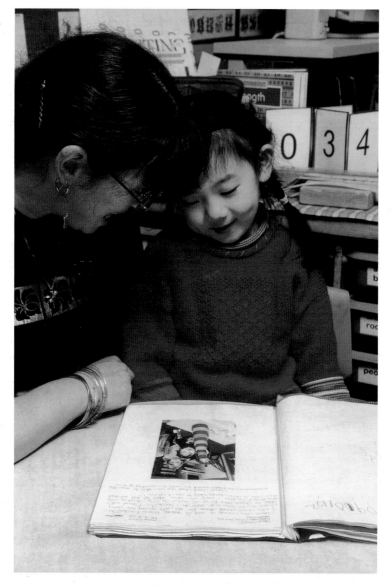

Being a good role model

Children learn more from how they see us act than they do from anything we may tell them. Children directly copy what adults do, so it is important that we nurture an environment which is free from any bias and which encourages equality of opportunity. Being a good role model involves:

- **Non-verbal communication:** Children pick up signals about how we think, feel and act from our body language, facial expressions, gestures, pauses etc.

- **Using appropriate language:** How you talk to children and respond to them is very important. You need to be able to adapt your language to the individual child and to be aware of any communication difficulties.

- **Co-operating with others:** Children need to see that you are pleasant and that you can get along with parents and other adults. Any conflicts between members of staff, for example, should be aired when in the staff room.

- **Showing respect:** learning how to pronounce difficult names and listening to other people's opinions are important in showing your respect for others.

- **Avoiding stereotypes and labels:** avoid using labels which result in children being stereotyped, e.g. 'the boy with glasses', 'the Asian girl' or 'the girl with the pretty dress'. Such labels devalue children, restricting their sense of self-worth. Always use the child's name.

- **Challenging discrimination:** Children pick on weaker children or 'different' children. If you see a child teasing, insulting or hitting another child – explain that such behaviour is hurtful. Criticise the *behaviour* rather than the *child*; for example, you could say; 'Kicking hurts. Carla is very upset because it hurt', rather than 'You're very naughty. Don't do that, I'm very cross with you'. This avoids children feeling that you don't like them or that they are worthless.

✏ ACTIVITY

Exploring assumptions and stereotypes

The following adjectives are often used to describe children:

bossy	*noisy*	*shy*
energetic	*competitive*	*helpful*
aggressive	*lively*	*gentle*
warm	*moody*	*quiet*
kind	*babyish*	*emotional*
strong	*lazy*	*sissy*
clinging	*cheeky*	

Use the headings: **girls**, **boys** and **either** to create three columns. Then put the adjectives from the list into the appropriate column, according to whether you think they describe girls, boys or either girls or boys. Compare your lists with those of a friend.

- How similar were your choices? Discuss the similarities and the differences.

- Discuss reasons why some adjectives are so closely related to gender.

- Do your lists really apply to all the children you work with or know?

Planning activities which promote equality of opportunity

Every child needs to feel accepted, and to feel that they belong, in the setting. Try to find out as much as possible about different cultures, religions and special needs. Activities should be planned which enable children:

✓ to feel valued as individuals;

✓ to explore a wide range of everyday experiences from different cultures and backgrounds, and

✓ to express their feelings.

Make sure that the books, posters and other resources include **positive images** of children with impairments, ethnic minority groups and that gender roles are **non-stereotyped** and reflect the diversity of family life.

Specific activities may include:

☐ Play with malleable materials such as play dough, sand or clay; drawing, painting and craft activities help children to express their feelings and are non-sexist activities; include examples from different cultures, e.g. papier mache, origami, weaving etc.

- Provide toys which offer a range of play opportunities rather than those which are aimed particularly at one sex or the other; e.g. provide a wide variety of dressing up clothes that can be used by girls and boys. Include dress from different cultures and make sure that superhero outfits are available for either sexes, i.e. Superwoman as well as Superman, Wonderwoman and Batman etc.

- Extend the home corner to provide a wide range of play situations; e.g. a home corner plus an office or shop or a boat.

- Using books and telling stories in different languages: invite someone whose first language is not English to come and read a popular story book – such as Goldilocks and the Three Bears – in their language to the whole group; then repeat the session using the English text, again to the whole group.

- Playing music from a variety of cultures – e.g. sitar music, pan pipes, bagpipes etc. and encouraging children to listen or to dance to the sounds.

- Plan a display and interest table around one of the major festivals from different cultures, e.g. Diwali, Hanukkah, Easter, Chinese New Year.

- Use posters which show everyday things from different countries, e.g. musical instruments, fruit and vegetables, transport and wildlife.

- Organise the home corner to include a variety of equipment commonly found in homes in different cultures, e.g. tandoor, wok, chopsticks etc.

- Provide dolls and other playthings which accurately reflect a variety of skin tones and features.

- Arrange cookery activities using recipes from other cultures and in different languages; contact the relevant organisations to find out how to promote cooking skills for children with special needs.

Promoting cultural diversity through music

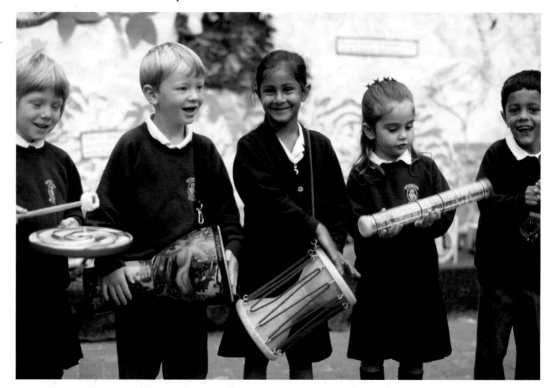

Personal and professional development

- taking responsibility for your own personal and professional development
- different types of personal and professional development, including further training
- the importance of receiving and acting upon feedback from other team members
- different forms of communication in other cultures

In any job the employer will be looking for personal and professional qualities. A system of **review** and **appraisal** helps you and your manager/employer to assess how you are performing in your job and whether you are happy. This provides an opportunity for both you and your employer to identify any aspects of the job that you are doing really well and any that need to be improved. It is on these occasions that you can raise any problems you have – about dealing with particular situations, children, parents or staff. When you are carrying out all your duties well you may be given more responsibility or moved to work in a different area to develop your experience with other age ranges or activities. This all forms part of your professional development but also contributes to your personal development by recognising and valuing your achievement and contribution to the team.

What qualities make a good early years worker?

Above all else you need to like children and to enjoy being with them. The main qualities needed when working with young children are:

☐ **Listening** – attentive listening is a vital part of the caring relationship. Sometimes a child's real needs are communicated more by what is left unsaid than what is actually spoken. You need to be aware of the different forms of **non-verbal communication**; when you are listening closely to a child, watch out also for the way they stand or sit and their facial expressions, as these give vital clues to a child's feelings.

☐ **Comforting** – this has both a physical and an emotional meaning. Physical comfort may be provided by hugging a child who appears distressed. Touching, listening and talking can all provide emotional comfort as well.

☐ **Empathy** – This should not be confused with sympathy. Some people find it easy to appreciate how someone else is feeling by imagining themselves in that person's position. A good way of imagining how a strange environment appears to a young child is to kneel on the floor and try to view it from a child's perspective.

☐ **Sensitivity** – You need to be able to be aware of, and to respond to, the feelings and needs of another person. Being sensitive to others' needs means you can anticipate their feelings; for example, when a child's mother has been admitted to hospital or their pet dog has just died, you may need to be ready with a friendly hug or a few words to show that you understand and that you really care.

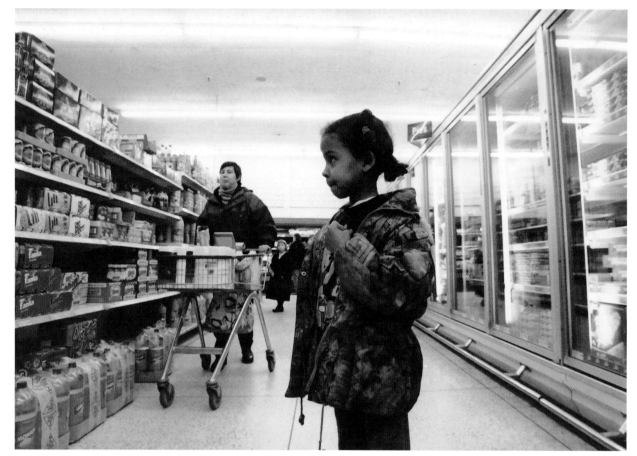

A child's eye view of the world

☐ **Patience** – You need to be patient and tolerant of other people's methods of dealing with problems, even when you feel that your own way is better! For example, letting a child develop independence by dressing himself even when you need to hurry.

☐ **Respect** – You need to be aware of a child's personal rights, dignity and privacy and must show this at all times; every child is unique and so your approach will need to take account of each child's individual needs;

☐ **Interpersonal skills** – A caring relationship is a two-way process. You do not have to *like* the child you are caring for, but being able to show warmth and friendliness helps to create a positive atmosphere and to break down barriers. Acceptance is important; you should always look beyond any disability or disruptive behaviour to recognise and accept the person.

☐ **Self-awareness** – You can become a better early years worker if you can judge what effect your behaviour has on other people, and be willing to adapt. When you are working as part of a team, you need to be aware of how others see you and to be prepared to change your behaviour to help the team to function well.

☐ **Coping with stress** – You need a great deal of energy when you are working in a caring profession; you need to be aware of the possibility of **professional burnout**. In order to help others we must first help ourselves; the carer who never relaxes or develops any outside interests is more likely to suffer 'burn-out' than the carer who finds his own time and space.

❑ **Knowledge and understanding** – you need to have an understanding of child development and basic child care in order to promote children's all-round development.

❑ **Learning from experience** – It is important to continue to learn and grow as professionals; observing babies and children helps you to avoid making assumptions about a child and helps you to identify any special need a child may have.

Professional development

You will have worked hard to obtain the Certificate in Child Care and Education and can then look forward to developing your career with babies and young children. This is called professional development and is important because it:

- enables you to develop greater knowledge and understanding in connection with your work;
- offers opportunities to improve skills or gain new ones;
- can enable you to experience new situations;
- can prepare you for different roles and responsibilities.

Some aspects of professional development are dealt with through training courses, often organised and paid for by your employer. You may receive the training from a member of your own staff or visit a college or recognised training organisation on a part-time basis. Courses can cover anything from dealing with a particular medical condition to developing ways of improving assessment and record-keeping. It is also important to keep abreast of all the changes in child care practice by reading the relevant journals, such as *Nursery World*, *Early Years Educator (EYE)*, *Child Education* and *Professional Nanny*.

Personal development

Your personal development includes your own 'growth' as a person. Your experiences at work and at home can change your attitudes, priorities and ambitions. Changes in home circumstances influence decisions you make about your work, for example the hours you work, where you work and the level of responsibility you take on. If you are without family responsibilities you may welcome the extra challenge of a training course to develop your career. However, if you have to strike a balance between career and home life and additional time is not available for training then this might seem a burden. Sometimes a personal interest will influence the course of your professional development. You may, personally, become interested in working with children with physical difficulties – perhaps you have become involved with the disabled child of friends – and would like to find a job in that field. The opportunity to gain experience or training would benefit you both personally and professionally.

Planning and keeping accurate records

You may be asked to plan an activity to implement in your work setting, for example, a story-telling session using props. (see Unit 2 for ideas and guidance.) Some work settings involve the whole team in planning a curriculum for the children; these plans can be made for the whole term, for three or four weeks or even on a daily basis. Records are kept in all work settings; these may be general information and attendance records or more detailed records about each child's progress. You need to be aware of your role in completing records, e.g. the Accident Report Book (see Unit 1, page 52).

ACTIVITY

Plans and records in the work setting

1 Find out how the day, week or term is planned in your work setting. Ask if you can

   a) see the plans in your workplace

   b) share the information with other school or college students

   Compare the differences between the plans made in nurseries, schools and day nurseries with your fellow students.

2 Find out what records are kept in your work setting – and what your responsibility is in adding to these records.

Conditions of employment

The Employment Protection Act (1978) and The Employment Acts (1980 and 1982) require that any employee who works for more than sixteen hours a week should have a **contract of employmen**t. This document must contain the following information:

* the name of the employer and employee
* the title of the job
* the date when employment commenced
* the scale of pay
* the hours of work

* entitlement to holidays
* sick pay provision
* pensions and pension schemes
* the length of notice required from employer and employee
* the procedures for disciplinary action or grievances

Responsibility for paying income tax and national insurance contributions will need to be decided; such payments are usually deducted from your **gross pay**. Those applying for jobs within the private sector may want to consider using a reputable nanny agency; such agencies are used to negotiating contracts that suit both employer and employee.

Date of issue: ....
This is a contract between .... (Employer's names) and .... (your name). .... (Your name) is contracted to work as a nanny by .... (Employer's name) at .... (Employer's address), starting on .... (Starting Date).

General information
The employers are solely responsible for accounting for the employer's and employees National Insurance and Income Tax contributions. Employers should ensure that they have employer's public liability insurance to cover them should the nanny be injured in the course of work.

Remuneration
The salary is .... per *week/month *before/after deduction of Income Tax and national Insurance payable on ....
The employers will ensure that the employee is given a payslip on the day of payment, detailing gross payment, National Insurance and Income Tax deductions and net payment. Overtime will be paid at £ .... net per hour or part thereof.

The salary will be reviewed *once/twice a year/on the date of ....

Hours of work
The employee will be required to work (hours) .... (days of the week) .... and may be called upon for baby-sitting up to (nights per week) .... In addition, the employee may be required to work overtime provided that .... days' notice have been given and agreed in advance. Overtime will be paid in accordance with the overtime detailed in the paragraph above. In addition, the employee will be entitled to .... *days/weeks paid holiday per year. In the first or final year of service, the employee will be entitled to holidays on a pro rata basis. Holidays may only be carried into next year with the express permission of the employers. Paid compensation is not normally given for holidays not actually taken. The employee will be free on all Bank Holidays or will receive a day off in lieu by agreement.

Duties
(Please specify)...

The employee shall be entitled to:
a) Accommodation
b) Bathroom *sole use/shared
c) Meals (please specify)
d) Use of car *on duty/off duty
e) Other benefits:

Sickness
The employer will pay Statutory Sick Pay (SSP) in accordance with current legislation. Any additional sick pay will be at the employer's discretion.

Termination
In the first four weeks of employment, one week's notice is required on either side. After four weeks continuous service, either the employer or the employee may terminate the contract by giving .... weeks notice.

Confidentiality
The employee shall keep all affairs and concerns of the employers, their household and business confidential, unless otherwise required by law.

Discipline
Reasons which might give rise to the need for disciplinary action include the following:

a) Causing a disruptive influence in the household.
b) Job incompetence.
c) Unsatisfactory standard of dress or appearance.
d) Conduct during or outside working hours prejudicial to the interest or reputation of the employers.
e) Unreliability in time keeping or attendance.
f) Failure to comply with instructions and procedures.
g) Breach of confidentiality clause.

In the event of the need for disciplinary action, the procedure will be firstly, an oral warning; secondly, a written warning, and thirdly, dismissal. Reasons which might give rise to summary dismissal include drunkenness, theft, illegal drug-taking, child abuse.

Signed by the employer ....
Date ....
Signed by the employee ....
Date ....

A specimen contract for a nanny

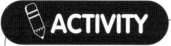 **ACTIVITY**

Read the contract on the previous page carefully, and answer the following questions:

1 Does it meet all the requirements for a contract of employment?

2 If you had been offered the post of Nanny, is there any additional information you would like?

3 Write a specimen advertisement stating what sort of job you would like; try to give a prospective employer a good idea of your personality and your abilities and be realistic in your demands.

Grievance and complaints procedures

If a dispute arises in the workplace, either among employees or between employers and employees, it *must* be settled; this is usually achieved at an early stage through discussion between colleagues or between the aggrieved person and the immediate superior. If, however, the grievance is not easily settled, then an official procedure is needed:

* All employees have a right to seek redress for grievances relating to their employment, and every employee must be told how to proceed.

* Except in very small establishments, there must be a formal procedure for settling grievances.

* The procedure should be in writing and should be simple and rapid in operation.

* The grievance should normally be discussed first between the employee and the immediate supervisor.

* The employee representative should accompany the employee at the next stage of the discussion with management if she so wishes.

* There should be a right of appeal.

Managers should always try to settle the grievance 'as near as possible to the point of origin', in the words of the Industrial Relations Code of Practice.

Trade unions and professional organisations

Trade unions and professional organisations exist to represent and protect members' interests. Their main functions are to:

* negotiate for better pay and conditions of service;

* provide legal protection and support;

* represent members at grievance and disciplinary hearings.

Two organisations which child care workers can join are:

● UNISON – a union for health workers;

● Professional Association of Nursery Nurses (PANN).

In addition to representing their members' interests, most trade unions and professional organisations publish newsletters and hold regular local meetings to discuss workplace issues.

THE PUBLIC SECTOR		
LOCAL EDUCATION AUTHORITY	**LOCAL GOVERNMENT SERVICES**	**HEALTH AUTHORITY**
Areas of work Nursery schools State nurseries Infant, lower and primary schools Schools for children with special needs	**Areas of work** Family centres Children's centres (run by Social Services) Holiday Playschemes	**Areas of work** Health visiting in the community Hospitals Hospital creches and nurseries Adventure Centres and One O'clock Clubs
Types of job Nursery Trained Teacher Nursery Assistant Classroom Assistant Special needs classroom assistant	**Types of job** Nursery Assistant in Family Centres and Children's Day Care Nurseries Playworker in Holiday Playschemes and Adventure Centres	**Types of job** Health Visitor Assistant in clinics and in clients' homes Play Assistant in hospital children's units Nursery Assistants in crèches and nurseries

THE VOLUNTARY SECTOR	
Areas of work Pre-school playgroups After-school clubs Holiday playschemes Nurseries	**Types of job** Nursery Assistants After-school club assistants Holiday playscheme workers Playworkers

THE PRIVATE SECTOR	
Areas of work Day nurseries Nursery schools Crèches (in workplaces, shopping centres or sports and leisure centres) Holiday companies: e.g. ski chalets, watersports, cruise ships, hotels Families	**Types of job** Nursery Assistants Playworkers or ski nannies Mother's help (looking after children and housework) Au pair – usually unqualified in child care; often young people from abroad who live with a family and offer childcare services Nanny – usually qualified in childcare; may live with the family or live out

Table 4.1 Working in the public, voluntary and private sectors

Preparing a C.V.

Preparing for employment through:

a preparing a curriculum vitae (C.V.);

b interview techniques.

A curriculum vitae (often referred to as a C.V.) is a record of your educational and employment history which charts 'the course of your life'. Many employers will ask for your C.V. when you apply for a job although some will require you to complete their own standard application forms which, generally, will ask for the same information.

It is a good idea to word-process your C.V. and 'save' it so it can be updated regularly to take account of new qualifications and experiences. You should be able to include all the necessary details on a maximum of 2 sides of A4 paper.

Personal details must always be provided, as should those for qualifications and employment. It is usual to list information in date order starting with the most recent first. If you are not sure what to include think carefully about what experiences you have had that particularly relate to the post you are applying for or which demonstrate your flexibility or personal strengths. Any part-time employment, even if it is not related to child care, may show that you have worked as part of a team, been punctual and reliable, handled money and been given responsibility – all of which may be important in a work setting.

There is no single way or format although it is usual to begin with personal details. Below are two suggested examples but your tutor will help you compile yours and it may follow a different format.

CURRICULUM VITAE

Name:	Mark Williams	**Date of Birth:**	04.04.1987
Address:	10 Station Road,	**Telephone No:**	01444 765432
	Castletown,		
	Hamptonshire,		
	CW1 1AB	**Nationality:**	Welsh
National Insurance No:	AB 1234 5678	**Marital status:**	Single

Education
September 2003–June 2004   Castletown College of Further Education, College Road, Castletown, CW1 7GT

Course: CACHE Certificate in Child Care and Education – One year full-time
Core units and Option Unit – Work with Babies

Placement Experience:

September–December 2003	Park Infant School	Age 4/6 yrs	36 days
January–April 2004	Sunny Day Nursery	Age 1/3 yrs	39 days
April–June 2004	Family home	Age 0/2+yrs	20 days
September 1998–June 2003	Castletown Community School, Main Road, Castletown, CW2 2YZ		

Qualifications – GCSE

Subject	Board	Date	Grade
English Language	AQA	June '03	D
English Literature	AQA	June '03	D
Mathematics	OCR	June '03	E
Science (Dual award)	OCR	June '03	E
Technology (Food)	OCR	June '03	D
French	AQA	June '03	F
Drama	AQA	June '03	C
Geography	OCR	June '03	D
History	OCR	June '03	E
Art	OCR	June '03	E

In addition: Duke of Edinburgh Bronze award – June '02
St John's Ambulance – Basic First Aid Certificate – April 2004

Work Experience
March 2004 – 2 weeks at Castletown Family Centre Nursery Unit

Employment

September 2003 to date:	Castletown Pet Shop	Saturdays only. Caring for pets, operating cash machine, dealing with customers.
March 2003 to date:	Mr and Mrs J. Smith	Casual babysitting for 3 children aged 9, 6 and 4 years.

Interests and hobbies: I am involved in the local theatre group productions and am also interested in animal welfare. I help with the St John's Ambulance 'Badgers'.

Referees
Ms A. Tutor (personal tutor), Castletown College of Further Education, College Road, Castletown, Hamptonshire. CW1 7GT
Tel: 01444 987654

Mr H. Jones (St John's Ambulance leader)
45 High Street, Castletown, Hamptonshire, CW2 8JA
Tel: 01444 654321

CURRICULUM VITAE

Name:	Harpreet Poonam	**Date of Birth:**	02.10.1977
Address:	25 Manor Road,	**Telephone No:**	01290 123456
	Hightown,		
	Buryshire,		
	HH17 2CD	**Nationality:**	British
National Insurance No:	CD 987654 S	**Marital status:**	Married

Education

September 2003–June 2004 Hightown Community College, Hill Road, Hightown, HH16 3FG

Course: CACHE Certificate in Child Care and Education – one year full-time
Core units and Option Unit – Work with Babies

Placement Experience:

Sept.–Dec. 2003	St Andrew's Primary School	Age 4/6 yrs	31 days
Jan.–Apr. 2004	St Andrew's Nursery Unit	Age 3/4+ yrs	37 days
Apr.–Jun. 2004	Family home	Age 0/2+yrs	20 days
September 1989–June 1994	Greenside Secondary School, Greenside Road, London, E24 8JY		

Qualifications – GCSE

Subject	Board	Date	Grade
English Language	MEG	June '94	C
English Literature	MEG	June '94	E
Mathematics	SEG	June '94	D
Science (Dual award)	SEG	June '94	E
Art & Design	AEB	June '94	E
German	AEB	June '94	F
Geography	SEG	June '94	C
History	MEG	June '94	E
I.T.	MEG	June '94	D

Work Experience

November 1993 – 2 weeks at Greenside Chemist Shop

Employment

July 1994–September 1999 Greenside Chemist Shop
Responsibility for ordering general stock, stocktaking, serving customers and working as cashier.

Voluntary Work Since the birth of my child (now aged 4 years) I have worked as a parent helper at the nursery unit he attends and been an active committee member for the school P.T.A. I also work as a fundraiser for the local branch of Dr Barnados.

Interests and hobbies: I enjoy sporting activities and swim and play badminton regularly.

Referees Ms C. Brown (personal tutor)
Hightown Community College, Hill Road, Hightown, HH16 3FG
Tel: 01290 876789

Mrs W. Taylor (Nursery Teacher)
St Andrew's Nursery Unit, St Andrew's Road, Hightown, HH17 0TY
Tel: 01290 543210

In addition to the information shown in the examples you may indicate your gender (there are many 'unisex' names e.g. Ashley), state that you are a non-smoker and say whether or not you can drive a car e.g.: Full, clean, driving licence since .... (date when test passed)

Many employers ask for a **letter of application** to accompany the C.V. It is from these two documents that they decide which applicants to interview for the vacancy. It is important to put time and effort into your application so that you have a chance to 'sell yourself' at an interview.

When writing your letter of application:

✓ Make sure you know the closing date for applications (if there is one)

✓ Use good quality, plain, A4 paper

✓ Do rough drafts first before copying out in your neatest handwriting OR

✓ Draft it on a word processor, save and edit (use a spellcheck) before printing

✓ Always keep a copy of your letter and application form (especially if you are applying for several posts with different employers)

✓ Check you address it to the right person using the correct title (Madam, or Dear Sir, if you do not know the person's name – e.g. where the advertisement asks you to apply to The Manager – end your letter Yours faithfully. Dear Mrs Taylor (or whatever, if you know the title and name), end with Yours sincerely. If you only have the full name for a female e.g. Wendy Taylor – you could address her Dear Ms Taylor)

✓ Remember to refer to the post for which you are applying and state where you saw the advertisement

✓ Explain why you are interested in the post (look carefully at the details and information you have been sent)

✓ Refer to aspects of your course and previous experience which are relevant to the job

✓ Explain how your personal qualities make you suitable for the job

✓ Sign your letter and print your name and title (e.g. Mark Williams, Mr) underneath

✓ Include a stamped s.a.e. if you want an acknowledgement for your application (this helps to prevent you worrying about whether they have received it if you hear nothing for a while!)

✓ Post your application in good time for the closing date

The interview

Employers have checked through applications and will interview those whom they believe have the right qualifications for the job. However, they are looking for 'the right person' for their particular team of staff so the interview gives them the opportunity to find out more about you. They are investing their time hoping to complete their team and want all the applicants to do themselves justice. They are not going to ask you 'catch' questions. Similarly, it is your opportunity to find out more about the work setting and the staff and decide if they suit you!

- ❑ Try to dress neatly, but appropriately for the work setting.

- ❑ Check the address and that you know how to get there. Make the journey beforehand if possible to judge how long it will take.

- ❑ Ensure you arrive in plenty of time.

- ❑ Try to take notice of what is going on while you are waiting – it may help you make relevant comments or ask appropriate questions during the interview.

- ❑ Take placement reports (PDPs), PER and any photographs or samples of children's work to show if there is time.

- ❑ During the interview sit comfortably without slouching.

- ❑ Look directly at the interviewer/s when answering questions.

- ❑ Try to avoid mumbling and fidgeting – e.g. pushing hair back or fiddling with clothing.

- ❑ Refer to your own experiences, giving examples (whenever they are relevant) to demonstrate your understanding.

Some questions which may be asked at interview for a post in a School Nursery Unit

- As a newly qualified Nursery Assistant can you tell us about your placement experience with 3 to 5 year olds?

- Describe a planned activity that you thought was successful.

- What do you particularly enjoy about working with this age range?

- What strategies might you use to deal with incidents of unwanted behaviour?

- What personal qualities do you think you have to make you a successful Early Years worker?

- What do you feel are your particular strengths?

- How do you think you would fit into our team?

- Thinking about confidentiality, children often share their concerns with us. How would you deal with this?

- Would you tell us more about the interests you have listed in your C.V.?

- Have you any questions?

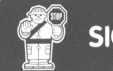

SIGNPOST: unit four

- Day care setting
- Nursery class
- School setting

1 For **each** of the above settings complete the following tasks:
  (a) Write a paragraph to describe the main function of the setting – include who the 'clients' or users are and who might fund it.
  (b) Explain briefly what job roles are found in the setting and draw a diagram to show how staff are organized. Show clearly where a Child Care and Education worker might fit into the organization and who has responsibility for him/her.
  (c) Describe the main duties and responsibilities of a Child Care and Education worker.

2 Explain clearly, with examples (from your own experience, if possible), the following terms:
  - Role model
  - Confidentiality
  - Stereotyping
  - Prejudice
  - Discrimination

3 What policies and Codes of Practice are commonly found in the three different work settings?

4 Explain, briefly, why they are necessary and give examples of what they contain.

5 Make a list of what you consider to be the most important qualities a Child Care and Education worker should possess.

6 Explain what type of professional development a Child Care and Education worker might expect in his/her first year of employment.

7 Create your own list of 10 'top tips' that you think would be helpful to a Child Care and Education worker about to begin his/her first job.

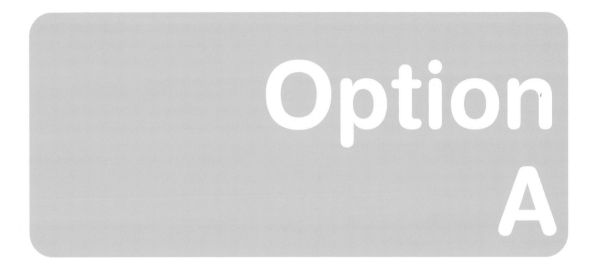

Option A

Work with Babies

1

The sequence of development of babies up to 12 months

- the stages and sequence of development
- the role of play in the development of the baby
- the variations in babies' personalities and rates of development
- effective communication and stimulation with babies
- effects that the lack of stimulation may have on babies
- how and when to encourage walking and other physical development

It is important to keep in mind that even a tiny baby is a person. People grow and develop physically and intellectually, but they are whole human beings from the very start. Every child is unique – the 'average' child or the 'normal' child does not exist. Learning about child development involves studying patterns of growth and development and these are taken as guidelines for normal.

The most important factor in caring for babies is **relationships**. So they need to be held, talked to, sung to and listened to.

Growth

Growth refers to an increase in physical size, and can be measured by height (or length), weight and head circumference. There are two main periods of particularly rapid growth: one in the first year, the next around puberty. Different parts of the body grow at uneven rates. Growth is determined by:

- heredity
- nutrition
- hormones
- emotional influences

Growth Charts

These charts are used to compare the growth pattern of an individual child with the normal range of growth patterns typical of a large number of children of the same sex; they are used to plot **height** (or, in young babies, length), **weight** and **head circumference**:

- the 50th centile (or percentile) is the median: it represents the middle of the range of growth patterns;
- the 10th centile is close to the bottom of the range; if the height of a child is on the 10th centile, it means that in any typical group of 100 children, 90 would measure more and 9 would measure less;

☐ the 90th centile is close to the top of the range; if the weight of a child is on the 90th centile, then in any typical group of 100 children, 89 would weigh less and 10 would weigh more.

a) Boys' weight 0–1 year,
b) Girls' length 0–1 year

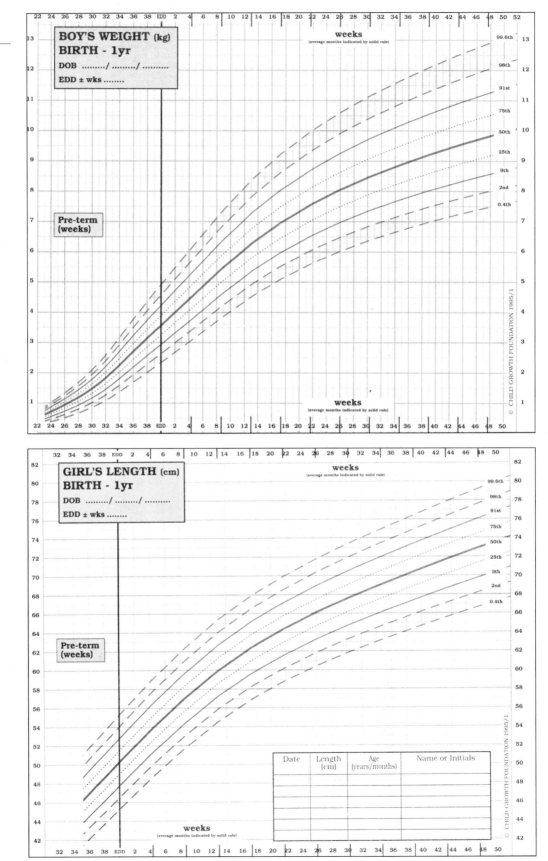

Development

Development is concerned with the possession of skills; **physical development** proceeds in a set order, with simple skills occurring before more complex skills – for example, babies sit before they can stand. The muscles involved in the act of standing require more complex involvement than those needed for sitting.

Stages of development

The newborn baby

Newborn babies display a number of automatic movements known as **reflexes**. These reflexes are a primitive response to the world outside the womb which help the baby to survive. By about 12 weeks these reflexes have disappeared as the baby gains voluntary control of her body.

- **The swallowing and sucking reflexes**: when anything is put in the mouth, babies at once suck and swallow; some babies make their fingers sore by sucking them while still in the womb.

- **The rooting reflex**: if one side of a baby's cheek or mouth is gently touched, the baby's head turns towards the touch and the mouth purses as if in search of the nipple.

- **The grasp reflex**: when an object or finger touches the palm of the baby's hand, it is automatically grasped.

- **The stepping or walking reflex**: when held upright and tilting slightly forward, with feet placed on a firm surface, babies will make forward-stepping movements.

- **Blinking reflex**: babies respond to light and touch by blinking. They also blink when a light is shone directly into the eyes.

- **The falling reflex (Moro reflex)**: any sudden movement which affects the neck gives babies the feeling that they may be dropped; they will fling out the arms and open the hands before bringing them back over the chest as if to catch hold of something.

Primitive reflexes in a newborn baby

Primitive reflexes in a newborn baby: **a** Swallowing and sucking reflex; **b** Rooting reflex

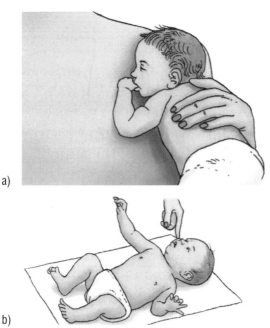

a)

b)

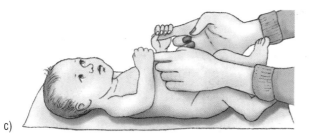

Primitive reflexes in a new-born baby: **c** Grasp reflex;
d Walking reflex; **e** Startle reflex; **f** Blinking reflex;
g Falling reflex

c)

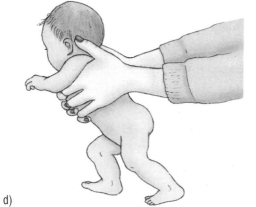

d)

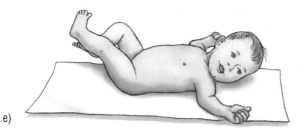

e)

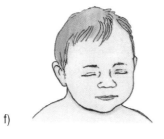

f)

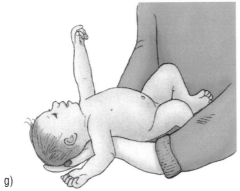

g)

The following charts show the patterns of development in babies from birth to one year of age.

Newborn baby

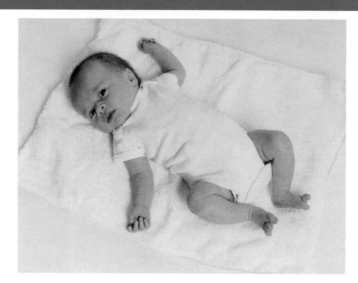

General development

Babies:
- will turn their head towards the light and stare at bright shiny objects
- are fascinated by human faces and gaze attentively at their carer's face when being fed or cuddled
- enjoy feeding and cuddling
- often imitate facial expressions
- respond to things that they see, hear and feel

Role of the adult

- Meet the baby's primary needs for milk, warmth and hygiene
- Provide plenty of physical contact and maintain eye contact
- Talk lovingly to babies and give them the opportunity to respond
- Feed on demand and talk and sing to them

Equipment and toys

- Pram or cot and bedclothes for sleeping
- Nappy changing mat and equipment
- Bathing equipment
- Clothes and laundry facilities
- Light rattles and toys strung over their pram or cot will encourage focusing and coordination
- Mobile hung over the nappy changing area or cot
- Use bright colours in furnishings

Safety points

- When playing with babies, always support the baby's head as their neck muscles are not strong enough to control movement.
- Always place babies on their back to sleep
- Keep the temperature in a baby's room at around 20°C (68°F)

Table A.1   From birth to 4 weeks

4–8 weeks

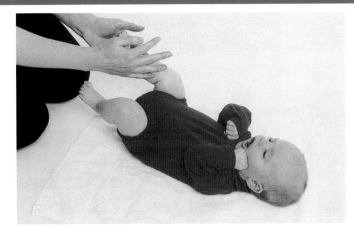

General development

Babies:
- can turn from side to back
- make jerky and uncontrolled arm and leg movements
- are beginning to take fist to mouth
- open hands to grasp an adult's finger
- show that they recognise their primary carers by responding to them with a combination of excited movements, coos and smiles
- love to watch movement: trees in the wind, bright contrasting objects placed within their field of vision etc.
- enjoy listening to the sound of bells, music, voices and rhythmic sounds

Role of the adult

- Meet the baby's primary needs for milk, warmth and hygiene
- Let them kick freely without nappies on
- Massage the baby's body and limbs during or after bathing
- Talk to and smile with the baby
- Sing while feeding or bathing the baby – allowing time for the baby to respond
- Learn to differentiate between the baby's cries and to respond to them appropriately
- Encourage laughter by tickling the baby

Equipment and toys

- Push chair or combination pram/pushchair
- Safety car seat
- Use a special supporting infant chair so that babies can see adult activity. Light rattles and toys strung over their pram or cot will encourage focusing and coordination

Safety points
- Never leave rattles or similar toys in the baby's cot or pram as they can become wedged in the baby's mouth and cause suffocation
- Do not leave a baby unattended on a table, work surface, bed or sofa; place them on the floor instead

Table A.2   From 4–8 weeks

3 months

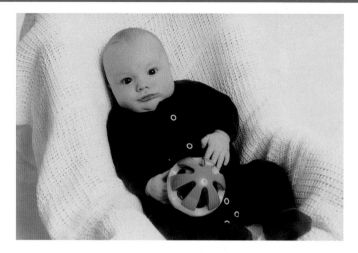

General development

Babies:
- can now lift both head and chest off the bed in the prone position, supported on forearms
- kick vigorously with legs alternating or occasionally together
- watch their hands and play with their fingers
- can hold a rattle for a brief time before dropping it
- are becoming conversational by cooing, gurgling and chuckling; exchange 'coos' with familiar person

Role of the adult

- Meet the baby's primary needs for milk, warmth and hygiene
- Provide brightly coloured mobiles and wind chimes to encourage focusing at 20 cm
- Place some toys on a blanket or play mat on the floor so that babies can lie on their tummies and play with them for short periods
- Give babies a rattle to hold
- Attach objects above the cot which make a noise when touched
- Change their position frequently so that they have different things to look at and to experience

Equipment and toys

- Rattles
- Chiming balls
- Cradle 'gym' to encourage focusing and reaching skills
- Wind chimes
- Pram toys which can be struck

Safety points

- Always protect babies of all skin tones from exposure to sunlight. Use a special sun protection cream, a sun hat to protect face and neck and a pram canopy
- Never leave small objects within reach as everything finds its way to a baby's mouth
- Always buy goods displaying an appropriate safety symbol

Table A.3   3 months

6 months

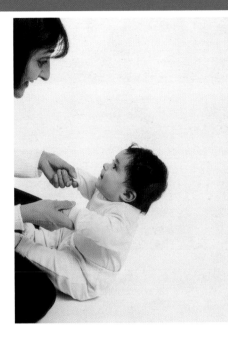

General development

Babies:
- when lying on their backs, can roll over – moving from back to stomach
- can sit with support; sometimes without support
- bounce their feet up and down when held on floor
- move arms purposefully and hold them up to be lifted
- reach and grab when a small toy is offered
- explore objects by putting them in the mouth
- understand 'up' and 'down' and make appropriate gestures, e.g. raising arms to be picked up

Role of the adult

- Meet the baby's primary needs for milk, warmth and hygiene
- Encourage confidence and balance by placing toys around the sitting baby
- Provide rattles and toys which can be hung over the cot to encourage the baby to reach and grab
- Encourage mobility by placing toys just out of the baby's reach
- Provide safe toys for babies to transfer to their mouths
- Look at picture books together and encourage the baby to point at objects with you

Toys and equipment

- Highchair with safety harness
- Stacking beakers and nesting toys
- Suction toys on table tops
- Provide cardboard boxes to put things into and take things out of
- Fabric books
- Simple musical instruments, e.g. a xylophone or wooden spoon and saucepan
- Safety mirror to develop the baby's recognition of self

Safety points

- Make sure that furniture is stable and has no sharp corners
- Always supervise a baby when trying 'finger foods' or at mealtimes
- Always supervise water play

Table A.4 6 months

9 months

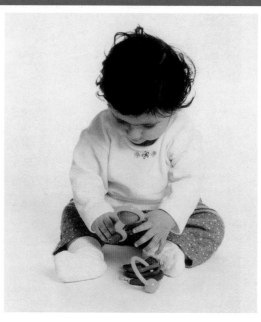

General development

Babies:
- sit alone without support
- stand holding on to furniture
- find ways of moving about the floor – e.g. by rolling, wriggling, or crawling on stomach
- grasp objects between finger and thumb in a pincer grip
- understand their daily routine and will follow simple instructions, e.g. 'kiss teddy'
- may drink from a cup with help
- enjoy making noises by banging toys

Role of the adult

- Meet the baby's primary needs for milk, warmth and hygiene
- Allow plenty of time for play
- Encourage mobility by placing toys just out of reach
- Provide small objects for babies to pick up; choose objects that are safe when chewed – such as pieces of biscuit, but always supervise
- Play peek-a-boo games and hiding and seeking
- Roll balls for the baby to bring back to you

Equipment and toys

- Highchair with safety harness
- Bath toys – beakers, sponges and funnels etc.
- Stacking and nesting toys
- Picture books
- Soft balls for rolling
- Pop-up toys

Safety points

- Always supervise eating and drinking
- Never leave babies alone with finger foods such as bananas, carrots, cheese etc.
- Use child-proof containers for tablets and vitamins and ensure that they are closed properly
- Use a locked cupboard for storing dangerous household chemicals, such as bleach, disinfectant and white spirit

Table A.5　9 months

12 months

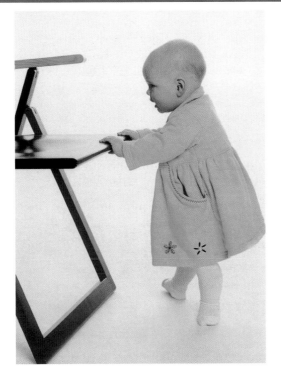

General development

Babies:
- crawl on hands and knees, bottom-shuffle or 'bear-walk' rapidly about the floor
- stand alone for a few moments
- 'cruise' along using furniture as a support
- point with index finger at objects of interest
- understand simple instructions associated with a gesture, e.g. 'come to Daddy', 'clap hands' and 'wave bye-bye'
- help with daily routines, such as getting washed and dressed

Role of the adult

- Meet the baby's primary needs for milk, warmth and hygiene
- Read picture books with simple rhymes
- Arrange a corner of the kitchen or garden for messy play, involving the use of water, play dough or paint
- Talk to the baby about everyday activities, and always allow time for a response
- Encourage creative skills by providing thick crayons and paint brushes and large sheets of paper (e.g. wall lining paper)

Equipment and toys

- Push-and-pull toys to promote confidence in walking
- Stacking toys and bricks
- Shape sorters
- Baby swing
- Cardboard boxes
- Use safety equipment, such as safety catches for cupboards and stair gates, ideally at top and bottom of stairs

Safety points

- As babies become more mobile, you need to be vigilant at all times. This is a very high-risk age for accidents
- Always supervise sand and water play

Table A.6 12 months

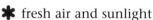 The needs of a young baby

Every baby depends completely on an adult to meet all their needs, but how these needs are met will vary considerably according to family circumstances, culture and the personalities of the baby and the caring adult. To achieve and maintain healthy growth and all-round (holistic) development, certain basic needs must be fulfilled:

* food
* shelter, warmth, clothing
* cleanliness
* fresh air and sunlight
* sleep, rest and activity

There are additional needs, which are not essential for survival, but are essential for healthy development and for well-being:

* The need for love and consistent and continuous affection
* The need for security
* The need for new experiences or play
* The need for praise and recognition
* The need for responsibility

The need for play

Babies need to play. Play is important because:

* it helps babies to learn about and to understand the world around them, and
* it helps them to socialise with their primary carers.

From a very early age babies learn best by exploring the world through their **senses** – of **touch**, **sight**, **hearing**, **taste** and **smell**; in other words they learn:

* by **doing**
* by **seeing**, and
* by **touching**.

During the first year of life, babies mostly play by themselves (**solitary play**) but there are many ways in which you can play with a baby. Even newborn babies respond to things that they see, hear and feel. Play for a newborn baby might include:

☐ **pulling face**s: Try sticking out your tongue and opening your mouth wide and the baby may copy you. Just leaving your tongue stuck out does not work – it seems to be seeing the movement which prompts the baby to imitate you.

☐ **showing objects**: Try showing babies brightly coloured woolly pompoms, balloons, shiny objects and black and white patterns. Hold them directly in front of the baby's face and give him or her time to focus before slowly moving them.

☐ **taking turns**: Talk with babies; if you talk closely to a baby and leave time for a response, you will find that very young babies react by a concentrated expression and later with smiles and excited leg kicking

As babies develop and learn to co-ordinate their arm and leg movements, they will be able to enjoy playing with rattles, soft toys and other playthings described in the charts on the preceding pages.

Each baby is unique

Just as some babies sleep for longer periods than others, so some babies cry and become bored or frustrated more often than others. Every child is different and will respond in his or her own unique way to the care and attention they receive. You need to be able to recognise when a baby is tired or frustrated and to respond to their feelings with sensitivity. Babies can suffer nearly as much from being over-stimulated as they can from being under-stimulated. Examples:

- **Over-stimulation**: A baby who is constantly being passed from one adult to another and tickled or bounced around may react by crying; the baby is missing out on the rest and 'personal space' that all babies need.

- **Under-stimulation**: A baby who is constantly left propped up in a chair in front of a playing television set will probably also react by crying; the baby is not receiving the intellectual, emotional and social stimulation that all babies need.

Finding the balance for the individual child between **too much** play or stimulation and *too little* is an important part of a carer's role; observing babies will help you to recognise these differences and to respond appropriately.

Promoting physical development

Babies master the physical skills of rolling over from front to back, crawling or bottom shuffling, bear-walking and standing during their first year. Some babies walk unaided by the age of one year, and 70% of babies walk by the age of 13 months. You can help babies in the following ways:

Sitting: By about 6 or 7 months, most babies can balance in the secure sitting position for a short while. You can help them:
  > by providing a protective 'ring' so that any sudden over-balancing is safe and painless. Place the baby on the floor with legs wide apart for balance and then place cushions or rolled-up blankets all around her.
  NB Never leave babies alone on the floor, even for a few minutes, as they could fall and trap their arms awkwardly.

Crawling: By about nine months, babies are usually starting to crawl, even if they cannot always control their direction. You can help by:
  > protecting their knees against friction on rough textured carpets etc. (for example, dressing them in light trousers or dungarees), and by foreseeing possible dangers, such as steps, splintery floors or unsuitable
  > objects left lying around. Follow the child-proofing advice in Unit 1.

Standing: Most babies can stand for a few moments at around ten months, but are not able to balance, and may suddenly sit down again. You can help them by ensuring that:
  > furniture is stable, i.e. not likely to topple over when babies hold onto them to pull themselves up
  > that there are no dangling cords, electrical flexes or tablecloths which the baby could pull on and cause themselves harm, and
  > by letting them go barefoot as much as is possible. (It helps when babies can feel the floor and so make sensitive adjustments with their toes to achieve balance).

Walking: Towards the end of the first year, babies are usually standing alone and able to cruise around the room holding onto furniture. You can help them by:
  > kneeling down one or two paces from the baby and encourage them to toddle into your arms;

> letting them walk in bare feet; whenever possible; avoid slippery floors and use socks with non-slip soles rather than shoes until the baby is walking confidently;

> protecting them from falls and keeping older, boisterous children out of their way when they are feeling unsteady and need to practise in a calm environment.

These milestones of physical development are all dependent on the individual baby's confidence and motivation, as well as on their muscles and co-ordination. You should never try to hurry a baby towards being able to stand or walk. You may actually hold their development back if, for example, they become afraid of falling over.

Providing toys and equipment for babies

Babies have no concept of danger, so it is important to supervise their environment for safety. Whether buying or making toys for babies, the following safety points should be applied:

✓ Materials should be durable, to avoid accidents from broken or splintered edges.

✓ Any painted items must be non-toxic paint.

✓ Toys should not contain small parts that could come loose and be swallowed.

✓ Strings or ribbons should never be used to attach anything around the baby's neck.

✓ Check soft toys – e.g. teddies and rag dolls – for safety (try to pull the eyes out of a teddy or to remove other small parts which could choke a baby or which may be put into their nose or ears).

✓ Always try to buy goods displaying the appropriate safety symbol.

✓ Note the manufacturer's guidelines with regard to age suitability and always follow any instructions.

✏️ ACTIVITY

Visit a toy shop and look at the range of toys for babies under one year old.

1 List the toys and activities under two headings:
  • Toys that strengthen muscles and improve co-ordination
  • Toys that will particularly stimulate the senses of touch and sight.

2 What safety symbols are shown on the toys?

3 If you were asked to suggest toys and activities for a baby with visual impairment, what specific toys could you suggest?

Communicating with babies

From the beginning, babies seem to want to communicate with other people. They have a built-in interest in listening to people's voices. Babies learn how to hold 'conversations' with their primary carers from a very early age. Although these are non-verbal conversations (i.e. not involving the use of words), they are important ways of communicating and interacting with others. Babies imitate adult gestures and facial signs and will naturally pause and 'take turns' with an adult, just as if the conversation were verbal. By about two or three months of age, babies begin to make their first language-like sounds. Parents copy these sounds back to their baby and use a high-pitched tone of voice, often called motherese.

Non-verbal conversation

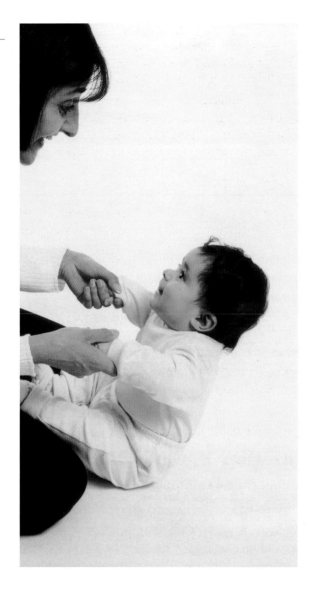

How you can help babies to talk

Talking to babies is easier for some people than for others; this applies to the baby's parents as well as to carers. Some people are naturally chatty; others are naturally quiet and may feel silly talking to a baby who cannot 'talk' back to them. Whilst you cannot change your personality, there are a number of ways in which you can help to communicate effectively with babies:

- Always listen to babies; when they smile at you or make cooing sounds, try to answer in words. You don't have to keep up a running commentary – you just have to be responsive to a baby's efforts to communicate.

- Try to talk naturally, without trying to simplify your language, so that it feels natural and like a real conversation with a friend.

- Tell babies what you are doing whenever you are handling them; e.g. if you are feeding a baby, talk about the food and about what will be the next course.

2

Preparing and feeding babies aged 0 to 1 year

- the nutritional needs of babies 0–1 year
- health and safety procedures when feeding babies
- methods of preparing feeds and cleaning feeding equipment
- communicating with babies before, during and after feeding
- the principles of weaning onto solid foods
- awareness of different milks or milk substitutes for cultural, religious or medical reasons
- specialist equipment for feeding babies with special needs
- consulting with parents and other carers

Nutritional needs of babies

The way babies and children are fed is much more than simply providing enough food to meet nutritional requirements; for the new-born baby, sucking milk is a great source of pleasure and is also rewarding and enjoyable for the mother. The ideal food for babies to start life with is breast milk and breast-feeding should always be encouraged as the first choice in infant feeding; however mothers should not be made to feel guilty or inadequate if they choose not to, or are unable to, breast-feed their babies.

Advantages of breast-feeding

✱ Human milk provides food constituents in the correct balance for human growth. There is no trial and error to find the right formula to suit the baby.

✱ The milk is sterile and at the correct temperature; there is no need for bottles and sterilising equipment.

✱ Breast milk initially provides the infant with maternal antibodies and helps protect the child from infection.

✱ The child is less likely to become overweight as overfeeding by concentrating the formula is not possible, and the infant has more freedom of choice as to how much milk she will suckle.

✱ Generally breast milk is considered cheaper despite the extra calorific requirement of the mother.

✱ Sometimes it is easier to promote the mother-infant bonding by breast-feeding, although this is certainly not always the case.

✻ Some babies have an intolerance to the protein in cows' milk.

✻ The uterus returns to its pre-pregnancy state more quickly, by action of oxytocin released when the baby suckles.

Breast-feeding

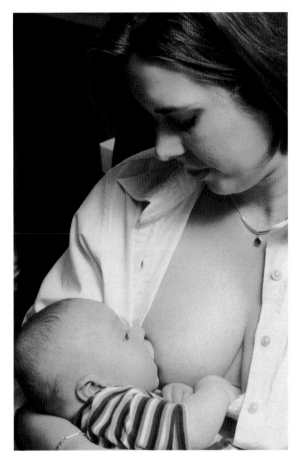

The advantages of bottle-feeding

✻ The mother knows exactly how much milk the baby has taken.

✻ The milk is in no way affected by the mother's state of health, whereas anxiety, tiredness, illness or menstruation may reduce the quantity of breast milk.

✻ The infant is unaffected by such factors as maternal medication. Laxatives, antibiotics, alcohol and drugs affecting the central nervous system can affect the quality of breast milk.

✻ Other members of the family can feed the infant. In this way the father can feel equally involved with the child's care, and during the night could take over one of the feeds so that the mother can get more sleep.

✻ There is no fear of embarrassment while feeding.

✻ The mother is physically unaffected by feeding the infant, avoiding such problems as sore nipples.

Bottle-feeding

Types of milk

Only commercially modified baby milks – known as formula milks – should be used for bottle-feeding babies from birth to 1 year old. The main types of formula milk for babies under 6 months are:

✳ **First stage formula milk**: normally used for babies from birth – the protein content has more whey in it than casein, which reflects the balance of whey and casein in breast milk

✳ **Second stage formula milk**: suitable for babies from birth, although usually promoted as being for 'hungrier' babies as it has a greater casein content, which is less easily digestible, and is intended to keep the baby feeling fuller for longer – this is sometimes called 'follow-on' milk

✳ **Soya formula**: is made from soya beans which, like cow's milk, are modified for use in formula with added vitamins, minerals, and nutrients. This is used for babies who are unable to tolerate cow's milk formula, or whose parents are vegans. Babies should only be given soya-based formula on the advice of a health professional, such as a health visitor, GP or dietician.

Some other specialist formula milks are used for babies who have other special needs, for instance pre-term babies.

NB Ordinary cow's milk, condensed milk, dried milk, goat's milk, evaporated milk, or any other type of milk should *never* be given to a baby under 12 months old.

Sterilising equipment

Babies are very vulnerable to germs and milk is an ideal breeding ground. Before giving a baby a bottle feed:

● ensure that bottles and teats are thoroughly washed after use with hot water and detergent, rinsed and then **sterilised**. Use a bottle brush to ensure the insides of the bottles are thoroughly clean and then squirt soapy water through the teats;

● remember to wash the locking rings, caps and bottle tops too;

● **always wash your hands** before handling feeding equipment.

There are four main ways of sterilising the baby's feeding equipment:

❑ **Steam sterilising:** steam sterilising units should be used as directed by the manufacturer. Bottles and teats will be very hot and should be left to cool down before use.

❑ **Microwave steam sterilising:** this special steam sterilising unit is placed in the microwave according to the manufacturer's instructions. Leave to cool down before making up the feeds.

❑ **Cold water chemical sterilising:** bottles, teats and all other feeding equipment must be submerged completely in the sterilising solution, checking no bubbles are trapped inside bottles and that teats are completely immersed.

❑ **Steriliser bottles and teats:** these are specially designed bottles with teats which can be sterilised in a conventional microwave oven. One bottle takes just 90 seconds; six bottles will be sterilised in about 6 minutes. Follow the manufacturer's instructions and make sure bottles are cooled before making up feeds.

Preparation of feeds

A day's supply of bottles may be made and stored in the fridge for up to 24 hours. A rough guide to quantities is: 150ml. of milk per kilogram of body weight per day; thus a baby weighing 4kg will require approximately 600ml in 24 hours. This could be given as 6 x 100ml. bottles.

Preparing a bottle feed

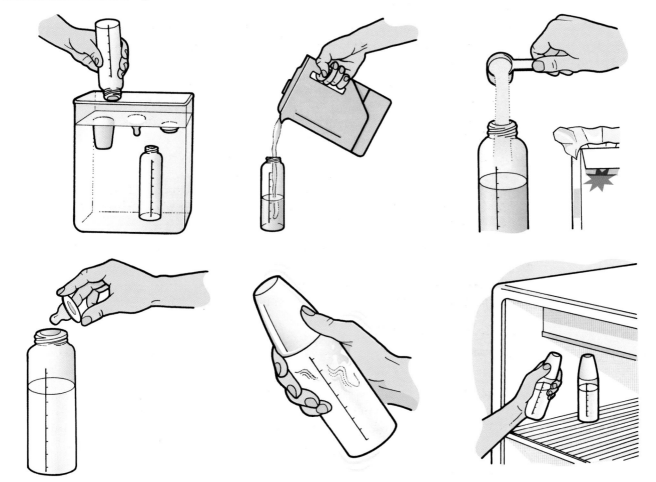

Guidelines on feeding a baby safely

✓ Always wash hands thoroughly when preparing feeds for babies.

✓ Never add sugar or salt to the milk, and never make the feed stronger than the instructions state – this could result in too high a salt intake that can lead to severe illness.

✓ Always check the temperature of the milk before giving it to a baby. Try a few drops on your wrist; it should feel neither hot nor cold to the touch.

✓ Do not use a microwave oven to warm the bottle as it may produce isolated hot spots. Expressed breast milk should not be microwaved because it breaks down the natural chemistry.

✓ Always check that the teat has a hole the right size and that it is not blocked.

✓ Never prop up a baby with a bottle – choking is a real danger.

✓ Always supervise siblings when feeding small babies.

Bottle feeding

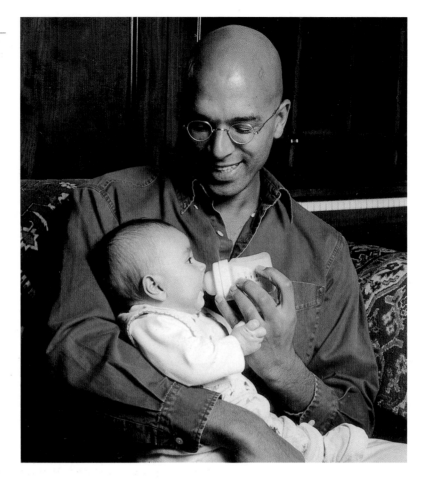

Giving a bottle feed

1 Collect all the necessary equipment before picking up the baby; the bottle may be warmed in a jug of hot water or in a bottle warmer; have muslin square/bib and tissues to hand.

2 Check the temperature and flow of the milk by dripping it onto the inside of your wrist (it should feel warm, not hot or cold).

3 Make yourself comfortable with the baby; do not rush the feed – babies always sense if you are not relaxed and it can make them edgy too.

4 Try to hold the baby in a similar position to that for breastfeeding and maintain eye contact; this is a time for cuddling and talking to the baby.

5 Stimulate the rooting reflex (see page 288) by placing the teat at the corner of the baby's mouth; then put the teat fully into her mouth and feed by tilting the bottle so that the hole in the teat is always covered with milk.

6 After about 10 minutes, the baby may need to be helped to bring up wind; this can be done by leaning her forwards on your lap and gently rubbing her back or by holding her against your shoulder. Unless the baby is showing discomfort, do not insist on trying to produce a 'burp' – the baby may pass the wind out in the nappy.

7 If the baby dozes off during a feed, she may have wind that is making her feel full. Sit her more upright and gently rub her back for a couple of minutes. Then offer her more milk. Remember to angle the bottle so that the teat is full of milk, with no air spaces.

8   When the baby has finished her feed, pull the bottle firmly away. If she still wants to suck, offer her your clean little finger. Release suction when a baby will not let go of the bottle by sliding your little finger between her gums and the teat.

✏️ **ACTIVITY**

Bottle feeding

Find out the average costs involved in bottle feeding a baby; include the following:

- the initial costs of equipment – sterilising unit, bottles, teats etc.
- the costs of formula milk and sterilising tablets for one year.

Bottles and teats

Most bottles today are made of clear plastic and are designed to be unbreakable. However, they can develop cracks with sharp edges so should be checked every time that they are washed. Disposable bottle systems require the use of a fresh plastic liner at every feed. Teats are made from latex or silicone. The latex teats last on average two to three months and should be discarded when they show signs of deterioration. Silicone teats tend to last up to a year.

Dummies

Babies are born with a strong sucking reflex and some babies are more 'sucky' than others are. If a dummy is used before the baby is weaned, it should be sterilised in the same way as teats are sterilised. For older babies careful washing and rinsing is sufficient. To prevent accidental strangulation, never hang a dummy from a ribbon or string around the baby's neck, nor from a cot rail.

The value of communicating with babies

Feeding a baby should be a special time for both you and the baby. Babies benefit emotionally from the feeling of being held securely and of being talked to:

- If possible, choose a place where you will not be disturbed.
- Make sure the baby can see your face, so you can make eye contact, smile and talk to the baby while you are feeding.
- Cuddle the baby close to you and talk gently.
- Talk to the baby if she stops sucking and give her a moment to gurgle, smile or wriggle in reply before she is encouraged to return to the bottle. (This is the start of turn-taking in conversation.)

Feeding problems

Babies often regurgitate small amounts of milk after a feed; this is known as **possetting** and is nothing to worry about. You should always inform the baby's parents if you are in a home setting, and your supervisor if you are in a group setting if you notice the following problems:

- **vomiting**: if the baby brings up large quantities of the feed; this could be due to trapped wind but there could also be an underlying illness.
- **refusal of a feed**: the baby may cry and draw her knees up to her chest – a sign of colic, or she may be hungry but unable to feed because of a problem with e.g. a blocked teat.

Always seek help if the baby you are caring for gives you cause for concern.

Weaning

Weaning is the gradual introduction of solid food to the baby's diet. The reasons for weaning are:

- to meet the baby's nutritional needs – from about six months of age, milk alone will not satisfy the baby's increased nutritional requirements, especially for iron;
- to develop the chewing mechanism; the muscular movement of the mouth and jaw also aids the development of speech;
- to satisfy increasing appetite;
- to introduce new tastes and textures; this enables the baby to join in family meals, thus promoting cognitive and social development;
- to develop new skills – use of feeding beaker, cup and cutlery.

Stages of weaning

Between three and six months is usually the right time to start feeding solids to a baby. Giving solids too early – often in the mistaken belief that the baby might sleep through the night – places a strain on the baby's immature digestive system; it may also make her fat and increases the likelihood of allergy.

- **Stage 1: (from 3–6 months)**

Pureed vegetables, pureed fruit, baby rice, finely pureed dahl or lentils. Milk continues to be the most important food.

- **Stage 2: (about 6–8 months)**

Increase variety; introduce pureed or minced meat, chicken, liver, fish, lentils, and beans. Raw eggs should not be used but cooked egg yolk can be introduced from 6 months; wheat-based foods e.g. mashed Weetabix™, pieces of bread. Milk feeds decrease as more solids rich in protein are offered.

- **Stage 3: (about 9–12 months)**

Cow's milk can safely be used at about 12 months; lumpier foods such as pasta, pieces of cooked meat, soft cooked beans, pieces of cheese, a variety of breads; additional fluids such as diluted unsweetened fruit juice or water. Three regular meals should be taken as well as drinks.

	4–6 months	6–8 months	9–12 months
You can give or add	Puréed fruit Puréed vegetables Thin porridge made from oat or rice flakes or cornmeal Finely puréed dhal or lentils	A wider range of puréed fruits and vegetables Purées which include chicken, fish and liver Wheat-based foods, e.g. mashed Weetabix Egg yolk, well cooked Small-sized beans such as aduki beans, cooked soft Pieces of ripe banana Cooked rice Citrus fruits Soft summer fruits Pieces of bread	An increasingly wide range of foods with a variety of textures and flavours Cows' milk Pieces of cheese Fromage frais or yoghurt Pieces of fish Soft cooked beans Pasta A variety of breads Pieces of meat from a casserole Well-cooked egg white Almost anything that is wholesome and that the child can swallow
How	Offer the food on the tip of a clean finger or on the tip of a clean (plastic or horn) teaspoon	On a teaspoon	On a spoon or as finger food
When	A very tiny amount at first, during or after a milk feed	At the end of a milk feed	At established meal times
Why	The start of transition from milk to solids	To introduce other foods when the child is hungry	To encourage full independence
Not yet	Cows' milk – or any except breast or formula mixed milk with other food Citrus fruit Soft summer fruits Wheat (cereals, flour, bread etc.) Spices Spinach, swede, turnip, beetroot Eggs Nuts Salt Sugar Fatty food	Cows' milk, except in small quantities Chillies or chilli powder Egg whites Nuts Salt Sugar Fatty food	Whole nuts Salt Sugar Fatty food

Table A.7 Introducing new solids to babies

Methods of weaning

Some babies take very quickly to solid food; others appear not to be interested at all. The baby's demands are a good guide for weaning; meal times should never become a battleground. Even babies as young as four months have definite food preferences and should never be forced to eat a particular food, however much thought and effort has gone into the preparation. Table A.7 gives guidelines on introducing new solids to babies. The best foods to start with are pureed cooked vegetables, fruit, and ground cereals such as rice. Chewing usually starts at around the age of six months, whether the baby has teeth or not and coarser textures can then be offered. The baby should be in a bouncing cradle or high chair – not in the usual feeding position in the carer's arms.

Baby being fed in a nursery

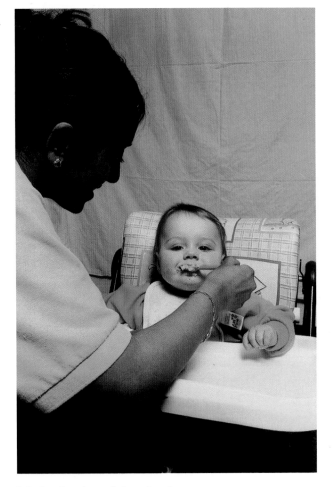

Methods of puréeing food

✱ rub through a sieve using a large spoon;

✱ mash soft foods such as banana or cooked potato with a fork;

✱ use a mouli-sieve or hand-blender;

✱ an electric blender (useful for larger amounts).

Guidelines on weaning

✓ try to encourage a liking for savoury foods;

✓ only introduce one new food at a time;

✓ be patient if the baby does not take the food – feed at the baby's pace, not yours;

✓ do not add salt or sugar to feeds;

✓ make sure that food is the right temperature

✓ avoid giving sweet foods or drinks between meals;

✓ never leave a baby when she is eating;

✓ limit the use of commercially prepared foods – they are of poorer quality and will not allow the baby to become used to home cooking.

✓ select foods approved by the baby's parents.

Baby feeding self

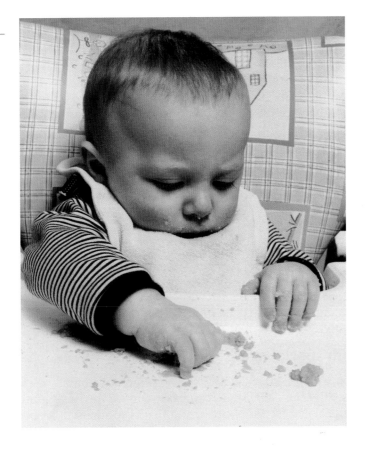

✏️ ACTIVITY

1 Prepare a booklet for parents on weaning. Include the following information:

- when to start weaning a baby;
- what foods to start with;
- when and how to offer feeds;
- a weekly menu plan which includes vegetarian options;

2 Visit a store which stocks a wide variety of commercial baby foods and note their nutritional content e.g. protein, fat, energy, salt, sugar, gluten and additives. Make a chart that shows:

- the type of food e.g. rusks and cereals, savoury packet food, jars of sweet and savoury food;
- the average cost in each category;
- the packaging – note particularly if manufacturers use pictures of babies from different ethnic backgrounds.

If possible, ask a parent who has recently used weaning foods what reasons they had for choosing one product over another.

Feeding babies with special needs

Food allergies and special diets

* **Cow's milk protein intolerance or allergy**: babies who have an intolerance to cow's milk or an allergy to it should be referred to a dietician, who may recommend a soya-based formula or a cow's milk-based formula that has been specially modified for babies with an allergy or intolerance.

* **Lactose intolerance**: lactose intolerance is an intolerance to lactose – the sugar found in milk. It is not an allergy, but babies will need to avoid milk; they may be given fermented milk products, such as yoghurt.

* **Gluten-free diet**: babies who have the rare condition, **coeliac disease**, must not be given any foods that contain gluten. This is found in cereals (wheat, rye, barley and oats) and all foods made with them, such as bread, cakes, pastries, biscuits and cakes. Gluten-free alternatives must be given. Dieticians will advise parents, and useful advice is given by The Coeliac Society (www.coeliac.co.uk)

* **Dairy-free diet**: some babies with severe eczema may be advised to avoid dairy products such as milk, cheese and butter. Again, a dietician will give advice about a suitable diet.

Babies with special needs

* **Cleft lip and palate**: feeding can be difficult in babies with this condition, as the gap caused by the cleft palate can cause milk to be regurgitated through the nose. Various specialist feeding bottles and teats can be used. A specially designed one-way valve and teat adjust milk flow to suit the baby's needs.

* **Down's syndrome**: some babies with Down's syndrome may have feeding problems in the first few weeks. They need to be able to sort out the complicated co-ordination necessary to suck, swallow and breathe at the same time and they may splutter and choke a bit. Try holding the baby fairly upright to feed and check first that the tongue is not sticking to the roof of the mouth. For a baby to suckle and obtain adequate milk the teat must be *on* the tongue (not under it). Specially adapted teats are available to help babies who have difficulty feeding. Do not hurry the feed. Babies with Down's syndrome often feed very slowly, so do not stop too quickly. If the baby falls asleep in the middle of a feed, try tickling her cheeks, chin and feet.

When caring for babies with special needs, try to find out as much as you can about the particular condition by consulting the relevant websites.

Consulting parents and other carers about feeding preferences

Parents usually have very definite ideas about what feed their baby should be given – and how often. You need to be aware of their preferences and to make sure that their instructions are followed. It is good practice to keep a record of when and how much food or milk is taken by babies in your care. You could record this information on a chart (see next page).

Feeding Chart

Name: Molly Bates

Date: 4/5/04

Time	Food/Drink	Comments
8.40 am	Baby rice and 100 ml milk	Both enjoyed
10.30 am	200 ml milk	Taken well
12.45 pm	Pureed sweet potato, carrot and lentils Half a small mashed banana 150 ml boiled water	Only ate 4 teaspoons Really enjoyed banana!
4.15 pm	200 ml milk	Taken well

Key worker: H. Charles

Bathing and changing babies

3

- the importance of bath time
- washing different parts of the baby in different ways
- use of nappies
- common and unusual skin conditions and reactions
- variations in bowel and bladder action
- the cultural differences in toileting and hygienic procedures
- importance of parent's wishes and advice

Caring for a baby's skin

A young baby does not have to be bathed every day because only her bottom, face and neck and skin creases get dirty. If a bath is not given daily, the baby should have the important body parts cleansed thoroughly – a process known as 'topping and tailing'. This process limits the amount of undressing. The newborn baby needs to be handled gently but firmly, and with confidence. Most babies learn to enjoy the sensation of water and are greatly affected by your attitude. The more relaxed and unhurried you are the more enjoyable will be the whole experience.

Topping and tailing

Babies do not like having their skin exposed to the air, so should be undressed for the shortest possible time. Always ensure the room is warm, not less than 20°C (68°F) and that there are no draughts. Warm a large, soft towel on a not-too-hot radiator and have it ready to wrap the baby afterwards. Collect all the equipment you will need:

- changing mat
- a small bowl of water that has been boiled and allowed to cool; this boiled water is important for a newborn baby, but from one month water may be used straight from the tap
- cotton wool swabs
- lidded buckets for soiled nappies, used swabs and clothes
- bowl of warm water
- a large soft towel
- clean clothes and a nappy
- protective cream e.g. Vaseline
- clean nappy and clothes
- brush and comb
- baby toiletries & nail scissors

1   Wash your hands

2   Remove the baby's clothes, leaving on her vest and nappy.

3   Wrap the baby in the towel, keeping her arms inside.

4   Clean the face: Use two separate pieces of cotton wool (one for each eye) squeezed in the boiled water and gently wipe the baby's eyes in one movement from the inner corner outwards (this will prevent any infection passing from one eye to the other).

5   Gently wipe all around the face and behind the ears. (Do not poke around inside her ears or nose; these areas are self-cleaning). Lift her chin and wipe gently under the folds of skin. Dry each area thoroughly by patting with a soft towel or dry cotton wool.

6   Unwrap the towel and take the baby's vest off; raise each arm separately and wipe the armpit carefully as the folds of skin rub together here and can become quite sore – again dry thoroughly and dust with baby powder if used.

7   Until the cord has dropped off, make sure that it is kept clean and dry using special antiseptic powder supplied by the midwife.

8   Wipe and dry the baby's hands.

9   Take her nappy off and place in lidded bucket.

10 Clean her bottom with moist swabs, then wash with soap and water; rinse well with flannel or sponge, pat dry and apply protective cream.

11 Put on clean nappy and clothes.

Bathing the baby

When the bath is given will depend on family routines, but it is best not to bath the baby immediately after a feed, as she may be sick. Some babies love being bathed; others dislike even being undressed. Bathtime has several benefits for babies:

Benefits of bath time

✓ the opportunity to kick and exercise

✓ cleansing and refreshing the skin and hair

✓ the opportunity for the carer to observe any skin problems – rashes, bruises etc.

✓ a valuable time for communication between the baby and the carer

✓ a time for relaxation and enjoyment

As for 'topping and tailing', ensure the room is warm and draught-free and collect all necessary equipment:

- small bowl of boiled water and cotton swabs (as for 'topping and tailing' procedure)

- baby bath filled with warm water – test temperature with your elbow, (not with hands which are insensitive to high temperatures); the water should feel warm but not hot

- changing mat

- 2 warmed towels

- 2 lidded buckets

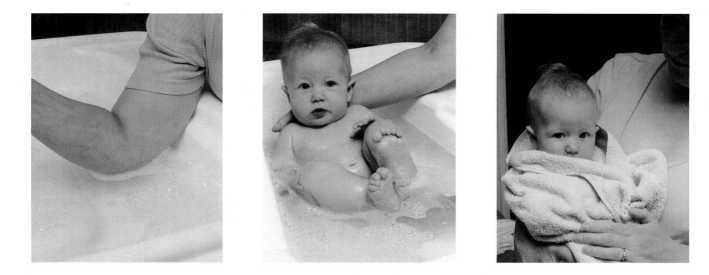

NB: Always fill any bath for a baby with cold water first, adding hot water until it feels just warm

1   Undress the baby except for her nappy and wrap her in a towel whilst you clean her face; clean face as for 'topping and tailing'.

2   Wash her hair before putting her in the bath; support her head and neck with one hand, hold her over the bath and wash her head with plain water or baby shampoo; rinse head thoroughly and dry with second towel.

3   Unwrap towel; remove nappy and place in bucket.

4   Remove any soiling from the baby's bottom with cotton wool; remember to clean baby girls from front to back to avoid germs from faeces entering the urethra or vagina.

5   Lay the baby in the crook of one arm and gently soap her body front and back with baby soap (if preferred, use baby bath liquid added to the bath beforehand).

6   To place her in the bath, remove the towel and, supporting her shoulders with your forearm, hook your hand around her shoulder and under her armpit. Cradle her legs with your other hand and gently lower her into the water.

7   Talk to the baby and gently swish the water to rinse off the soap; pay particular attention to all skin creases – under arms, between legs and behind knees. Allow time for the baby to splash and kick but avoid chilling.

8   Lift the baby out and wrap in warm towel; dry her thoroughly by patting, not rubbing.

9   Baby oil or moisturizer may now be applied to the skin; do not use talcum powder with oils as it will form lumps and cause irritation.

10 Dress the baby in clean nappy and clothes.

Guidelines for bathing

✓ Cultural preferences in skin care should be observed; cocoa butter or special moisturisers are usually applied to babies with black skin and their bodies may be massaged with oil after bathing.

✓ Collect equipment and test temperature of water with your elbow or the inner side of your wrist; always put cold water in the bath before adding hot – many babies have been severely scalded by contact with the hot surface of the bath.

✓ Do not top up with hot water while the baby is in the bath; make sure that taps are turned off tightly as even small drops of hot water can cause scalds.

✓ Do not wear dangling earrings or sharp brooches and keep your own nails short and clean.

✓ Never leave a baby alone in the bath – even for a few seconds. A small baby can drown in a few inches of water.

✓ From a few months old, babies may be bathed in the big bath, keeping the water shallow and following the same guidelines regarding temperature and safety. A non-slip mat placed in the bottom of the bath will prevent slipping.

✓ Avoid talcum powder because of the risk of inhalation or allergy; if it is used, place on your hands first and then gently smooth it onto completely dry skin.

✓ Do not use cotton wool buds – they are not necessary and can be dangerous when poked inside a baby's ears or nose, which are self-cleansing anyway.

✓ Nail care should be included in the bathing routine. A young baby's nails should be cut when necessary after a bath when they are soft. Some parents use their own teeth to bite them gently off.

✓ Hair should be washed daily in the first few months, but shampoo is not necessary every day. A little bath lotion added to the bath water could be gradually worked into the baby's scalp until a lather forms and may then be rinsed off using a wrung out flannel.

✓ If the baby dislikes having her hair washed, try to keep hair washing separate from bath time so that the two are not associated as unpleasant events.

Common skin problems in babies

A newborn baby's skin has a unique tender quality, as it has not been exposed to the environment and its ultraviolet radiation. There are certain common disorders that may affect the newborn child.

Dry skin

Some babies have dry skin that is particularly noticeable in cold weather. It can be treated by using a water-soluble cream (e.g. Unguentum Merck) instead of soap for washing and by applying vaseline to lips, cheeks or noses – the most commonly affected skin areas.

Urticaria

Neonatal urticaria are red, blotchy spots, often around a small white or yellow blister. They usually appear from around the second day and disappear within a few days. They are harmless to the baby.

Sweat rash

Sweat rash is caused by the sweat glands being immature and not allowing heat to evaporate from the skin. A rash of small red spots appears on the face, chest, groin and armpit. The baby should be kept cool and the skin kept dry; calamine lotion will soothe the itch.

Milia

Milia – often called 'milk spots' – occur in fifty per cent of all newborn babies. They are firm, pearly-white, pin-head sized spots which are really tiny sebaceous cysts, and are felt and seen mostly around the baby's nose. They will disappear without scarring in three to four weeks.

Peeling

Most newborn babies' skin peels a little in the first few days, especially on the soles of the feet and the palms. Post-term babies – i.e. babies born after the expected delivery date – may have extra-dry skin, which is prone to peeling. Babies of Asian and Afro-Caribbean descent often have drier skin and hair than babies of European descent. No treatment is necessary.

Cradle cap

This is a type of **seborrhoeic dermatitis** of the scalp and is common in young babies. It is caused by the sebaceous glands on the scalp producing too much sebum or oil. The scalp is covered with white or yellowish brown crusty scales, which although they look unsightly, rarely trouble the baby. It may spread as red, scaly patches over the face, neck, armpits and eyebrows. Sometimes it is caused by inefficient rinsing of shampoo. Treatment is by applying olive oil to the affected area overnight to soften the crusts and by special shampoo.

Infantile eczema

Infantile eczema (or atopic dermatitis) presents as an irritating red scaly rash, usually on the baby's cheeks and forehead, though it may spread to the rest of the body. It is thought to be caused by an allergy and appears at 2–3 months. It causes severe itching, made worse by scratching. It should be treated by rehydrating the skin with short, cool baths using an unscented cleanser and frequent application of special moisturisers. If the eczema is severe, the doctor may prescribe special cortisone creams. The baby's finger nails should be kept short and scratch mittens worn. Cotton clothing should be worn and antibiotics may be used to treat any infection. It is not contagious.

Nappies

The choice of nappies will depend on several factors: convenience, cost, personal preference and concern for the environment. There are two main types of nappy:

- ☐ **Fabric nappies**: these are made from terry towelling and come in different qualities and thickness. Two dozen are required for everyday use. Fabric nappies may be squares or shaped to fit. The latest style is similar in shape to the disposable nappy and has popper fastenings. If using fabric squares, you will also need special nappy safety pins, six pairs of plastic pants. Disposable one-way liners may be used with towelling nappies to keep wetness from the baby's skin and to make solid matter easier to dispose of down the toilet.

▢ **Disposable nappies**: these are nappy, liner and plastic pants all in one and are available in a wide range of designs. Some have more padding at the front for boys and there are different absorbencies for day and night time use. Some makes have resealable tapes so that you can check if the nappy is clean.

▢ Some cultures have alternative customs regarding toileting needs of babies. For example, babies may be placed over a potty at regular intervals and placed on an absorbent cloth at other times. In settings other than the child's own home, nappies must be worn to minimise the risk of infection.

Changing a nappy

Young babies will need several changes of nappy each day – whenever the nappy is wet or soiled. As with any regular routine, have everything ready before you begin:

- a plastic-covered padded changing mat
- nappy sacks for dirty nappies
- a bowl of warm water (or baby wipes)
- cotton wool
- baby lotion
- baby bath liquid
- barrier cream e.g. zinc and castor oil
- new, clean nappy
- disposable gloves if in a nursery setting

Safety point: If you are using a special changing table or bed, make sure the baby cannot fall off. Never leave the baby unattended on a high surface. As long as there are no draughts and the room is warm, the changing mat can be placed on the floor.

Cleaning a girl

1   First wash your hands and put the baby girl on the changing mat.

2   Wear disposable gloves if in a nursery setting. Undo her clothing and open out the nappy.

3   Clean off as much faeces as possible with the soiled nappy.

4   Use wet cotton wool or baby wipes to clean inside all the skin creases at the top of her legs. Wipe down towards her bottom.

5   Lift her legs using one hand (finger between her ankles) and clean her buttocks and thighs with fresh cotton wool, working inwards towards the anus. Keep clear of her vagina and never clean inside the lips of the vulva.

6   Dry the skin creases and the rest of the nappy area thoroughly. Let her kick freely and then apply barrier cream.

Cleaning a boy

1   First wash your hands and place the baby boy on the changing mat. It is quite common for baby boys to urinate just as you remove the nappy, so pause for a few seconds with the nappy held over the penis.

2   Wear disposable gloves if in a nursery setting. Moisten cotton wool with water or lotion and begin by wiping his tummy across, starting at his navel.

3   Using fresh cotton wool or a wipe, clean the creases at the top of his legs working down towards his anus and back.

4   Wipe all over the testicles holding his penis out of the way. Clean under the penis. Never try to pull back the foreskin.

5   Lift his legs using one hand (finger between his ankles) and wipe away from his anus, to buttocks and to back of thighs.

6   Dry the skin creases and the rest of the nappy area thoroughly. Let him kick freely and then apply barrier cream.

Methods of folding fabric nappies

There are two main ways of folding fabric nappies:

☐ the triple absorbent fold: this is the most suitable method for a newborn baby and is a neat shape. It is unsuitable for larger babies. Start with a square nappy folded into four to make a smaller square with the open edges to the top and to the right.

☐ the kite fold: this is suitable for a larger baby and the depth of the kite can be adjusted to suit the size of the baby.

a) (Triple absorbant fold) a) Lift the top layer of the nappy by the right-hand corner; b) Pull the corner to the left to make a triangle; c) Turn the nappy over so the point is at the top right; d) Fold in the middle layers twice to make a thick panel

b) (Kite fold) a) Fold the sides in to the centre to make a kite shape; b) Fold the point at the top down to the centre. Fold the bottom point up to fit the size of the baby

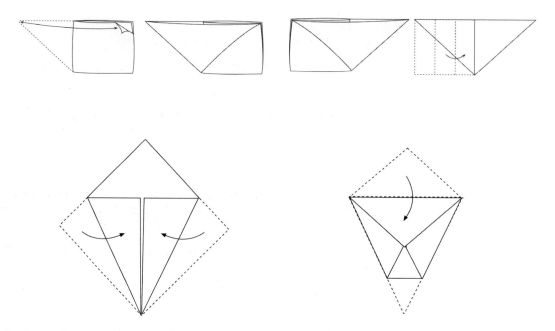

Nappy rash

Almost all babies have occasional bouts of redness and soreness in the area of their nappies; it may be caused by leaving wet and dirty nappies on too long, poor washing techniques, infections, skin disorders such as eczema or seborrhoeic dermatitis or reaction to creams or detergents.

The most common types of nappy rash are:

☐ candidiasis or thrush dermatitis;

☐ ammonia dermatitis.

Thrush dermatitis

This is caused by an organism *candida albicans*, a yeast fungus that lives naturally in many parts of the body. The rash is pink and pimply and is seen in the folds of the groin and around the anus and genital area; it is sometimes caused in breast-fed babies whose mothers have taken a course of antibiotics, or in bottle-fed babies where the teats have been inadequately cleaned and sterilised.

Treatment

- Use a special anti-fungal cream prescribed by the doctor at each nappy change.

- Do not use zinc and castor oil cream until clear of infection as the thrush organism thrives on it.

- If oral thrush is present a prescribed ointment may be used.

Ammonia dermatitis

This produces the most severe type of nappy rash and is caused by the ammonia present in the baby's urine and stools reacting with the baby's skin. It is more common in bottle-fed babies because their stools are more alkaline and provide a better medium for the organisms to thrive. The rash is bright red, may be ulcerated and covers the genital area; the ammonia smells very strongly and causes the baby a lot of burning pain.

Treatment

✱ Wash with mild soap and water and dry gently.

✱ Expose the baby's bottom to fresh air as much as possible.

✱ Only use creams if advised and leave plastic pants off.

✱ If using towelling nappies, a solution of 30ml vinegar to 2 litres of warm water should be used as a final rinsing solution to neutralise the ammonia.

Differences in bowel and bladder function

The first 'stool' or motion a newborn baby passes is **meconium** – a greenish-black treacle-like substance that is present in the baby's bowels before birth and is usually passed within 48 hours of birth. Once the baby starts to feed on milk, the stools change:

✱ a breast-fed baby has fluid, yellow mustard-coloured stools which do not smell unpleasant;

✱ a bottle-fed baby has more formed stools which are browner and may smell slightly.

Bottle-fed babies tend to pass stools more often than breast-fed babies, possibly because there is little waste. As the baby is weaned onto solid foods and starts to eat a more varied diet, her stools will alter in colour and consistency. Each child develops his or her own pattern of bowel movements; some may have a movement once or twice a day, or every two days.

Changes in bowel movements

It is quite normal for a baby's stools to look different from one day to the next. If the baby is being breast-fed any food eaten by the mother will affect the baby and may show a difference in the stools.

Constipation

Constipation means that there are long or irregular intervals between bowel movements. When a motion is passed, it is accompanied by pain and abdominal discomfort and the stools are hard and dry. In babies, these may look like little marbles. (Some babies will grunt and go red when they pass a motion – this is normal.) Constipation is more common in bottle-fed babies than in breast-fed babies

NB If the baby is severely constipated, or passes blood in her stools, seek medical advice.

✱ A young baby may be given extra boiled water between feeds

✱ Older babies should be given plenty of fluids and more fibre-rich foods such as fruit and vegetables, wholemeal bread and cereals in their diet.

✱ Do not give a laxative without first consulting a doctor.

✱ Do not add sugar to the baby's bottle.

Blood in the stools

This should always be taken seriously, although the cause may be minor, for example, a small crack in the skin around the anus. Seek medical advice in case the presence of blood is an indication of an intestinal infection.

Diarrhoea

Diarrhoea is caused by food passing through the intestines too quickly, not leaving enough time for it to be digested; the baby will pass frequent, loose watery stools. They may look greenish and smell different from the baby's usual stools. It should always be taken seriously in a young baby, especially if accompanied by vomiting, as there is the risk of **dehydration**. Seek medical advice and:

- give cooled, boiled water only;
- bottle feeding of formula milk should be stopped, but breastfeeding may continue if the baby wants it.

If the baby is dehydrated the **fontanelles** will be sunken and she may be fretful and refusing feeds.

Bladder function

Once food has been absorbed into the bloodstream, waste is removed from the blood by the kidneys and eliminated from the body as urine. A young baby's bladder will empty itself automatically and frequently; as soon as it contains a little urine, the bladder wall stretches and the emptying action is stimulated. As she grows the baby's bladder will become capable of holding more urine for longer periods of time.

If the baby's urine is strong and concentrated, this is an indication of dehydration. If the urine remains strong after giving extra fluids, or if the smell is offensive, there may be a urinary infection. Seek medical advice.

Care of the teeth

Although not yet visible, the teeth of a newborn baby are already developing inside the gums. A baby's first teeth are called primary teeth or milk teeth and start to appear at around six months.

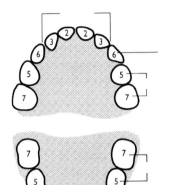

There are 20 primary teeth in all and they are of three types:

☐ incisors: tough, chisel-shaped teeth with a sharp edge to help in biting food;

☐ canines: pointed teeth which help to tear food into manageable chunks;

☐ molars: large, strong teeth that grind against each other to crush food.

Rarely, a baby is born with the first tooth and it may have to be removed, if loose. Most children have 'cut' all twenty primary teeth by the age of 3 years; the two front teeth on the lower jaw are usually the first, followed by those on the upper jaw.

Teething

Some babies 'cut' their teeth with no ill effects; others may experience:

- general fretfulness and rubbing mouth or ears
- a bright red flush on one or both cheeks and on the chin
- red or sore patches around the mouth
- dribbling
- diarrhoea

Teething should not be treated as an illness, but babies will need comforting if in pain. Teething rings and hard rusks usually provide relief, but teething powders and gels are not advised, as they are dangerous if given in large quantities. Infant paracetamol may be helpful in relieving pain but is unsuitable for babies under three months unless advised by the doctor.

Caring for teeth

Teeth need cleaning as soon as they appear, because plaque sticks to the teeth and will cause decay if not removed. Caring for the temporary first teeth is important because:

☐ it develops a good hygiene habit which will continue throughout life;

☐ if milk teeth decay, they may need to be extracted; this could lead to crowding in the mouth as the natural gaps for the second teeth to fill will be too small;

☐ painful teeth may prevent chewing and cause eating problems;

☐ clean, white shining teeth look good.

Healthy teeth require:

✓ a healthy well-balanced diet by the mother during pregnancy, especially foods rich in protein, calcium and vitamin D

✓ fluoride (see below)

✓ avoidance of sugary foods, drinks and medicines

✓ routine care of teeth; the baby should have her own toothbrush, kept clean and separate from others

Cleaning a baby's teeth

Use a small amount of baby toothpaste on a soft baby toothbrush or a piece of fine cloth (e.g. muslin) to clean the plaque from the teeth. Gently smooth the paste on to her teeth and rub lightly. Rinse the brush in clear water and clean her mouth. Brush twice a day – after breakfast and before bed. After the first birthday, children can be taught to brush their own teeth – but will need careful supervision. They should be shown when and how to brush, that is, up and down away from the gum; they may need help to clean the back molars.

Fluoride

Some toothpastes contain fluoride, which is a mineral that can help prevent dental decay. Some waterboards in the UK add fluoride to the water supply; in areas where the fluoride level is low, dentists recommend giving fluoride drops daily to children from six months of age until teething is complete (usually by age 12). If water in your area has added fluoride, do not give drops or tablet supplements as an excess of the mineral can cause mottling of the teeth.

Diet

Healthy teeth need calcium, fluoride, vitamins A, C and D, and foods that need chewing, such as apples, carrots and wholemeal bread. Sugar causes decay and can damage teeth even before they have come through. 'Dinky feeders' and baby bottles filled with sweet drinks are very harmful, because the teeth are kept bathed in sugar for a long time. It is better to save sweets and sugary snacks for special occasions only, or at least after meals, and to clean teeth thoroughly afterwards.

Visiting the dentist

The earlier a child is introduced to the family dentist, the less likely she is to feel nervous about dental inspection and treatment. Try to arrange for her to accompany a parent or carer when they visit the dentist. NHS dental treatment is free for children and for women during pregnancy and during the child's first year. Once the child is about two, she should visit the dentist regularly to make sure her teeth are healthy and growing properly.

Care of the feet

❑ Feet should always be dried thoroughly between the toes and clean socks put on every day.

❑ All-in-one baby suits must be large enough not to cramp the baby's growing feet.

❑ Toenails should be cut straight across, not down into the corners.

✏ ACTIVITY

Describe the daily routine for a baby. You should identify the baby's needs during a twenty-four hour period and show how each need is met by each part of the daily routine.

4

Dressing babies

- different types of baby clothing and fabrics used
- the importance of hygiene and cleanliness
- cleaning and disinfectant materials for baby clothing and nursery equipment
- laundry methods/techniques for different types of materials

Clothing and equipment

Families are under a lot of pressure from friends, from advertising companies and from television programmes to provide the very best clothing and equipment for their new baby. You are in an important position to be able to advise on the basic principles when choosing equipment. The idealised picture of happy, smiling parents cuddling their precious bundle of joy is hard to resist; advertisers use these images to bombard the new parents with a dazzling array of objects that are deemed 'essential' to happy parenthood. Parents should prioritise their needs by considering all factors relevant to their circumstances:

- **Cost**: How much the parents can afford to spend; what may be available on loan from friends who have children past the baby stage; can some equipment, e.g. the pram, be bought second-hand or hired cheaply?

- **Lifestyle**: Is the family living in a flat where the lifts are often out of action, in bed and breakfast accommodation, or in a house with a large garden? These factors will affect such decisions as pram vs. combination model or buggy – or where the baby will sleep.

- **Single or multiple use**: will the equipment be used for a subsequent baby e.g. the priority may be to buy a large pram on which a toddler can also be seated? It may be worth buying new, quality products if they are to be used again.

- **Safety and maintenance**: does the item of equipment chosen meet all the British Safety Standards? What if it has been bought second-hand? How easy is it to replace worn out parts?

Clothing and footwear

The layette is the baby's first set of clothes; some shops specialising in baby goods supply complete layettes. There is a vast range of clothing available.

Baby clothes should be:

✓ **loose and comfortable** to allow for ease of movement; as babies grow rapidly, care should be taken that all-in-one stretch suits do not cramp tiny feet – there should always be growing space at the feet to avoid pressure on the soft bones;

✓ **easy to wash and dry**, as babies need changing often; natural fibres (e.g. cotton and wool mixtures) are more comfortable;

✓ **non-flammable**: all garments for babies up to three months old must carry a permanent label showing that it has passed the low flammability test for slow burning;

✓ **easy to put on and take off** – avoid ribbons, bows and lacy-knit fabrics which can trap small fingers and toes;

✓ **non-irritant** – clothes should be lightweight, soft and warm; some synthetic fibres can be too cold in winter as they do not retain body heat, and too hot in the summer as they do not absorb sweat or allow the skin pores to 'breathe';

✓ **appropriate for the weather** – e.g. in cooler weather a hat is necessary to prevent the loss of heat from the baby's head; in hot weather, a hat with a wide brim will protect her from the sun.

Note also that:

✱ several layers of clothing are warmer than one thick garment;

✱ outside shoes should not be worn until the baby has learned to walk unaided; socks and shoes should be carefully fitted and checked every three months for size;

✱ babies hate having their faces covered, so choose clothes with front fastenings or with wide envelope necks;

✱ tights are practical and warm for both boys and girls. Most babies love to kick their way out of socks and woollen bootees;

✱ clothing needs will vary according to the season, and the baby will need protective clothes such as pram suits, bonnet or sun hat, mittens, and bootees;

✱ Every parent enjoys dressing a baby up, but there is no need to spend a fortune as babies do grow out of their clothes very quickly.

Equipment for a young baby

Babies will need somewhere to sleep, to be bathed, to feed, to sit, to play and to be transported.

For sleeping

Cradles and Moses baskets (wicker baskets with carrying handles) can be used as a bed for a young baby, but are unsuitable for transporting the baby outside or in a car.

Prams and carrycots come in a wide variety of designs; safety mattresses are available which are ventilated at the head section to prevent the risk of suffocation. Prams can be bought second-hand or hired for the first year of a baby's life; they must meet safety standards

Cots

Often a baby will move into a cot for sleeping when he has outgrown his carrycot, but they are suitable for newborn babies. Cots usually have slatted sides, which allow the baby to see out with one side able to be lowered and secured by safety catches. Safety requirements are:

✓ bars must be no more than 7 cm apart;

✓ safety catches must be child-proof;

✓ the mattress should fit snugly with no gaps;

✓ cot bumpers (foam padded screens tied at the head end of the cot) are not recommended

✓ if it has been painted, check that lead-free paint has been used.

Blankets and sheets

These should be easy to wash and dry as they will need frequent laundering; the ideal fabric for sheets is brushed cotton and blankets are often made from cellular acrylic fabric, which is both lightweight, warm and easily washable.

For bathing

Baby baths are easily transportable (when empty), plastic basins which can be used with the fixed base bought for a carrycot, or within the adult bath. After a few months, the baby can be bathed in the adult bath – carers should guard against back strain, cover hot taps because of the risk of burns and always use a non-slip rubber mat.

Safety note: Never leave a baby alone in any bath, even for a few seconds.

For feeding

If the baby is being bottle-fed, 8–10 bottles and teats, sterilising equipment and formula milk will be required. If she is being breast-fed, one bottle and teat is useful to provide extra water or fruit juice. A high chair, with fixed safety harness, is useful for the older baby.

For sitting

Bouncing cradle

This is a soft fabric seat, which can be used from birth to about six months; babies and their carers generally appreciate it as it is easily transported from room to room, encouraging the baby's full involvement in everyday activities. It should always be placed on the floor – never on a worktop or bed as even young babies can 'bounce' themselves off.

High chair

A high chair may be used for a baby who is able to sit unaided. It should always be used with a safety harness, preferably a fitted harness.

Safety harness

A harness should always be used to strap babies into a pram, pushchair or high chair to prevent them falling out. It should have straps for the shoulders as well as the waist and crotch.

For transport

Baby slings

Baby slings, used on the front of the carer's body enable close physical contact between carer and baby, but can cause back strain if used with heavy babies; child 'back carriers' which fit on a frame like a rucksack are suitable for larger babies when out walking.

Pram, push-chair or buggy

A newborn baby can be transported in a special buggy with a tilting seat which can be used for as long as the baby needs a pushchair. The buggy has the advantage of being easier to handle than a pram, easier to store at home and can be taken on public transport. It is not possible to carry heavy loads of shopping on a buggy or pushchair and they should not be used for long periods of sleeping.

Car seats

A baby should never be carried on an adult's lap on the front seat of a car. Small babies can be transported in a sturdy carrycot with fixed straps on the back seat or in a rearward facing baby car seat; for babies under 10kg, these seats can also be used as a first seat in the home.

Care and maintenance of equipment

You need to make sure that any equipment used with babies is kept safe and hygienic. This means that you should regularly:

* check equipment with moving parts, such as prams, push-chairs and buggies both for cleanliness and safety

* check high chairs for splits in the plastic trays and for hygiene; high chairs should always be cleaned after each use

* check rattles and other playthings for damage and hygiene; always sterilise babies' toys and store in a clean, dry area

* wash and disinfect soft toys and bedding according to manufacturer's instructions

* follow the health and safety procedures in the setting.

ACTIVITY

Design a leaflet for a parent which explains the **equipment**, **toiletries** and **clothes** that would be required for a newborn baby. Include the cost of each item.

Points to consider when selecting clothes are:

* the ease of washing and drying;

* the design and colours used: are you reinforcing the stereotypes of pink for girls and blue for boys?

* the safety aspects – no fancy bows or ties etc.

* the suitability of the fabrics used.

Points to consider when selecting equipment are:

* safety;

* ease of cleaning;

* versatility and durability.

Toiletries should be specially formulated for babies – hypo-allergenic and kind to sensitive skins.

5

The provision of a safe and stimulating environment for babies

- importance of providing a safe, stimulating and caring environment for babies
- health and safety procedures of the setting for babies from 0–1 year
- health and safety measures in the disposal of body waste or body fluids
- equipment and materials appropriate to the care and education of babies 0–1 year
- the importance of partnerships with parents

Creating a safe, stimulating and caring environment for babies

In Unit 1, the factors which make up a safe, stimulating and caring environment were described. The same principles apply when caring for babies in nursery settings. **The key worker** system is particularly important in providing continuity of care. Babies need to be cared for by just one other person most of the time so that they can form a close relationship with them. This also helps to minimise the difficulty of separation for babies from their parents or primary carers.

The importance of routines

Having routines for everyday activities is reassuring for both babies and their carers and also ensures that care is consistent and of a high quality. This does *not* mean that caring for babies is, or should be, in itself a routine activity. Anyone looking after babies needs to be able to adapt to their individual needs which will change from day to day. Therefore you need to be flexible in your approach and allow, whenever feasible, the individual baby to set the pattern for the day – as long as all the baby's needs are met.

Respecting differences

All babies need respectful care. Within the day care or nursery setting, physical care arrangements should allow for individual differences; for example:

✱ Provide a variety of foods – not expecting each child to eat the same thing.

✱ Allow babies to sleep when they need to, rather than having a set group time.

✱ Books, toys and ceremonies should reflect the cultural diversity of the nursery and should be positively non-sexist and non-violent.

✱ Staff must avoid stereotyping language.

The pressures on family life

Many parents of young babies find themselves under pressure in all sorts of ways. Factors leading to stress include:

- **Financial**: If both parents have to go out to work, they may need to reduce the hours of work or need to pay for child-care.

- **Age of parents and support available**: very young parents or parents who are at the upper end of the child-bearing scale may have less support from their peers and find the adjustment to parenthood more stressful.

- **Tiredness**: Having a young baby can disrupt parents' sleeping patterns; this is particularly stressful if both parents have to get up to go to work.

- **Responsibility**: Some parents find the responsibility of looking after a young baby overwhelming; they may worry that they cannot cope or find that 'the baby' has completely taken over their life.

Causes of crying

Hunger:	This is the most common cause of crying. It is quite likely unless the baby has just been fed. Breast-fed and bottle-fed babies should be fed on demand in the early weeks. By the age of four months, the baby will probably need solid foods.
Being undressed:	Most new babies hate being undressed and bathed, because they miss the contact between fabric and bare skin. One solution is to place a towel or shawl across the baby's chest and tummy when she is naked.
Discomfort:	Until they can turn themselves over, babies rely on an adult to change their position; babies show marked preferences for sleeping positions.
Nappy needs changing:	Some babies dislike being in a wet or dirty nappy and there may be nappy rash.
Twitches and jerks:	Most new babies make small twitching and jerking movements as they are dropping off to sleep. Some babies are startled awake and find it difficult to settle to sleep because of these twitches. Wrapping a baby up firmly – or swaddling – usually solves the problem.
Over-tired or over-stimulated:	Some babies can refuse to settle if there is too much bustle going on around them e.g. loud noises, too much bouncing or bright lights in a shopping centre; take her somewhere quiet and try rhythmical rocking, patting and generally soothing her.
Pain or illness:	A baby might have a cold or snuffles and be generally fretful or may have an itchy rash, such as eczema. (For signs and symptoms of illness in babies, see page 331)
Allergy:	An intolerance of cow's milk could cause crying; seek medical advice.
Thirst:	In particularly hot weather, babies may be thirsty and can be given cool boiled water. Breast-fed babies may be offered an extra feed as breast milk is a good thirst-quencher.
Feeling too hot or too cold:	Temperature control is not well developed in the young baby; if too hot, she will look red in the face, feel very warm and may be sweaty around the neck folds; loosen clothes and wrappings and remove some layers of bedding, but watch for signs of chilling. If too cold, she may also have a red face or may be pale; to check, feel the hands, feet, tummy and the back of the neck; cuddle the baby, wrap a blanket around her and try a warm feed.
Boredom/need for physical contact:	Babies find being cuddled or carried reassuring; talk to her and provide interesting objects for her to look at and a mobile; put pram under a tree or near a washing line so that she can see movements (NB: remember to fix a cat net to prevent insects and other unwanted visitors).
Colic:	If the baby cries after being fed or has long bouts of crying especially in the evening, she may be suffering from colic.
Child abuse:	A baby who has been abused in any way may cry and the carer should seek help from appropriate professionals.

Table A.8   Causes of crying

Crying in young babies

An important part of creating a caring environment for babies is learning how to respond when they cry. Crying is a baby's way of expressing her needs; babies never cry for no reason at all, although in the first few weeks some babies cry from what appears to be a generalised feeling of discomfort as they adjust to life outside the womb. The average healthy baby cries for a total of three hours a day during the first three months. Finding out why a baby is crying is often a matter of elimination, so it is important that you understand the physical and emotional needs of a baby at each stage of development. The way in which you respond to crying is important. Research has shown that those mothers who respond quickly to their baby's crying have babies who are contented and secure, whereas babies whose cries are ignored tend to cry even more.

Crying caused by pain

If a baby is fretful, off her food and generally miserable, she may be in some kind of pain. A short, spasmodic pain will usually produce bouts of distressed, shrill crying; a more continuous, generalised pain will produce a more grizzly, intermittent cry.

A high-pitched and persistent cry accompanied by drowsiness, floppy limbs, a bulging fontanelle (soft areas between the skull bones) or a rash, which does not disappear when pressed, can indicate a serious infection such as meningitis.

Any crying which you think is caused by pain should be dealt with by taking the baby to the doctor without delay.

Persistent crying

Some babies do cry a great deal more than others and are difficult to soothe and comfort. Parents and carers can feel quite desperate through lack of sleep, personal problems and a baby who won't stop crying; they may suffer guilt at not being able to make their baby happy or lack confidence in caring for her. Such feelings of desperation and exhaustion can result in possible physical violence to the baby – throwing her into the cot, shaking her or even hitting her.

Help list for a crying baby

- ❑ Make sure the baby is not hungry or thirsty.
- ❑ Check that the baby is not too hot or cold.
- ❑ Check that the baby is not physically ill (see page 331 for signs of illness in babies).
- ❑ Check if the baby's nappy needs changing.
- ❑ Treat colic or teething problems.
- ❑ Cuddle the baby and try rocking gently in your arms. (**Note**: the most effective rate of rocking a young baby is at least 60 rocks a minute; the easiest way to achieve this rapid and soothing rocking without getting exhausted is to walk whilst rocking her from side to side.)
- ❑ Rock the baby in a cradle or pram.
- ❑ Talk and sing to the baby.
- ❑ Take the baby for a walk or a car ride.
- ❑ Leave the baby with someone else and take a break.
- ❑ Play soothing music or a womb sounds recording.

☐ Talk to a health visitor, GP or a parent's helpline.

☐ Accept that some babies will cry whatever you do.

☐ Remember that this phase will soon pass.

If the crying ever feels too much to bear:

- Take a deep breath and let it out slowly. Put the baby down in a safe place, like a cot or a pram. Go into another room and sit quietly for a few minutes, perhaps with a cup of tea and the TV or radio on to help take your mind off the crying. When you feel calmer, go back to the baby.

- Ask a friend or relative to take over for a while.

- Try not to get angry with the baby as she will instinctively recognise this and will probably cry even more.

- Never let things get so bad that you feel desperate. There are lots of organisations that can help at the end of a telephone line.

Help and advice

Often just talking to others helps the carer to feel less isolated. Self-help groups such as Serene (formerly Cry-sis), Parentline UK or the National Childbirth Trust Post-natal Support System can help by offering support from someone who has been through the same problem. Talking to the health visitor or GP may help, and some areas run clinics that help to devise a programme to stop the 'spiral' of helplessness.

Never shake a baby

A baby's head is big and heavy compared with the rest of her body. Unless supported, the head flops around because the neck muscles aren't yet strong enough to hold it still.

Shaking can cause serious, permanent injuries or even death

Shaking makes the head move back and forth very quickly and with great force. When this happens, tiny blood vessels can tear and bleed inside the baby's brain causing one or more of the following: blindness, deafness, seizures, learning difficulties, brain damage or even death.

Why would anyone shake a baby?

Some parents or carers may lose control and shake their baby in a moment of frustration or anger. This is particularly likely if the baby will not stop crying. Most people do not realise the damage that shaking can do; some may even think that it is preferable to smacking the baby.

Signs of illness in babies

Raised temperature	The baby may look flushed or be pale, but will feel hot to the touch (black babies may look paler than usual and the eyes may lose sparkle); occasionally a high temperature may trigger a seizure (fit) or febrile convulsion.
Loss of appetite	The baby may refuse feeds or take very little; an older baby may only want milk feeds and refuse all solids.
Diarrhoea	Persistent loose, watery or green stools can quickly dehydrate a baby.
Vomiting	If persistent or projectile in nature and not the more usual possetting.
Excessive and persistent crying	If the baby cannot be comforted in the usual way or if the cry is very different from usual cries.
Lethargy or 'floppiness'	The baby may appear to lack energy and lack the normal muscle tone.
Dry nappies	If her nappies are much drier than usual because she has not passed urine, this may indicate dehydration.
Persistent coughing	Coughing in spasms lasting more than a few seconds; long spasms often end with vomiting.
Difficulty with breathing	If breathing becomes laboured or noisy with a cough, the baby may have bronchitis or croup.
Discharge from the ears	Ear infections may not show as a discharge but the baby may pull at her ears and may have a high temperature.
Sunken anterior fontanelle	A serious sign of dehydration, possibly after diarrhoea and vomiting.
Seizures (also called convulsions or fits)	During a seizure a baby either goes stiff or else jerks her arms or legs for a period lasting up to several minutes. Her eyes may roll up, she may go blue, may dribble and will be unresponsive to you.

Table A.9   Signs and symptoms of illness

Signs of illness in babies

The responsibility of caring for a baby who becomes ill is enormous; it is vital that you recognise the signs and symptoms of illness and when to seek medical aid.

Your role in caring for a sick baby

When any child is unwell, you should proceed as follows:

1   Inform the next-of-kin; always make sure you have a contact number

2   Seek medical advice. This may be the family doctor; or, in an emergency, phone 999 for an ambulance and inform the next-of-kin as soon as is possible.

3   Stay with the baby at all times; you will be able to report on any examinations carried out and will be a reassuring presence to the baby.

4   Observe the baby carefully and note any changes; record the temperature and take steps to reduce a high temperature (see Unit 1 page 85).

5   Give extra fluids if possible and carry out routine skin care. The baby may want extra physical attention or prefer to rest in their cot.

Sudden Infant Death Syndrome

Sudden Infant Death syndrome is often called 'cot death'. It is the term applied to the sudden unexplained and unexpected death of an infant. The reasons for cot deaths are complicated and the cause is still unknown. Although cot death is the commonest

Preventing SIDS: the feet-to-foot position: 1) incorrect, 2) correct

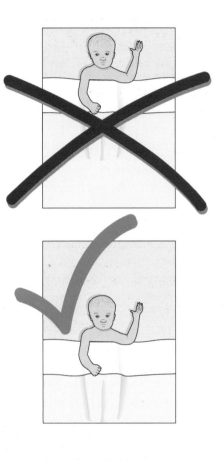

The feet-to-foot position

Side sleeping is not as safe as sleeping on the back, but it is much safer than sleeping on the front. Healthy babies placed on their backs are not more likely to choke. To prevent a baby wriggling down under the covers, place the baby's feet at the foot of the cot and make the bed up so that the covers reach no higher than the shoulders. Covers should be securely tucked in so that they cannot slip over the baby's head. Duvets or quilts, baby nests and pillows have the potential to trap air and may increase the risk of overheating.

cause of death in babies up to one year, it is still very rare, occurring in approximately two out of every 1000 babies. Recent research has identified various risk factors and the Foundation for the Study of Infant Deaths has written the following guidelines for parents:

✓ Place your baby on the back to sleep.

✓ Cut smoking in pregnancy – fathers too!

✓ Do not let anyone smoke in the same room as your baby.

✓ Do not let your baby get too hot or too cold.

✓ Keep baby's head uncovered – place your baby in the 'feet to foot' position to prevent from wriggling under the covers.

✓ If your baby is unwell, seek medical advice promptly.

Preventing the spread of infection (cross-infection)

Babies are particularly vulnerable to infections and can become ill quite rapidly. To minimise the risks of infection, you should:

Wash your hands:

Before preparing bottles or feeds
Before changing nappies or bathing babies
After blowing your nose or sneezing
After using the toilet and handling animals
After changing nappies and disposing of them

Dispose of waste materials safely

Nappies should be wrapped and be disposed of in special double-lined sealed bags – never flushed down the toilet
In nursery and day care settings, disposable gloves should be worn during hygiene routines and then disposed of in the same way as nappies
Used cotton wool, baby wipes and tissues should be disposed of carefully, according to the policies of the setting

Personal hygiene items

Babies each need to have their own toothbrush, flannel and towel
Items for personal hygiene should be kept clean and separate from others feed
In nurseries, towels etc. should be named

Nursery toys and equipment

Follow the nursery's policy for washing toys and playthings
Mop up all spills immediately
Wash down high chairs after each meal

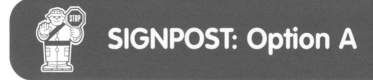

SIGNPOST: Option A

1 For each of the ages 3 months, 6 months and 9 months, describe the stage of physical development most babies will have reached. Use the photocopiable chart (page 377) for your work.

2 For each of the ages 3 months, 6 months and 9 months, describe the stage of emotional and social development most babies will have reached. Use the photocopiable chart for your work.

3 In relation to babies and young children, what is meant by the term 'stimulation'? Explain why it is important and give examples of ways in which parents can stimulate babies of:
(a) 3 months
(b) 6 months
(c) 9 months

4 Make a list of all the physical needs of babies aged 3 months, 6 months and 9 months. *NB. Remember, many of them will be the same for all three ages – look back at your chart for task 1 and think about the ways in which the needs change in relation to improving skills and abilities.*

5 Taking each item from your list in task 4, one at a time, describe how parents may care for the baby's needs. *Choose just one of the ages – 3 months* **or** *6 months* **or** *9 months.* Safety is of concern to all parents. Identify all aspects of health and safety that need to be considered when caring for babies – remember to include personal and food hygiene, clothing, toys, sleep, equipment and the general environment.

6 For **one** of the ages – 3 months, 6 months and 9 months – write some health and safety 'DOs and DON'Ts' as advice and guidance for parents.

NB Remember that in all of these tasks, for some aspects, there may be different advice for boy and girl babies and also think about different cultural practices.

Option B

Parents and Carers

1

The role of parents in the care and education of the child

- the role of parents as the primary carers and educators of their children
- parenting styles and attitudes, family structures and arrangements
- parents wishes and differing values

In this chapter the use of the term 'parents' also applies to the guardians or primary carers of children.

All children need to form a deep attachment with one or more adults on whom they can depend to ensure their basic needs are met. For most children their relationship with their parents is the most important. It is from their parents that they:

☐ learn about themselves and the world around them;

☐ develop values and attitudes which shape their lives and actions; and

☐ gain confidence to try new things.

Similarly, it is parents who know their children best and can share their knowledge and experience with those involved with their upbringing. As 'part-time' – and non-primary – carers, staff in a care or education setting must first acknowledge parents' prime role in children's lives and recognise that they are working in partnership for the children's benefit.

Family structures

In today's society there are many different types of family structure and the children in a work setting are likely to come from a range of home backgrounds. Many children will live with parents who co-habit but are not legally married. They may have been given either (sometimes both) of the parents' surnames as their own.

There are many different types of family:

☐ **the nuclear family** – one which has a father, a mother and their 'joint' biological children;

☐ **the reconstituted family** – one which has two parents, each of whom may have children from previous relationships, but has re-formed into a single unit;

☐ **the extended family** – one which includes grandparents and/or aunts and uncles (usually living in the main family home);

☐ **the single-parent family** – one in which there is only one parent living with the children – it is often assumed that this is the mother but in many instances it is the father;

❏ **the adoptive family** – one in which a child has been adopted resulting in the parents have assumed legal responsibility for the child;

❏ **the foster family** – one which is temporarily caring for a child and may, or may not have 'parental responsibility' (see – the Children Act 1989 page 231).

These represent patterns of family life which are commonly found, but within any of them there will be variations. Examples:

● A reconstituted family may have not only step parents and step children but also children from the new adult partnership who become half-siblings (half-brothers or sisters) to the existing children.

● In single-parent families the absent parent may remain in contact with, and have access to, the children but may have formed new relationships and had more children. This means that the original children are part of ***both*** a single-parent family ***and*** a step family.

● There is an increasing number of homosexual and lesbian couples who have children and live as family units.

Other family types which are less common include:

✱ The nomadic family – one which has no permanent town or village. A nomadic family may live in a 'mobile' home and travel to different sites, settling in any one place for only a short period of time;

✱ The communal family – one in which children live in a commune where, in addition to their parent or parents, they are cared for by other people who share the home.

A family with a boy and twin girls

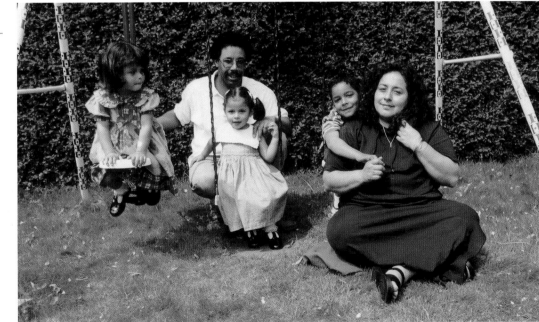

CASE STUDY

Samantha is 19 and lives in a first floor flat in a large inner-city area. She has one child, Jamie, who is two and a half years old. Jamie's father, Kevin, lived with Samantha until Jamie was two years old but has now returned to his mother's home because he felt he couldn't cope with all the arguments over money and child care. Kevin's mother dislikes Samantha and feels that she 'trapped' her son by becoming pregnant. Samantha is very close to her parents who live around the corner. Her mother has a full-time job but helps out by babysitting. Samantha has the opportunity to return to study to take GCSEs. Kevin has offered to look after Jamie for one day a week and will take him to the college nursery the following morning. Samantha is excited by the prospect of this new opportunity but anxious about Kevin caring for Jamie overnight because of his mother's feelings. Identify some of the difficulties that each person may have. How can the staff at the nursery support Jamie and all the family members involved in his care?

ACTIVITY

Group discussion

Within the confidentiality of your group, find out the types of family structure which your own experiences reflect.

- What can you identify as positive and negative aspects of them? Make two columns and write your ideas under the headings: Positive aspects and Negative aspects.

- Look at the different types of family structure and choose one example to **research** and present to the group.

- Identify any positive aspects a child in this situation might experience. How might staff in a work setting build on these?

Regardless of family structure, all families develop their own customs and practices, even in small daily events such as mealtimes. For some it is always a 'sit at the table' affair, for others it is always 'eat on your lap', for many it is a mixture of formal and informal depending on the time and occasion. Similarly some regular family activities, like walking the dog or going shopping, often follow a pattern and a routine is developed which will be very different from another family's. Special occasions (perhaps birthday celebrations or other cultural festivals) often have highly developed routines which are followed every time and, as they are passed down through families become traditions or even rituals.

Every family develops its own customs and traditions – often handed down from generation to generation. The extract from Flora Thompson's evocation of a country childhood in the 1870s and 1880s shows how a small village community came together to help parents and families around the birth of a new baby.

'The Box'

A familiar sight at Lark Rise was that of a young girl – any young girl aged between ten and thirteen – pushing one of the two perambulators in the hamlet around the Rise with a smallish-sized, oak clothes box with black handles lashed to the seat... She had been to the Rectory for THE BOX, which appeared almost simultaneously with every new baby, and a gruelling time she would have had pushing her load the mile and a half, keeping it from slipping from its narrow perch. But, very soon, such small drawbacks would be forgotten in the pleasure of seeing it unpacked. It contained half a dozen of everything – tiny shirts, swathes, long flannel barrows, nighties, and napkins, kept in repair, and lent for every confinement by the clergyman's daughter. In addition to the loaned clothes, it would contain, as a gift, packets of tea and sugar and a tin of patent groats for making gruel . . . The little garments on loan were all good quality and nicely trimmed with embroidery and hand tucking. The clergyman's daughter also kept two christening robes to lend to the mothers, and made a new frock, as a gift, for every baby's 'shortening'. Summer or winter, these little frocks were made of flowered print, blue for the boys and pink for the girls, and every one of the tiny, strong stitches in them were done by her own hands . . .

Taken from *Lark Rise to Candleford* by Flora Thompson

A Buddhist blessing

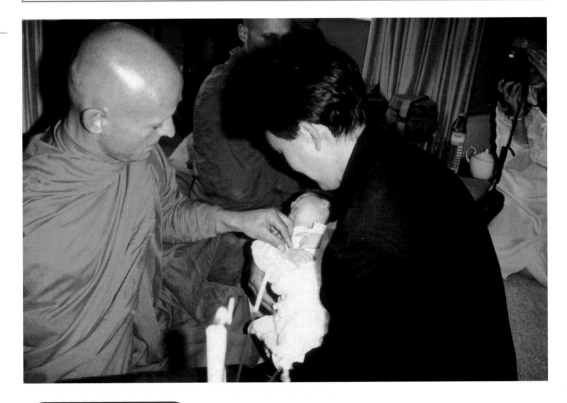

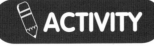 **ACTIVITY**

Think of one or more customs or traditions peculiar, or special, to your family and share them with your group.

Parents and partnership

Practices in child-rearing vary around the world and many cultures have strong traditions as to the role of each parent and in relation to discipline.

Whatever the children's backgrounds, the parents are their earliest educators. While some parents will have looked at many different care/education facilities before deciding which suits them and their child best, others will have had little choice. It is likely that they will have read the prospectus or brochure which explains the aims and **ethos** of the work setting but that does not necessarily mean that they share all those views and attitudes.

It is not the job of staff in a work setting to tell parents how to raise their children. They can, however, offer suggestions and support, when appropriate, in the best interests of the child. To be able to do this effectively a good, trusting relationship between parents and staff needs to be established. Parents need to feel able to express anxieties and difficulties in confidence and without feeling their parenting skills are being judged.

CASE STUDY

An infant school clearly states in its prospectus that there is a uniform and gives reasons why it wishes pupils to wear it. Four-year-old Ryan has just started in the reception class and his parents believe that:

- uniforms prevent children from being seen as individuals and
- it is inappropriate for very young children, anyway.

Ryan's teacher believes that Ryan has noticed that he is the only child in the class not in a school sweatshirt and keeps asking when he will be given his.

Discussion: Think about and discuss the following questions:

- What reasons might the school have for wanting its pupils to wear a uniform?
- What should the teacher's first step be?
- How can the situation be resolved to everyone's satisfaction?
- What are your views about uniforms, generally, and why?
- List the advantages and disadvantages.

Parental rights and responsibilities

With an increasingly wide range of family structures and fewer people choosing legal marriage, problems arise when families break up. In order to focus on the rights of children new legislation was introduced (The Children Act 1989).

The Children Act 1989

This Act identifies the needs of children as **paramount** (that is, of the greatest importance) and attempts to support them in the family by giving '**parental responsibility**' to one, or more, appropriate person(s).

Parental responsibility is automatically given to married parents or to the natural mother, if unmarried. In cases of parents co-habiting the natural father can be made a legal guardian by applying through the courts. Divorced parents may have joint 'parental responsibility' or, in some circumstances adults other than the parents may be given it – perhaps grandparents or foster parents. Where a child is the subject of a care order (there are many reasons for this e.g. at risk from abuse, parental ill-health etc.) then the **local authority** has 'parental responsibility'.

Parental responsibility under the Act includes:

* naming and registering the child at birth;
* deciding where the child should live;
* making decisions about the child's education – how and where – and making sure the child receives education from 5–16 years;
* consenting to medical care and treatment;
* choosing the faith/religion in which the child will be raised;
* maintaining the child;
* protecting the child;
* applying for a passport for the child.

The Children Act 1989 also identified the right of parents to be involved in decisions about education and care where a child was deemed to be 'in need'. It highlighted the importance of respecting parents as partners and of developing positive relationships with them.

Factors giving rise to pressure or difficulties within families

Every family undergoes periods of strain or difficulty from time to time. For some it is short-term while for others it is prolonged and gives rise to tensions which affect

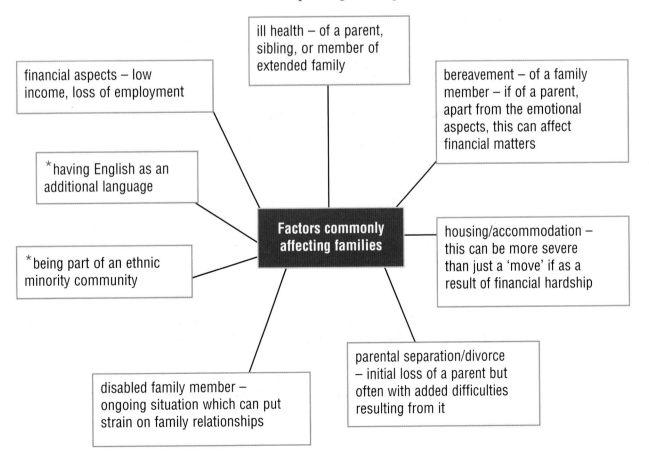

children's daily lives. When working with children and their families you need to be understanding of the needs of individuals as well as the whole family unit in order to support them effectively.

Many families experiencing any of the above factors will cope well with the difficulties, finding support among relatives and friends and other organisations. Indeed, some of the factors (particularly those marked with an *) can have very definite positive aspects to them.

ACTIVITY

In pairs, choose one factor and create an imagined situation for a family with a young child in a work setting. Try to use different aged children for each factor. Then identify:

- the different ways in which staff might know about the situation
- what extra provision might be needed for the child
- how staff might approach the parent(s) to talk about how the child is behaving/progressing
- what other support would be available to them from state or voluntary organisations.

Present the results of your discussions and research to the rest of your group.

2

Effective communication with parents

- establishing good relationships with parents
- passing on only appropriate information to parents
- importance of providing parents with regular information about their child, both positive and negative
- barriers to communication
- sources of help when communication is difficult

Establishing good relationships with parents

Working with parents is an essential aspect of work with young children. Parents are the first and primary educators of their children. You can strengthen and build on this responsibility so that parents experience an increase in enjoyment of their children and an understanding of child development. Remember that it takes time and regular communication to build good relationships with parents that are founded on mutual trust and respect.

Making parents welcome in the setting

Parents start off in an unequal relationship with child care staff. Some parents may feel very anxious, as they are not familiar with the building, the staff or the rules and relationships within the setting. Other factors may increase their uncertainty and feelings of helplessness, for example:

✱ they may speak a different language from that spoken in the setting;

✱ they may be under emotional pressure about leaving their child;

✱ they may have other worries – e.g. about getting to work, financial problems, etc.

Welcome to Parkside Nursery

Parents and carers are very welcome to spend time in the nursery. You may like to read a story, work with a small group, accompany us on a visit, cook, garden or support a creative activity. It really is up to you, but we are there to guide and support you. Please watch the notice boards in the entrance hall, which will keep you up-to-date on school activities, local events and other important issues.

You need to be able to see things from a parent's point of view and to do everything possible to make them welcome in the setting. Some useful ideas include the following:

- **Names accurately recorded**: first of all, make sure that you have the parents' names accurately recorded. Find out how they want to be addressed – do not assume that their surnames will be the same or, necessarily, the same as the child's

- **Greeting**: make a point of greeting parents and smiling at them

- **Name badges**: these are useful so that parents know to whom they are talking and who their children are talking about

- **Photos**: a board with staff names and regularly updated photos could be put in the reception area and in newsletters

- **Key worker**: parents need to know which staff member will be working most closely with their child. Most nursery settings have an identified key worker, who will be responsible for keeping notes and records of progress for a small number of children; these key workers will be the main point of contact for the families of those children.

In many nursery settings the children are cared for in groups according to age and/or development and there may be one supervisor for each group. The manager or supervisor of a nursery or the headteacher in an infant school would still retain overall responsibility.

Ways of communicating with parents

Ongoing communication with parents is essential if children's needs are to be met. For many parents there can be regular and informal communication when children are brought to, or collected from, the work setting. However, it is unusual for both parents to perform this task and, therefore, it is often the same parent who has contact. The methods below can usually work for both parents and care workers.

Finding ways to communicate with parents can sometimes be difficult, especially when staff may not feel confident themselves.

- ☐ **Regular contact with the same person:** always meet and greet parents when they arrive. At the start, it is very important that parents meet the same care worker – preferably their child's teacher or key person/worker – on a daily basis.

- ☐ **A meeting place for parents:** ideally, there should be a room that parents can use to have a drink and a chat together.

Exchanging routine written information

Written information	How and when it is used
Formal letter	Welcome letter prior to admission to the setting To give information about parent's evenings or meetings To alert parents to the presence of an infectious disease within the setting To advise parents about any change of policy or staff changes
Newsletters	To give information about future events – fundraising fairs, open forums and visiting speakers, etc.
Notice boards	To give general information about the nursery, local events for parents, support group contact numbers, health and safety information, daily menus, etc.
Activity slips	To inform parents about what their child has been doing
Admission form	All parents fill in an admission form when registering their child (see sample below). This is confidential information and must be kept in a safe place where only staff have access to it
Home books	To record information from both staff and parents. Home books travel between the setting and the home and record details of the child's progress, any medication given, how well they have eaten and slept, etc.
Accident slips	To record information when a child has been ill or is injured when at the setting
Suggestions box	Some settings have a suggestions box where parents can contribute their own ideas for improving the service
Policy and procedure documents	These official documents should be openly available, and parents should be able to discuss them with staff if they have any concerns

- Information which affects the longer term should, ideally, be given in writing – e.g. concerning food allergies or medical conditions. As well as telling staff, notices may need also to be attached to a child's own equipment, lunchbox or displayed in particular areas e.g. food preparation, nappy-changing. In a school setting the class teacher should ensure any other adults involved in the child's care know information as appropriate.

Copies of all letters received and sent and a record of all communication should be kept for future reference.

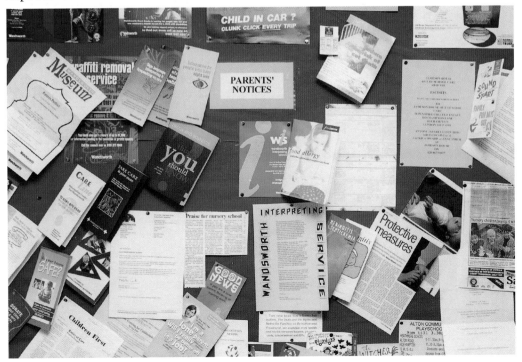

Parents' notice board

Verbal information

Routine information can be – and often is – exchanged verbally. This usually happens at the start and end of the session, when parents and their child's key worker chat informally.

☐ **Talking with parents**: always tell parents about their child's positive behaviour and take the opportunity to praise the child in front of their parents. If you wish to share a concern with them, they already understand that you are interested in their child's welfare and are not being judgemental. (Many adults associate being called in to see the person in charge with their own experiences of a 'telling-off'.)

☐ **Recording information and passing on messages**: you will need to record some information the parent has talked to you about – especially if you are likely to forget it! You should always write down a verbal message that affects the child's welfare, so that it can be passed on to other members of staff; for example, if someone else is collecting the child, if a favourite comfort object has been left at home, or if the child has experienced a restless night. The person delivering the message needs confirmation that it will be acted upon. Where there are shift systems in operation a strict procedure for passing on messages needs to be established.

☐ **Telephone calls**: information received or delivered by telephone should be noted in a diary so that action can be taken.

Greenfield Day Nursery

ADMISSIONS FORM

Child's Name:

Date of birth: Sex:

Child's first language:

Religion: Ethnic Origin:

Disabled? Y/N   Access Requirements

Address:

Telephone number:

Mother's name: Occupation:

Name and address of workplace:

Telephone number:

Father's name: Occupation:

Name and address of workplace:

Telephone number:

In an emergency, please contact:

Name

Relationship to child   Telephone number

People authorised to pick up child:

Name

Relationship to child   Telephone number

Sessions required:

Required starting date:

Signed: Date:

Barriers to communication: how you can help

☐ **Time constraints**: there may be several children arriving together, which puts pressure on staff at a busy time. Parents may be in a rush to get away when bringing their children. Do not interpret this as a lack of interest. Greet them with a friendly nod and pass on any information briefly.

☐ **Not seeing parents regularly**: when someone other than the parents brings and fetches the child, staff will need to find other ways to maintain regular communication.

☐ **Body language and non-verbal communication**: be aware of how parents may be feeling at a particular time, even when they do not mention anything; for example, if a parent does not make eye contact, it may be that they are depressed.

☐ **Written communication**: unless sent in the post, there is a chance that some letters and other written notes may not reach the parent. Also some parents might have difficulty reading and writing and not want to seek help. The notice board can also be used to display a general letter sent to all parents.

☐ **Making messages clear**: remember that we understand messages not only from what is said but also from how it is said – tone of voice, gestures and facial expressions can change the meaning of a message. The person on the receiving end of a written message has no such clues. It is important to give careful consideration to the wording of any letter and try to make sure that it cannot be misinterpreted.

☐ **When English is not the parent's first language**: you can help by signing or – where possible – by involving bilingual staff or translators. Notice boards can display signs in picture form – for example, showing the activities their child will be doing during the session. Having **written information** in a number of different languages is also helpful.

Confidentiality

In order to establish a relationship of mutual trust and respect, you must ensure that you practise confidentiality at all times. Details of your responsibilities are given on page 356. Most settings have a Confidentiality Policy – see below.

Parkside Nursery

Confidentiality Policy

To ensure that all those using and working in the nursery can do so with confidence, we will respect confidentiality in the following ways:

- Parents will have ready access to the files and records of their own children but will not have access to information about any other child.

- Nursery staff will not discuss individual children, other than for purposes of curriculum planning/group management, with people other than the parents/carers of that child.

- Information given by parents/carers to the nursery supervisor or key worker will not be passed on to other adults without permission.

- Issues concerning the employment of staff, will remain confidential to the people directly involved with making personnel decisions.

- Any anxieties/evidence relating to a child's personal safety will be kept in a confidential file and will not be shared within the nursery except with the child's key worker, the nursery supervisor and the chair of the management committee.

- Students or volunteers working in the nursery will be advised of our confidentiality policy and required to respect it.

3

Admission/settling-in procedures

- settling-in policies and procedures for different settings
- importance of the settling-in period for the child and the parent
- involving parents in the settling-in procedures
- reactions to separation by parents and children

Settling-in policies

Most work settings will have a **settling-in policy** to make the transition from home to day care/nursery/school or from one care setting to another as smooth as possible. Unit 3 has dealt with these in considering the children and their needs. Here we need to think about them from the viewpoint of the parents.

Helping a distressed or concerned parent to separate from their equally unhappy child is one of the main issues in nursery settings. This particular age group (under 4 years) finds it particularly hard to separate. This is not helped by a system of irregular attendance that makes continuity of settling difficult. Some children sail through this process, most do not.

Good practice in settling-in procedures

- **Training**: training should be provided to enable staff to gain skills in interacting with and settling babies and children for whom they are not the key person/worker.

- **Arrival and greeting**: a child's key person or key worker should greet parents each time their child attends and leaves the setting. The key person should always ensure time is allowed for two-way communication to take place with each parent on these occasions.

- **Key worker or key person**: parents need to meet and get to know the adults who will be caring for their child. They need to know that their anxieties will be taken seriously and that they can trust staff to support them.

- **Policies, procedures and routines**: parents should be given full information about how the nursery or other setting operates when they apply for a place, both verbally and in booklet form. The policies and procedures should be openly available and parents should be able to discuss them with staff if they have any concerns.

- **Child's preferences**: parents should be given the opportunity to explain their child's likes/dislikes, routines, etc., so that the work setting may take them into account. Ideally a home visit is made by the setting's staff. Encourage parents to provide the child's favourite teddy or comfort object.

- **Parental preferences**: it is important to find out, in the event of the child becoming upset, whether the parents would prefer to be fetched immediately or would be happy for staff to persist with trying to settle her a bit longer. Find out how and when they can be contacted if there is a problem with settling in.

- **Communicating with parents**: the needs of parents whose first language is not English should ideally be met through translation services, interpreters and staff language skills. The local Early Years Development and Childcare Partnership (EYDCP) can offer useful advice.

- **Supporting parents**: staff should also be skilled in identifying ways in which all parents, including those with disabilities or learning difficulties, can be supported in their contribution to their child's learning and development.

- **Keeping parents informed**: parents need to be reassured that they will be told about their child's day and progress, with the opportunity to check that she or he has settled. This is particularly important in the early stages of settling in.

Parkside Nursery

Settling-in Policy

Parkside Nursery wants children to feel safe and happy in the absence of their parents/carers, to recognise other adults as a source of authority, help and friendship and to be able to share with their parents/carers afterwards the new play and learning experiences enjoyed at nursery.

In order to accomplish this we will:

- Encourage parents/carers to visit the nursery with their children during the weeks before an admission is planned

- Introduce flexible admission procedures, if appropriate, to meet the needs of individual families and children

- Make clear to families from the outset that they will be supported in the nursery for as long as it takes to settle their child there

- Reassure parents/carers whose children seem to be settling into the nursery

- Introduce new families into the group on a staggered basis rather than a large number of new children all at once

- Encourage parents/carers, where appropriate, to separate from their children for brief periods at first, gradually building up to longer absences.

Children cannot play or learn successfully if they are anxious and unhappy. Our settling-in procedures aim to help parents/carers to help their children to feel comfortable in the nursery, to benefit from what it has to offer, and to be confident that their parents/carers will return at the end of the session/day.

Understanding and respecting the needs of parents

You need to be aware of the wide variety of parenting and family approaches.

* **Full-time employment**: some parents, who are in full-time employment, may have a different attitude towards their child settling-in from those who have chosen to place their child in a nursery or playgroup on a part-time basis to widen the child's experience.

✱ **Individual needs**: every situation and family must be treated individually and its needs met through a flexible approach; for example, parents who are dealing with a large family or with disabled family members will have different priorities from a lone parent family with one child.

✱ **Transition to school**: schools often have to deal with children who have had no experience of early childhood education or nursery care, as well as with those who have been in day nurseries from a few months old. Some parents whose children have been in full-time day care find the school's 'staggered' intake – when children attend on a part-time basis at first – both unnecessary and inconvenient, especially if they work. However, most children take time to adapt to a full school day, which includes a long lunch-time period with less supervision than they are used to and no facilities for an afternoon rest.

✱ **Referral by Social Services**: when children have been placed in a child care setting on the advice of a social worker, there may be some resentment from parents. They may feel that their rights and responsibilities have been overridden. It is important that a positive relationship between parents and the setting is established as soon as possible, with a clear understanding that the interest of the child is everyone's main concern. In these situations there will usually be regular meetings involving parents, staff and other professionals to discuss the child's progress.

The role of the key worker

A key worker is a designated member of staff who is responsible for the care of one or more children within the nursery. Their responsibilities might include:

✱ planning the child's day;

✱ monitoring and recording the child's development;

✱ liaising with the child's parents, and

✱ welcoming and settling-in the child and returning the child to the parent at the end of a session.

The key worker system helps children to cope with separation and change; it also enables the key worker and the child to form an attachment. Parents who have to work full-time may not be able to spend time settling their children in to the nursery and the key worker needs to adapt their practice to fit in with the parent's needs.

This information is confidential and should be kept in a safe place where only staff members may have access to it. The supervisor or manager must check that all staff are aware of medical conditions or cultural issues which affect the day-to-day care of a child. It is also important to ensure that these details are updated regularly.

ACTIVITY

1 The parents of three-year-old Thomas have been anxious about their son's appetite since he was ill with a virus. The staff at the day nursery have been observing Thomas, keeping written records and taking photographs, at snack and mealtimes over a period of a week. They have made sure the food is attractively presented, includes some of Thomas' favourite items and offered small portions. They have noticed a great improvement and want to share their findings with his parents and discuss how he is at home.

2 Five-year-old Charlotte has recently become withdrawn from both adults and other children. For the past week or so she has needed encouragement to complete work tasks which are within her capability and when she has had free-choice activity she has tended to sit alone in the home corner with a soft toy. This represents a change in Charlotte's behaviour and the teacher wants to discuss her concerns with the parents.

- In each case, what method would you use to contact the parents?

- Explain what you would say/write and what you would arrange in order to deal with each situation.

ACTIVITY

Design a newsletter for parents of a reception class child. It should include information about the topic being studied for the forthcoming half term, suggest what items the children might like to bring in, what parents could do to support the topic or get involved in school. Include some reminders about days when children need their P.E. kit and school fundraising events coming up.

- value of involving parents in the work setting
- using skills and abilities of parents
- encouraging parents to become interested in the children's activities
- why parents may not want to participate in the work of the setting

The value of involving parents in the work setting

There are many reasons why it is valuable to involve parents or carers in the work setting:

✓ Parents know their children better than anyone else

✓ Children benefit from the extra attention, particularly one-to-one help

✓ A range of different skills can be brought to the work setting, e.g. music, sewing, drawing, cooking, etc.

✓ Parents who do not share the same language or culture as the work setting can extend the awareness and knowledge of both staff and children about the way other people live, cook and communicate

✓ Parents and carers can help by sharing lots of books with children from an early age, and by hearing and helping their child read when they start school

✓ Involving parents in the play and learning experiences of their children can help to counteract any negative feelings parents may have about education systems, arising perhaps from memories of their own school days.

Some work settings have produced a policy for parental involvement. See the example on the next page.

Meadway Nursery School Policy for Working in Partnership with Parents

(In this policy 'parents' includes the child's parents, legal guardians, close relatives or other carers who look after the child on a regular basis)

Meadway Nursery School aims to make all parents and carers feel comfortable and welcome in the group. We recognize that parents are their child's first and most important educators; by working together the results can have a positive effect on children's learning and development.

- We welcome the involvement of parents in the nursery school, but appreciate that parents may have family or work commitments, or may simply want a well-deserved break.
- Parents are welcome to visit the nursery school at any time and participate in nursery school events.
- Parents are welcome to help during a session, either for the whole time or just for a short period.
- We welcome comments about our provision and any suggestions for topics, visitors to the group or improvements in our procedures will be given serious consideration.
- Parents will be encouraged to share their knowledge and expertise to support the learning opportunities we provide. This includes sharing family celebrations.
- Wherever possible parents will be given choice concerning the sessions their child attends.
- The nursery school realizes that family life can sometimes be stressful and will offer support to parents where needed. This will include a flexible approach to the payment of fees.
- We will continually consider ways to improve our communication with parents and provide opportunities for parents to discuss together relevant issues concerning child care.

Information for parents

- Information about the nursery school will be given to parents who enquire about a placement for their child in the form of a brief introductory leaflet. Further information including our curriculum, policies and procedures will be given to parents in the form of a 'Welcome Pack' once their child is due to start.
- Where there is a need, we will aim to give this information to parents in their home language, in Braille or by use of audiotape, interpreters, etc.
- A meeting will be arranged with parents prior to their child starting at the group to discuss the contents of the 'Welcome Pack', which will include the personal details and consent forms we require, together with procedures for collecting children, if a child is missing and making complaints.

Exchanging information

- The nursery school will give parents regular newsletters to keep them informed of the nursery school activities. Information will also be displayed on our notice boards.
- Staff will be available at the beginning and end of the sessions to talk to parents.
- Parents will be given the opportunity to discuss their child's progress at least once a term and a 'home links' diary will enable staff and parents to share information on a more regular basis.
- The nursery school will hold 'Open Days' for parents to come and talk to staff about the work we do and see our resources.
- Books and other information relating to early years education, child development, health matters and other child care issues will be available for parents to borrow.
- A copy of our OFSTED report and Action Plan will be available to all parents.

Parental access to records

- Parents will be informed about the records we keep concerning their child, where they are kept and who has access to them.
- Parents will be able to see the records at any time and will be invited to contribute to the record of their child's development.
- The nursery school is registered under the Data Protection Act.

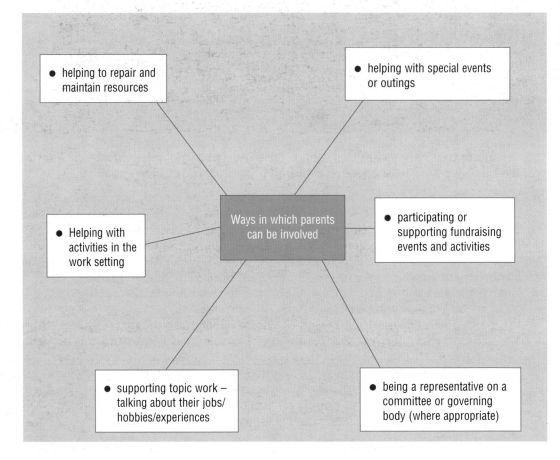

- helping to repair and maintain resources
- helping with special events or outings
- Helping with activities in the work setting
- Ways in which parents can be involved
- participating or supporting fundraising events and activities
- supporting topic work – talking about their jobs/hobbies/experiences
- being a representative on a committee or governing body (where appropriate)

Reasons why parents may not want to become involved

Many parents will want to become involved in their child's setting, especially if there is an open, welcoming atmosphere and a place to meet other parents. There will always be some parents who do not want to participate. There could be a number of reasons for this reluctance. These include:

✳ working full-time or having other daytime commitments;

✳ feeling that they have nothing of value to contribute;

✳ not being interested in spending time with other people's children;

✳ lacking confidence or feeling shy.

It is important that parents do not feel pressured into becoming involved. You should always respect parents' decisions and not assume that this shows a lack of interest in their children.

Some early years settings have a drop-in facility for parents which helps support those feeling isolated and experiencing problems, while a family support group, with a skilled family worker on hand, can help people with parenting skills and other issues.

Your role within the work setting

- your role in the work setting and the boundaries of that role
- the roles of others and lines of management
- confidentiality and why it is important to maintain it

In most instances you will be working under the supervision of others and it is likely that parents will pass confidential information directly to a staff member. However, there may be occasions on which you are given information and asked to pass it on, or that you may hear or be told confidential information in the course of the daily routine. This issue is dealt with in the section on Confidentiality (page 357) and so long as you follow guidelines, procedures and practices which apply to the work setting you will not go far wrong.

Remember that there are lines of management in place in most work settings and you should follow them if you need to check your understanding or to ask advice. Try to be aware of the ways in which staff members relate to, and communicate with, parents and try to identify which methods seem to be most effective.

Training Placements

- What are training placements and how many will there be?
- How are placements arranged?
- What are the placement responsibilities?
- What are the student responsibilities?

What are they and how many?

During the course, you will be allocated a range of placements, which may include nurseries, schools and families. These are arranged by your study centre and should enable you to carry out all the requirements set out in your PER. You are likely to need at least two placements to cover both core age ranges. For those taking the 0–1 year Option Module (Work with Babies) there may be a third placement. The variety of placements available will depend on your locality and the structure of early years care and education provision.

What are the placement responsibilities?

Many training placements have a wealth of experience in helping students on a number of courses and may have a designated person (e.g. **a placement supervisor**) to liaise with the study centre:

☐ They welcome well-motivated students and will afford time and advice for those willing and keen to accept it.

☐ They understand that there are course requirements which you need to be able to implement but they will also expect you to carry out tasks they have planned and arranged and to follow policies and procedures laid down in their setting.

Take advantage of any extra opportunities you may have to attend special events or outings as these provide valuable experience in seeing children in a range of situations and environments.

Before starting a new placement

Many students are nervous when starting in a new placement, and staff will be aware of their concerns. The following checklist will help you to feel more confident and to feel settled more quickly:

- Before I start – making contact: Find out exactly where the placement is – practise the route beforehand so that you allow enough time; make sure you have the telephone number and that you know who to report to. (Many placements will be happy to show you around prior to starting work.) At this first visit you could ask the following questions:

- What hours will I be working?

- What should I wear?

- What sort of things will I have to do?

- What shall I do if I am ill or cannot attend?

- What shall I do at lunchtime?

- What happens at the end of a placement period?

What are the student responsibilities?

☐ Attendance	☐ Co-operation
☐ Appearance	☐ Professionalism
☐ Paperwork	

1 *Attendance*

☐ *Check attendance times*: Make sure you have checked the following with your supervisor: your starting time, break and lunch times and finishing time. There is sometimes some flexibility if you have limited transport choices or have unavoidable appointments.

☐ *Be flexible:* Always offer to make up missed time and be prepared to stay longer on some occasions, if possible, to help complete a job and prepare for the following day, for example when displays are being changed – much easier to do without children around!

☐ *Reliability and punctuality*: these are very important and poor performance in these aspects can lead to tensions between you and staff. Their main concern must be the children in their care and they will be less likely to co-operate with you and to give responsibility for tasks if you cannot be relied upon to arrive on time and be prepared.

☐ *Absence from placement:* If, for some good reason, you cannot attend then you must contact your placement and inform them as soon as possible (preferably before the children arrive) so alternative arrangements can be made, indicating whether you are likely to be able to attend on the next scheduled date. You should also inform your study centre to avoid a visiting tutor making an unnecessary journey. Whenever possible, missed days should be 'made up'.

2   *Appearance*

Your study centre will give guidance for appearance, particularly if there is a uniform (often a sweatshirt over dark trousers).

- Choose clothing carefully, bearing in mind the types of activity you are likely to be involved in.

- Footwear should be comfortable and not too heavy.

- Avoid long fingernails and have no nail varnish – flakes chipping off into the snack you are preparing is not at all appetising or hygienic!

- Similarly avoid jewellery other than a watch – small children pull on chains and earrings and heavy rings and bracelets are inappropriate for dealing with playdough, paint or for changing nappies.

3   *Paperwork*

Although time is always precious, try to identify a time each week or fortnight when you can sit down with your supervisor and discuss your progress. You should discuss:

✳ what competencies you feel you have achieved

✳ how you might achieve those which do not occur during the normal daily routine

✳ what activities you have planned and need to carry out

✳ forthcoming plans and events which involve you.

Keeping a log or diary: This will help you to recall things you have done and match them to the competencies in the **PER**. It is **your responsibility** to do this, not your supervisor's. Try to become familiar with the requirements and make a pencil mark next to those you believe you have carried out competently – if you can show a date, or dates, and refer to your log, then your supervisor is more likely to remember it and may sign it off.

The Practice Evidence Record (PER): Remember that your **PER** is your record of achievement in placement and is vital evidence for you to earn the Certificate.

✳ *Do not lose it!* It is important to keep a record of signed competencies throughout the course and check it regularly with your tutor in case the worst should happen.

✳ *Keep your PER in a safe place*: Try to avoid leaving your PER with your supervisor – this may seem sensible but often leads to disaster if you or he/she is absent, the book gets mislaid or damaged or the placement comes to an end followed by a long holiday!

✳ *Attendance record:* Your study centre may require you to keep an **attendance sheet** which logs the time and dates of placement attendance. This needs to be regularly signed by your supervisor and kept by you.

✳ *Getting signatures*: In addition to your attendance record and PER competencies you will also need to obtain your supervisor's signature to **authenticate** (show it is genuine) displays, observations and portfolio activities.

4   *Co-operation*

No two training placements, nor supervisors, will be the same. It is important, therefore, to settle as quickly as possible into new and different routines and practices. Gathering the placement information as suggested on page 356 should speed up this process.

Co-operating with other professionals and recognising their contributions are areas which are assessed through the PDP at the end of each placement. For students who attend for two or three days a week it can be difficult to pick up the threads of what has happened on the days you have been at your **study centre**. The opportunity to attend your placement for a **block week** will give you the chance to experience the full range of activities including P.E., music, cookery and other topic work which you may otherwise be missing.

As you are attending on the same days each week it may seem that you are always given the same jobs to do – Fridays usually involve washing paint pots! These have to be done and, if they are carried out by other staff members or helpers on other occasions then it is not unreasonable for you to be expected to do them too as part of your training.

It only becomes a problem if you are given tasks which are always, or often, away from the children and you are not having the opportunity to carry out the requirements of the course. If this is the case you need to speak to your tutor who may visit and discuss these issues with your supervisor.

5 *Professionalism*

This is something you will develop as you gain experience. The PDPs in the back of your PER cover all the aspects of professionalism on which you will be judged and assessed.

Perhaps the most important is **confidentiality**.

* You will be entrusted with personal information about children, parents and staff, either directly (being told or being given written information) or indirectly (hearing staffroom discussions, parental comments or children's conversations) and it is important that you do not repeat any of it at home or to friends.

* There have been embarrassing, not to say unpleasant, incidents, sometimes resulting in students' placements being cancelled, through thoughtlessness. In small communities such as schools or nurseries it is easy for a parent or family member to overhear confidential information relating to daily events (e.g. an incident involving aggressive behaviour or swearing) or individual children (personal or family difficulties affecting the child concerned) if it is mentioned to a neighbour or the person you babysit for, even if it is through concern.

* The incidents may be discussed in your teaching sessions amongst your student group but you should not identify the children concerned and it must be agreed that they are not talked about beyond the group.

The next important aspect of professionalism is that of being a good **role model**.

● Children are likely to treat you as any other adult on the staff – assuming that you can help them and are there to care for them as well as discipline them.

● This means that by your behaviour, language and attitudes you set an example for the children you are working with and caring for.

● **Being a good role model** involves:

✓ showing consideration for others

✓ taking care over hygiene and appearance

✓ using appropriate language (you must address the children and adults politely and using the correct terms – avoid referring to the children as kids!)

✓ supporting other staff and parents and following set procedures and policies.

Use of **initiative** is one of the aspects some students struggle with. It involves trying to anticipate (see in advance) situations and taking appropriate action.

☐ *Have confidence:* Using initiative effectively requires confidence on your part and reassurance from your supervisor that you can (and should) deal with many incidents yourself if you happen to be the nearest adult.

☐ *Safety issues*: It is vital that you take steps on your own initiative when matters of safety are concerned – e.g. spilt sand/water, a blocked fire exit etc.

☐ *Handling disputes*: Additionally you will be expected to deal with children's disputes and maintain behaviour according to your placement guidelines when you are supervising groups.

Remember – nobody will expect you to know everything at first. Staff are there to help you to get the most out of each placement and your tutor will discuss any concerns you may have. Most students thoroughly enjoy this aspect of the course.

SIGNPOST: Option B

- **Day care setting**
- **Nursery class**
- **School setting**

1 (a) For **each** of the above, and **working in pairs**, make a list of the **main** concerns parents might have about their baby/child starting and settling into the setting.
   (b) Compare your list with another pair and discuss similarities and differences.

2 Working in small groups, choose **one** of the settings and write a list of the ways in which the setting would welcome baby/child and parents and how the settling-in period can be eased. *NB. Try to use your own practical experiences in placement to help you – what information do parents provide about their child? is there a key-worker system? etc.*

3 The amount of parental involvement varies from setting to setting and depending on the age of the children concerned. Thinking about your answers to questions 1 and 2, and using the same setting you chose for question 2, explain how a parent will be involved in the settling-in process.

4 Complete a chart (see photocopiable sheets in Appendix) as below to show the role of the Child Care and Education worker during the settling-in process in relation to the child **and** to the parent(s).

Role in relation to child	Role in relation to parent
Learn child's name quickly	Greet by name
Always welcome child by name	Make time to discuss any concerns
Be ready to give reassurance and attention	Etc . . .
Etc . . .	

5 A strong partnership between parents and carers helps a child to develop and make good progress. Most settings provide parents with information about various policies (for example discipline or behaviour) and explain why they have certain procedures and how **they** will care for, and educate, the children.

As a member of staff (in the setting chosen in question 2) some parents have asked you what they should be doing to ensure their child's care and education progresses well and how they can support you and your work.

Create a leaflet to give to parents identifying their role. It must suggest **what** they can do to support different areas of your work (for example feeding/mealtimes, behaviour, politeness, getting enough sleep, etc.) and explain **how** it helps the child, the parents and you!

Appendix

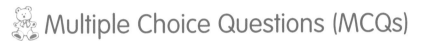 Multiple Choice Questions (MCQs)

Set One

1 **Children are particularly vulnerable to infection because they:**
   a) Have not always been immunised
   b) Do not wash their hands properly
   c) Play outside with other children
   d) Have immature immune systems

2 **Child care and education workers can BEST help to ensure the safety of children at home time by:**
   a) Teaching children about 'stranger danger'
   b) Helping them to cross the road
   c) Only letting children be collected by a known adult
   d) Producing a written procedure for collecting children

3 **A child who you know has asthma is becoming breathless. You must FIRST:**
   a) Dial 999 and ask for an ambulance
   b) Put the child in the recovery position
   c) Sit the child down and reassure them
   d) Telephone the health visitor

4 **Which of these is the normal body temperature for a child?**
   a) 36.9°C
   b) 38.5°C
   c) 33°C
   d) 35.5°C

5 **A child in your care has scalded herself with a cup of hot coffee. The correct first aid measure is to:**
   a) Cover the scalded area with a clean, non-fluffy dressing
   b) Reassure the child and notify her parents
   c) Rub the scalded area with butter
   d) Immerse the scalded area in cold water

6 **The MAIN benefits of outdoor play for children are**:
1 Helping obese children to reduce weight
2 The opportunity to share and take turns
3 Improving muscle tone and co-ordination skills
4 Teaching them about the weather
5 Promoting healthy lung development
6 Helping the digestion of food

a) 1, 2, 4, 6
b) 2, 3, 5, 6
c) 1, 2, 3, 6
d) 2, 3, 4, 5

7 **Children's gross motor skills can BEST be stimulated by**:
a) Playing with wooden bricks
b) Catching balls
c) Jumping from a low bench
d) Threading beads onto a lace

8 **Which of the following activities will BEST promote fine manipulative skills in a child of three years?**
a) Threading beads
b) Playing with water
c) Playing with sand
d) Pushing a truck

9 **Sam can kick a ball hard, stand and walk on tiptoe, walk upstairs with one foot to a step and ride a tricycle using the pedals. Sam is aged**:
a) 18 months
b) 2 years six months
c) Three years
d) 2 years

10 **Successful bowel and bladder control can best be achieved by**:
a) Rewarding the child every time he or she uses the potty
b) Taking the child to the toilet regularly
c) Ignoring the child's distress when he or she has an 'accident'
d) Waiting until the child shows he or she is ready to be toilet trained

11 **The MOST important factors to consider when choosing clothes for children are**:
1 Ease of washing
2 Fashion
3 Comfort
4 Warmth
5 Cost
6 Easy fastening

a) 1, 3, 4, 6
b) 1, 2, 5, 6
c) 2, 3, 5, 6
d) 1, 2, 4, 5

12 **Carbohydrate is an essential part of children's diets because it**:
a) Helps in the formation of haemoglobin
b) Aids the formation of bones
c) Provides heat and energy
d) Provides material for growth

13 Which vitamin may be found in dairy products and is helpful in bone formation?
    a) C
    b) D
    c) K
    d) A

14 Which of the following foods must be avoided by a child who has coeliac disease?
    a) Gluten (found in bread flour and cereals)
    b) Pork sausages
    c) Milk and cheese
    d) Peanuts

15 An appropriate definition of plaque is:
    a) Painful teeth
    b) A sugary substance in the mouth
    c) Dental caries
    d) A film of bacteria on the teeth

16 If a child refuses to eat green vegetables you should:
    a) Keep the child at the table until he or she has eaten them
    b) Encourage the child to eat them but do not force him or her
    c) Refuse to give the child a pudding until he or she has eaten them
    d) Be firm with the child

17 When caring for a child who is unwell at the nursery, you should:
    1 Isolate the child
    2 Keep the child company
    3 Provide challenging play
    4 Give practical help
    5 Provide reassurance
    6 Relax their expectations

    a) 1,2,3,5
    b) 1,4,5,6
    c) 2,4,5,6
    d) 2,3,5,6

18 Play is described as 'solitary' when a child plays:
    a) Interactively with a small group of children
    b) Alone with toys
    c) Alongside another child but without interacting
    d) At the same activity and communicates with another child

19 A two-and-a-half year old child comes to the day nursery with a comfort blanket. The BEST response from the early years worker is to:
    a) Allow the child to keep the blanket with them
    b) Ask the parent or carer to take the blanket home
    c) Gently explain to the child that they will be too busy to need the blanket
    d) Keep the blanket in the staff room in case it is needed

20 In creative activity, demonstrations of how to copy and use materials, and the use of patterns cut from templates are:
    a) Unhelpful
    b) Essential
    c) Good practice
    d) Desirable

21 **Non-verbal communication includes**:
   a) Body language, singing, talking
   b) Asking questions, gestures, reading aloud
   c) Talking, singing, gestures
   d) Facial expressions, eye contact, gestures

22 **Which of the following activities is most likely to promote communication skills in a three-year-old child?**
   a) A varied messy play area
   b) A variety of good construction toys
   c) Jigsaw puzzles
   d) Discussion and review time

23 **Gender stereotyping may**:
   a) Encourage girls to do technology
   b) Affect the choices which boys and girls make
   c) Help boys to enjoy music and dancing
   d) Encourage good parenting skills

24 **Promoting equality of opportunity in a school includes**:
   a) Providing the same facilities for all children
   b) Treating everyone the same
   c) Recognising differences and enabling all children to participate
   d) Ignoring the differences that exist between children

25 **When separated from his or her main carer, a two-year-old child will benefit MOST from nursery care that includes**:
   a) A set routine that is applied to all the children in the nursery
   b) A key worker system that has a high ratio of carers to children
   c) A group of children of a wide variety of ages
   d) A large, lively, stimulating group of young children

26 **A group of four-year-old children argue about sharing a doll's pram. The adult should**:
   a) Put the pram into the toy store
   b) Leave the children to sort out the argument
   c) Start a discussion about sharing
   d) Tell the children to take turns

27 **A partially sighted six-year-old child wears spectacles. When taking part in physical education the child should**:
   a) Do the same as the other children but with the spectacles securely fastened
   b) Be offered easier activities
   c) Be encouraged to do the same activities as other children
   d) Take off the spectacles and do the same activities as other children

28 **The primary value of role play for young children is that it stimulates**:
   a) Intellectual and conceptual skills
   b) Imaginative and imitative skills
   c) Gross and fine motor skills
   d) Sensory development

29 **In reaction to a stranger, a child of one year is most likely to**:
   a) be happy as long as the stranger is kind
   b) Not mind being with the stranger
   c) Show positive interest in the stranger
   d) Be shy and cling to their carer

30 **Between which years are children characteristically possessive and tend to extreme swings of mood and behaviour?**
   a) 1 and 2 years
   b) 2 and 3 years
   c) 3 and 4 years
   d) 4 and 5 years

31 **Early years workers are MOST likely to have realistic expectations of children's behaviour if they:**
   a) Read many books and articles
   b) Are stricter with children to start with
   c) Understand age-appropriate behaviour
   d) Provide few boundaries for children

32 **Children are most likely to develop socially acceptable behaviour patterns if they are:**
   1 Praised when they behave acceptably
   2 Given adult attention as they work and play
   3 Punished when they are aggressive
   4 Given clear boundaries
   5 Given attention when they demand it
   6 Told off each time they behave in an unacceptable way

   a) 1,3,6
   b) 2,3,5
   c) 1,2,4
   d) 4,5,6

33 **When settling a child into a new setting, it will be MOST helpful if the early years worker:**
   a) Makes sure that the child's peg is labelled
   b) Sends the parent information
   c) Tells the other children about the new child
   d) Settles the child in gradually

34 **Which of the following is NOT a voluntary organisation?**
   a) NSPCC
   b) DSS
   c) RNIB
   d) MENCAP

35 **An early years worker who is trying to promote self-help skills and independence in young children will be more successful if she or he says:**
   a) 'Come on, you're a big boy now; you can do it by yourself'
   b) 'See – everyone else has done it. You can do it too'
   c) 'You'll have a present if you do it all by yourself'
   d) 'That's clever. Shall I help you with this bit if you can't manage?'

36 **Any written records about children and their families and carers should be:**
   a) Available to the head teacher/nursery manager only
   b) Stored securely and confidentiality maintained
   c) Kept in the office to which only staff have access
   d) Freely available to all the staff

37 **The commonest cause of death amongst toddlers and young children is:**
   a) Infections
   b) Accidents
   c) Cancers
   d) Child abuse

38 **A lone parent experiencing difficulties could obtain practical help and advice from**:
a) Gingerbread
b) Barnardos
c) Childline
d) Shelter

39 **In which year was The Children Act passed by Parliament?**
a) 1989
b) 1986
c) 1999
d) 1993

40 **The main work of the National Childbirth Trust is concerned with**:
a) Giving education for parenthood
b) Campaigning for changes in the law relating to abortion
c) Arranging for mothers to have babies in hospital
d) Closing down maternity wards

Set Two

1 **An obstetrician specialises in the**:
a) Care of children from the time they are born
b) Function and disorders of the female reproductive system
c) Health care of the mother and her unborn child
d) Treatment of obstructions of the digestive system

2 **The most important reason for immunising children is to prevent**:
a) Absence from school
b) Side-effects of the disease
c) Spread of the disease
d) The disease occurring

3 **The MOST EFFECTIVE methods for preventing the spread of infection in early years settings are**:
1 Encouraging children to wash their hands regularly
2 Good ventilation
3 Excluding children with an infection
4 Preventing outdoor play
5 Reducing the heating temperature
6 Cleaning out pet cages regularly

a) 2, 4, 5
b) 1, 2, 3,
c) 3, 4, 6
d) 2, 4, 6

4 **The spread of head lice could be reduced if children had their hair**:
a) Cut short
b) Inspected regularly
c) Washed frequently
d) Combed regularly and after every nursery session

5 **When planning an outing the MOST IMPORTANT considerations are**:
1 Choosing a destination
2 The cost of transport
3 Parental consent
4 Taking spare clothes

5 Adequate adult/child ratios
6 First Aid Kit

a) 2,3,4
b) 1,3,5
c) 1,4,6
d) 1,4,5

6 **If an early years worker finds an unconscious child, their FIRST action should be to**:
a) Send for their immediate supervisor
b) Contact the parents
c) Check for breathing
d) Send for an ambulance

7 **Most children will be able to tie their own shoelaces by the age of**:
a) 3 years
b) 4 years
c) 5 years
d) 6 years

8 **What are the necessary procedures for the safe and hygienic care of animals?**
1 Provide secure housing
2 Make sure that children wash their hands after handling pets
3 Provide children with unsupervised access to the animals
4 Provide clean bedding on a regular basis
5 Allow children to take the pets home in the holidays
6 Supervise children when handling animals

a) 1,2,3,4
b) 1,2,4,6
c) 2,4,5,6
d) 3,4,5,6

9 **A safe adult/child ratio for 2–5-year-old children on an outing is**:
a) 1 adult to 54 children
b) 2 adults to 5 children
c) 1 adult to 3 children
d) 1 adult to 2 children

10 **At 3 years of age, most children are able to**:
a) Build a tower of 9 or 10 bricks, cut with scissors, copy a circle
b) Build three steps with six bricks, thread small beads, copy a square
c) Catch a ball, draw recognisable pictures, thread a needle
d) Draw a diamond shape, sew neatly with needle and thread, tie shoelaces

11 **When dealing with a bleeding wound, the early years worker should wear disposable gloves**:
a) If the child is, or you think may be, HIV positive
b) If the child has haemophilia
c) Every time a child is treated
d) If the child has leukaemia

12 **Which vitamin helps the absorption of iron?**
a) D
b) K
c) B
d) C

13 **How can an adult encourage a three-year-old child who has been ill to eat?**
   a) By giving baby foods
   b) By offering small portions, attractively presented
   c) By waiting until the child is hungry
   d) By giving favourite foods

14 **Which religion forbids its followers to eat beef?**
   a) Muslim
   b) Christian
   c) Greek Orthodox
   d) Hindu

15 **Koplik's spots can be seen in the mouth if a child has**:
   a) Measles
   b) Rubella
   c) Chicken pox
   d) Impetigo

16 **The most common type of worm infestation found in young children in the UK is**:
   a) Hookworm
   b) Threadworm
   c) Roundworm
   d) Tapeworm

17 **Insulin is given to children who have the condition of**:
   a) Coeliac disease
   b) Phenylketonuria
   c) Diabetes
   d) Anaemia

18 **The interval between the onset of infection and the first signs and symptoms of an infectious disease is called**:
   a) Isolation period
   b) Incubation period
   c) Quarantine period
   d) Convalescent period

19 **A child should first be fitted for shoes when he or she**:
   a) Learns to crawl
   b) Is able to stand unaided
   c) Starts to play outdoors
   d) Starts to walk

20 **Displays are important for children because they**:
   1 Show adults' work
   2 Encourage sensory exploration
   3 Increase their self-esteem
   4 Decorate the environment
   5 Increase knowledge
   6 Promote discussion

   a) 1, 2, 3, 4
   b) 2, 3, 5, 6
   c) 2, 3, 4, 5
   d) 3, 4, 5, 6

21 **Which of the following practices discriminates unfairly?**

a) Children only being allowed to go on an outing if their parents can pay for it
b) Children only being allowed to play outside in winter if their coats are fastened
c) Children not being allowed to go to school when they have an acute infectious illness
d) Children not being allowed to go swimming if they have a bad cold

22 **How can an early years worker BEST use a home corner to promote language development in a group of three-year-old children?**
a) Sit in the home corner and talk to one of the children
b) Dress up in a hat and take the part of a visitor
c) Leave the children alone to develop their play
d) Join in the play and direct questions to the children

23 **A three-year-old child invents an imaginary person. This can BEST be dealt with by**:
a) Gently explaining that this person is not really there
b) Telling the child that you can see the person too
c) Saying kindly that you do not like lies
d) Listening and accepting whatever the child says

24 **Young children's thinking can be described as egocentric. This means that they**:
a) Are selfish and intolerant
b) Are conceited and difficult to handle
c) See the world from their own viewpoint
d) Have no feelings for other people

25 **The MAIN benefits of providing musical activities for young children are to promote**:
a) Spatial awareness, emotional development, listening skills
b) Emotional development, sequencing skills, fine motor skills
c) Social development, fine motor skills, spatial awareness
d) Sequencing skills, social development, listening skills

26 **The MOST important aspects of the adult role when providing play for young children are**:
1 Planning activities
2 Participating appropriately
3 Producing good results
4 Putting things away
5 Preventing damage
6 Preparing materials
7 Providing opportunities
8 Preventing disruption

a) 1, 2, 6, 7
b) 1, 2, 3, 6
c) 2, 3, 6, 8
d) 1, 4, 5, 7

27 **The term given to the group of a similar age with whom children spend a lot of their time is**:
a) Friendship group
b) Status group
c) Peer group
d) Role group

28 **A young child is noticeably upset and tells you that her family's pet cat died at the weekend. The BEST way to help the child would be to**:
   a) Listen and let her talk to you
   b) Tell her about when your cat died
   c) Offer her a stimulating activity to distract her
   d) Encourage her to play with a lively group of children

29 **When using behaviour modification techniques, the best way to discourage unwanted behaviour is to**:
   a) Reward the child when he or she behaves negatively
   b) Use physical restraint whenever it is needed
   c) Give the negative behaviour little open attention
   d) Give the child lots of attention when he or she behaves negatively

30 **When communicating with parents, it is ESSENTIAL that early years workers ensure that**:
   a) Parents receive regular newsletters
   b) Communication is a two-way process
   c) There is a parents' noticeboard
   d) An information booklet is available

31 **The 'antecedent' to a child's behaviour is**:
   a) What happens afterwards
   b) What happened before the behaviour occurred
   c) What the child actually does
   d) The acceptable parts of the behaviour

32 **In a situation where there is conflict with parents, an early years worker should**:
   a) Explain to the parents why they are wrong
   b) Tell the parents that professionals know best
   c) Make a note of any complaints
   d) Take their concerns seriously

33 **Many employers have a code of practice concerning equal opportunities. The most important aspect of this is that it makes clear statements about**:
   a) The policy towards early retirement
   b) The amount of holiday each employee is entitled to
   c) The treatment of employees within the organisation
   d) The pay structure of the organisation

34 **Which combination of equipment will best stimulate gross motor skills when used by a young child?**
   a) Balls, hoops, bats
   b) Jigsaws, collage activity, beads and thread
   c) Hats, dolls, small bricks
   d) Bicycles, trucks, climbing frame

35 **To work successfully with children and their parents/carers, early years workers should acknowledge that parents**:
   1 Are the main educators of their children
   2 Know and understand their children
   3 Need to be told how to care for their children
   4 Prefer to leave educating their children to professionals
   5 Will value being involved in the education of their children
   6 Can share knowledge with staff to benefit their children

a) 1, 3, 4, 6
b) 1, 2, 5, 6
c) 2, 4, 5, 6
d) 3, 4, 5, 6

36   The term 'normal behaviour' best describes:
   a) The behaviour of a child at school
   b) Any behaviour that is acceptable at home
   c) The age-appropriate behaviour of a child
   d) Behaviour that is very mature for the age of the child

37   The political framework for the provision of services in Britain is democratic. This means that decisions about what services will be provided are made by:
   a) Politicians who are voted into office by citizens
   b) Members of the armed forces
   c) One leader who rules the country
   d) A self-appointed committee

38   An example of a statutory organisation is:
   a) Childline
   b) Citizens Advice Bureau
   c) Social Services Department
   d) Barnardo's

39   A question that is open-ended:
   a) Requires a monosyllabic answer
   b) Is easiest for children to answer
   c) Does not have one particular answer
   d) Gives the opportunity for several different answers

40   Statutory services are MAINLY funded from:
   a) Voluntary donations
   b) Taxes and national insurance
   c) Fundraising events
   d) Profits from business

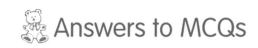 Answers to MCQs

Set One

1	d	15	d	29	d
2	c	16	b	30	b
3	c	17	c	31	c
4	a	18	b	32	c
5	d	19	a	33	d
6	b	20	a	34	b
7	b	21	d	35	d
8	a	22	d	36	b
9	c	23	b	37	b
10	d	24	c	38	a
11	a	25	b	39	a
12	c	26	c	40	a
13	b	27	a		
14	a	28	b		

Set Two

1	c	15	a	29	c
2	d	16	b	30	b
3	b	17	c	31	b
4	d	18	b	32	d
5	b	19	d	33	c
6	c	20	b	34	d
7	d	21	a	35	b
8	b	22	b	36	c
9	d	23	d	37	a
10	a	24	c	38	c
11	c	25	d	39	d
12	d	26	a	40	b
13	b	27	c		
14	d	28	a		

Age/Aspect	Growth	Gross motor skills	Fine motor skills	Sensory skills
1 year	Wt: Ht:			
2 years	Wt: Ht:			
3 years	Wt: Ht:			
4 years	Wt: Ht:			
5 years	Wt: Ht:			
6 years	Wt: Ht:			
7 years	Wt: Ht:			

Age range	Activity	Aspect(s) of sensory development	Aspect(s) of intellectual development
1–2 years			
2–4 years			
4–7 years			

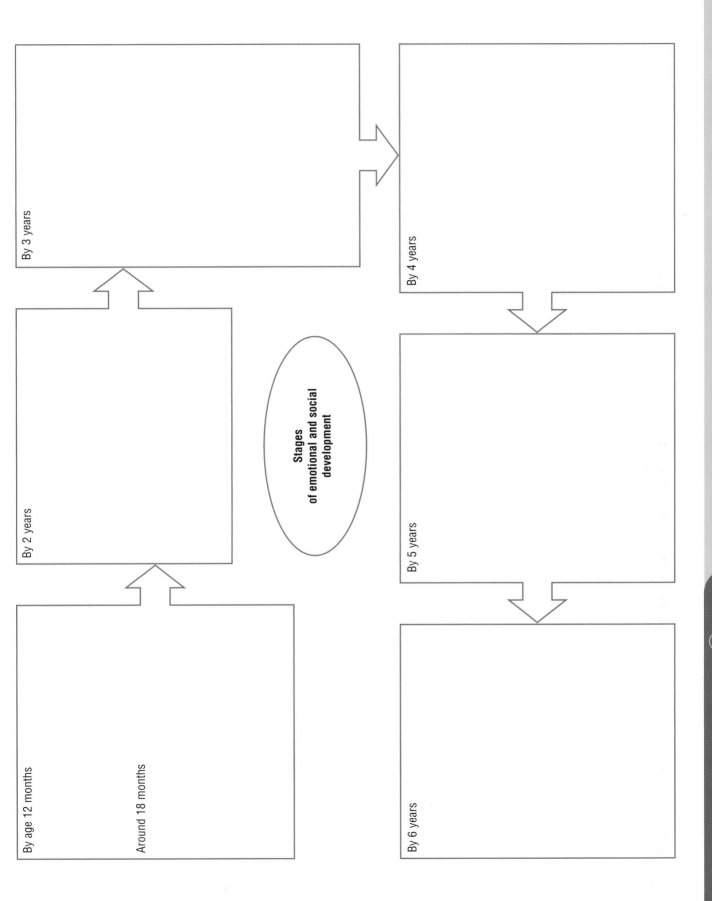

By 3 years

By 4 years

By 2 years

Stages
of emotional and social
development

By 5 years

By age 12 months

Around 18 months

By 6 years

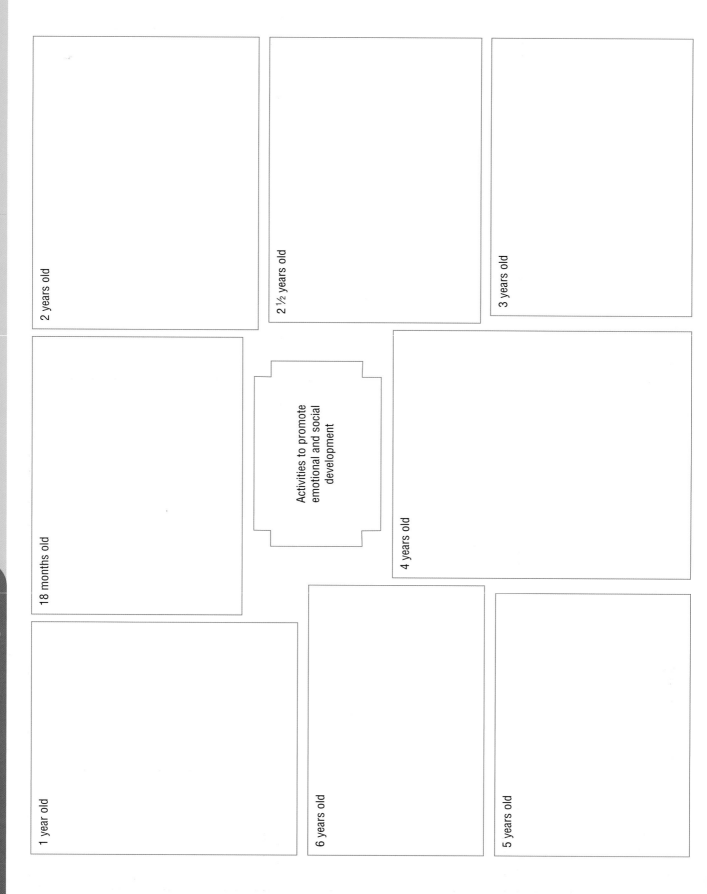

2 years old

2 ½ years old

3 years old

18 months old

Activities to promote emotional and social development

4 years old

1 year old

6 years old

5 years old

Age/Aspect	Emotional development	Social development
3 months		
6 months		
9 months		

Age/Aspect	Growth	Gross motor skills	Fine motor skills	Sensory skills
3 months	Wt: Length:			
6 months	Wt: Length:			
9 months	Wt: Length/Ht:			

Role in relation to child	Role in relation to parent

Glossary

aerobic exercise	activity which results in physical exertion, which increases oxygen consumption and so benefits the lungs, heart and circulation
ageism	discrimination against an individual or group on account of their age
anterior fontanelle	a diamond-shaped soft area at the front of the head, just above the brow; it closes between 12 and 18 months of age
autism	a rare developmental disorder which impairs children's understanding of their environment
benefit system	benefits are the statutory amounts of money which are issued and distributed via the Benefits Agency to those members of society who need this support
Benefits Agency	the agency within the Department of Social Security which is responsible for the assessment and payment of social security benefits
body language	the language of non-verbal communication, body language also covers the way the body, face, eyes and hands look and move
calorie	unit of energy obtained from foods
chromosome	a thread-like structure in the cell nucleus which carries genetic information in the form of genes
Code of Practice	a document which states how a Policy e.g. Equal Opportunities Policy, is put into place
cognitive/intellectual development	these words both refer to the ideas and thinking of the child. Cognition emphasises that children are aware, active learners, and that understanding is an important part of intellectual life. Intelligence is about the ability to profit from experience
colic	an attack of acute abdominal pain caused by spasms in the intestines as food is being digested; sometimes called '3-month colic'
convulsions	uncontrolled movements of the muscles which may be accompanied by loss of consciousness
dehydration	the loss of fluid or water from the body
disablism	discrimination against an individual or group on account of their disability
discrimination	treating a person or group unfairly, usually because of a negative view of certain of their characteristics
Down's syndrome	a genetic disorder resulting from the presence of an extra chromosome; children usually, but not always, have learning difficulties
eczema	a skin condition which can give rise to cracked and sore patches of skin
egocentric	self-centred or viewing things from one's own standpoint
equality of opportunity	the principle that all people should be provided with an equal opportunity to succeed, irrespective of their age, sex, ethnic or religious group, physical abilities or sexual orientation
ethos	characteristics/beliefs and attitudes of a community (in this case, work setting)
first-hand experience	one which is 'lived' through personally rather than experienced by someone else and seen or heard about
fontanelles	the soft spots on the top of the new born baby's head; when they are sunken, they are a sign of dehydration

gene	unit of the chromosome containing a pattern which is passed on through generations (Genes influence hair and eye colour and blood group, etc.)
glue ear	a build-up of sticky fluid in the middle ear; this usually affects children under 8 years old
gross pay	the pay you receive before any deductions, such as tax or National Insurance, are made
implement	to carry out or put into effect; to execute … your plan
jaundice	yellow coloration of the skin and the whites of the eye caused by the interference with the production of bile
key-worker	a member of staff (usually in a nursery setting) who spends more time with a small number of identified children, builds a close relationship with them and is the main contact person for their families
meconium	the first 'stool' or motion that a new born baby passes: a greenish-black tarry substance usually passed within 48 hours of birth
motherese	when adults (often mothers) talk to babies in a high-pitched tone about what is happening
nature/nurture	nature: the features, characteristics, abilities one is born with; nurture: one's upbringing including health, emotional, social, educational factors
non-verbal communication	everything which is not actual words; it can include body language, posture, tone of voice, etc.
pejorative	insulting or derogatory
plaque	a rough, sticky coating on the teeth that consists of saliva, food debris and bacteria
Policy document	a document which covers areas of ethical concern and good practice, e.g. health and safety policy
possetting	when a baby regularly vomits small amounts of her feeds but has no sign of illness. Usually caused by a weakness of the muscle at the opening of the stomach.
prejudice	to prejudge somebody on the basis of their membership of a particular category or group
pulse	in musical terms this is the regular, underlying beat of a tune or rhythm
racism	discrimination against an individual or group on account of their race or ethnic group
reconstituted family	a family unit which is made up of members of two or more 'original' families
rhythm	the pattern of beats or sounds of varying lengths. When clapping to 'Baa Baa Black Sheep' there is a steady underlying beat as follows — '**Baa** Baa **Black** Sheep, **Have** you any **Wool**?'
role model	an individual whose behaviour may be copied or aspired to.
sexism	discrimination against an individual or a group on account of their biological sex
self-esteem	the way you feel about yourself — good or bad — leads to high or low self-esteem
self-image/self-concept	how you see yourself, and how you think others see you
sibling	term for a brother or sister
socialisation	the lifelong process by which we learn about ourselves, others and the world around us
social referencing	babies and young children look at adults to see how they react, as a guide to how they should react to a situation themselves
statementing	a formal process of negotiation between an education authority and parents; it aims to identify the child's needs and to specify the educational provision required
statutory services	central government services and local government services e.g. the NHS, Social Services, Local Education Authority, etc.
stereotyping	the process whereby individuals or groups are characterised in simple and often **pejorative** terms, so that all members within the category are seen in one particular way
voluntary organisation	an association or society which has been created by its members rather than having been created by the state e.g. a charity
welfare state	a society in which the state (i.e. the government) accepts responsibility for ensuring a minimum standard of living for all people. It was set up in 1948 following the Beveridge Report and is supported by a **benefit system**.

Bibliography and references

Apusskido (1996) 2nd edition. London: A&C Black.

Bruce, Tina (1991) *Time to Play*. London: Hodder & Stoughton.

Bruce, Tina (1996) *Helping Young Children to Play*. London: Hodder & Stoughton.

Bruce, Tina (1997) *Early Childhood Education*. London: Hodder & Stoughton.

Bruce, Tina (2001) *Learning Through Play: Babies, Toddlers and the Foundation Years*. London: Hodder & Stoughton.

Bruce, Tina (2004) *Cultivating Creativity in Babies, Toddlers and Young Children*. London: Hodder & Stoughton.

Bruce, Tina and Meggitt, Carolyn (2002) *Child Care and Education* 3rd ed. London: Hodder & Stoughton.

Beaver, M., Brewster, J., Keene, A. (1997) *Child Care and Education for CCE and NVQ2*. Cheltenham: Stanley Thornes.

Bruce, Tina (1996) *Helping Young Children to Play*. London: Hodder & Stoughton.

Davies, M. (1995) *Helping Children to Learn Through a Movement Perspective*. London: Hodder & Stoughton.

Einon, Dorothy (1985) *Creative Play*. London: Penguin.

Einon, Dorothy (1985) *Child Behaviour*. London: Penguin.

Flanagan, Cara (1996) *Applying Psychology to Child Development*. London: Hodder & Stoughton.

Gura, P. (1996) *Resources for Learning*. London: Hodder & Stoughton.

Holland, P. 'Is Zero Tolerance Intolerance? An Under Fives Centre takes a fresh look at their policy on war/weapons/superhero play'. *Early Childhood Practice: The Journal for Multi-Professional Partnerships*, 1999, Volume 1, No. 1, pp. 65–73.

Lyus, Verna (1998) *Management in the Early Years*. London: Hodder & Stoughton.

MacGregor, Helen (1999) *Bingo Lingo*. London: A&C Black.

Matterson, Elizabeth (compiler) (1991) *This Little Puffin . . .* (revised edition). London: Penguin.

Meggitt, Carolyn (2001) *Baby and Child Health*. Oxford: Heinemann.

Meggitt, Carolyn (1997) *Special Needs Handbook for Health and Social Care*. London: Hodder & Stoughton.

Meggitt, Carolyn (1999) *Caring for Babies*. London: Hodder & Stoughton.

Meggitt, Carolyn and Sunderland, Gerald (2000) *An Illustrated Guide to Child Development*. Oxford: Heinemann.

Nolte, Dorothy Law (1998) *Children Learn What They Live*. Workman Publishing Company, Inc.: New York.

Richards, Judy (1999) *The complete A–Z Health & Social Care handbook*. London: Hodder & Stoughton.

RNIB (1995) Play it My Way. RNIB/HMSO.

Ta-ra-ra boom de-ay (1977) London: A&C Black.

Tinder-box (1982) London: A&C Black.

Umansky, Kaye (1994) *Three Singing Pigs*. London: A&C Black.

Umansky, Kaye (2000) *Three Tapping Teddies*. London: A&C Black.

Whiting, M. and Lobstein, T. (1992) *The Nursery Food Book*. London: Edward Arnold.

Young, S. and Glover, J. (1998) *Music in the Eary Years*. London: Falmer Press.

Equality of opportunity

There is a wealth of information available which will help you to understand equal opportunity issues and to create a positive environment for children. Many cheap and authentic artefacts can be collected by asking parents and friends going abroad on holiday to bring back specific items for the nursery or school, e.g. traditional costumes, dolls, greetings cards, photographs, cooking utensils, etc.

The following organisations are particularly relevant, and some of them have their own websites. If you do write off for information, please remember to enclose a stamped address envelope for their reply.

An Equal Start: Guidelines for working with the under eights
A guide available from:
Equal Opportunities Commission
Overseas House
Quay Street
Manchester M3 3HN

CRE (Commission for Racial Equality)
Elliott House
10–12 Allington St
London SW1E 5EH
www.cre.gov.uk

EYTARN
Early Years Anti-Racist Network
www.decet.org

Royal National Institute for the Blind (RNIB)
224 Great Portland Street
London W1N 6AA
(020) 7388 1266
www.rnib.org.uk

Royal National Institute for the Deaf (RNID)
19–20 Featherstone Street
London EC1Y 8SL
(020) 7296 8060
www.rnid.org.uk

Minority Group Support Service
Southfields
South Streeet
Coventry CV1 5EJ

SCOPE
12 Park Crescent
London W1N 4EQ
(020) 7636 5020
www.scope.org.uk

National Autistic Society
393 City Road
London EC1V 1NE
(020) 7833 2299
www.carryon.oneworld.org/autism

Down's Syndrome Association (E & W)
155 Mitcham Road, Tooting,
London SW17 9PG
(020) 8682 4001
www.downs-syndrome.org.uk

MENCAP (Royal Society for Mentally Handicapped Children and Adults) MENCAP National Centre

123 Golden Lane
London EC1Y 0RT
(020) 7454 0454
www.mencap.org.uk

National Asthma Campaign

Providence House, Providence Place,
London N1 0NT
(020) 7226 2260
0345 010203 Asthma helpline
(9am–9pm each day)
www.asthma.org.uk
Posters which promote multi-cultural awareness
are available from:

Pictorial Wall Charts Educational Trust (PCET)

27 Kirchen Road
London W13 0UD

A comprehensive listing of materials, including
posters, videos, books and toys may be found at the
end of Chapter 1 in *Child Care and Education* 3rd
Edition by Tina Bruce and Carolyn Meggitt (see
Resources section on page 350)

UNISON

1 Mabledon Place,
London WC1H 9AJ
Phone 020 7388 2366
www.unison.org.uk

Professional Association of Nursery Nurses (PANN)

2 St James' Court,
Friar Gate,
Derby, DE1 1BT.
Tel: 01332 343029
www.pat.org.uk

CACHE – Council for Awards in children's Care and Education)

8 Chequer Street
St Albans
Hertfordshire AL1 3XZ
Tel. 01727 847636
www.cache.org.uk

EDEXCEL (for BTEC)

www.edexcel.org.uk

Videos

RNIB (1995) One of the Family, No. 4, Play It My
Way.

Froebel Block Play Project (1991) Building a Future.
(Available from Community Playthings,
Robertsbridge, East Sussex.)

National Children's Bureau
8 Wakeley Street,
London EC4 7QE:
(a) Treasure Baskets (for sitting babies)
(b) Heuristic Play (for toddlers)

BBC Horizon on ADHD.

Useful Addresses

Learning to Landscape Trust (advice on outdoor
environments)

Wendy Titman Associates Ltd.
PO Box 283
Elton
Peterborough

Clear Vision Project (for sharing braille and dual
textbooks)

Linden Lodge School
61 Princes Way
London SW19 6JB

Index